Szabo and Demetrovics have written a very clever book that clears up some conceptual ambiguities and methodological weaknesses in exercise addiction research. *Passion and Addiction in Sports and Exercise* is compulsory reading for anyone interested in the subject, whether as a researcher, coach or athlete.

Dr. Robert Gugutzer, *Professor for Social Sciences of Sports, Goethe University Frankfurt am Main, Germany*

Passion and Addiction in Sports and Exercise

Passion and Addiction in Sports and Exercise is about the bright and dark aspects of sports and exercise behavior and revolves around two closely related yet distinct concepts. Passion is a joyful and healthy reflection of one's enjoyment and dedication to an adopted sport or exercise. At the same time, exercise addiction is an obligatory and must-be-done training regimen. This book is the first to attempt to explain the significant differences between passion and addiction in sports and exercise, as well as the relationship between the two.

This book presents an overview of three dimensions of passion and offers a new frame to contextualize exercise addition. The work also addresses the misinterpretation of certain aspects of training (e.g., intensity, frequency, and commitment) often related to the risk of exercise addiction. After introducing the health benefits of exercise, the book looks at the passion for sports and exercise training and the transition into maladaptive practice. Then it presents definitions and theoretical models for exercise addiction. It then examines exercise addiction cases while also illustrating how excessive or high exercise volumes could be beneficial instead of problematic. The last chapter offers a new approach for a better understanding of exercise addiction.

Passion and Addiction in Sports and Exercise is helpful for students, researchers, and clinicians interested in sport and exercise psychology, athletic training, behavioral addictions, and physical education. As well as being valuable reading for all regular exercisers and physically active individuals, including athletes competing at various levels in different sport disciplines.

Attila Szabo, PhD, DSc, is Doctor of the Hungarian Academy of Sciences and Professor of Psychology at ELTE Eötvös Loránd University in Budapest, Hungary. He completed his undergraduate and postgraduate education at Concordia University (BSc in Psychology and MSc in Biology) and University of Montreal (PhD in 'Sciences de l'activité physique') in Montreal, Canada. He served the sport science teaching and research teams at Nottingham Trent University, first as Senior Lecturer then as Reader for nearly nine years. His research interest is in behavioral addictions and placebo effects in sports and exercise.

Zsolt Demetrovics, PhD, DSc, is Clinical Psychologist and Cultural Anthropologist. Until 2021, he was the Dean of the Faculty of Education and Psychology, and Director of the Institute of Psychology, as well as Head of the Department of Clinical Psychology & Addiction at the ELTE Eötvös Loránd University, Budapest, Hungary. Currently, Zsolt is Chair of Centre of Excellence in Responsible Gaming at the University of Gibraltar. He is former president of the Hungarian Association on Addictions and funding Editor-in-Chief of the Journal of Behavioral Addictions. Furthermore, Zsolt is the president of the International Society for the Study of Behavioral Addictions. He is board member of the International Collaboration on ADHD and Substance Abuse (ICASA), and the European Association of Substance Abuse Research (EASAR).

Routledge Psychology of Sport, Exercise and Physical Activity
Series Editor: Andrew M. Lane
University of Wolverhampton, UK

This series offers a forum for original and cutting edge research, exploring the latest ideas and issues in the psychology of sport, exercise, and physical activity. Books within the series showcase the work of well-established and emerging scholars from around the world, offering an international perspective on topical and emerging areas of interest in the field. This series aims to drive forward academic debate and bridge the gap between theory and practice, encouraging critical thinking and reflection among students, academics, and practitioners. The series is aimed at upper-level undergraduates, research students and academics, and contains both authored and edited collections.

Available in this series:

For more information about this series, please visit:
Routledge Psychology of Sport, Exercise and Physical Activity – Book Series – Routledge & CRC Press

Passion and Addiction in Sports and Exercise

Attila Szabo and Zsolt Demetrovics

Routledge
Taylor & Francis Group
NEW YORK AND LONDON

First published 2022
by Routledge
605 Third Avenue, New York, NY 10158

and by Routledge
4 Park Square, Milton Park, Abingdon, Oxon, OX14 4RN

Routledge is an imprint of the Taylor & Francis Group, an informa business

© 2022 Attila Szabo and Zsolt Demetrovics

Library of Congress Cataloging-in-Publication Data
A catalog record for this book has been requested

ISBN: 978-1-032-00300-9 (hbk)
ISBN: 978-1-032-00301-6 (pbk)
ISBN: 978-1-003-17359-5 (ebk)

DOI: 10.4324/9781003173595

Typeset in Baskerville
by Apex CoVantage, LLC

To my sons, Sébastien and Olivér.

– Attila Szabo

Contents

Figures

Tables

Foreword

It gives me great pleasure to write the Foreword for the book *Passion and Addiction in Sports and Exercise* by two of my long-time friends and research colleagues, Attila Szabo and Zsolt Demetrovics.

I have been researching behavioral addictions for 35 years. Little did I know that over three decades after starting my own PhD that I would still find myself irresistibly hooked into researching a fascinating and interesting area of human behavior. Thankfully, other researchers like Attila and Zsolt have joined me in carrying on researching that passion.

The academic and scholarly study of exercise addiction has come a long way in 30 years. In many parts of the world, exercise addiction has become an area of increasing research interest. Arguably, both Attila and Zsolt have been at the center of that growing interest. Over the past couple of decades, Attila and Zsolt have been relentless in trying to get problematic exercise on many research and policymaking agendas including on those working in the mental health field. Many may question whether exercise in its most extreme forms can be genuinely addictive, and this book demonstrates that it can be and that there is a clear distinction between passionate exercise and addictive exercise. Exercise addiction is one of the growing number of 'mixed blessings addictions,' a term coined by Brown (1993) to describe activities (along with activities such as work and sex) that are very positive and of necessity in the lives of the overwhelming majority of individuals but when taken to excess can be problematic and addictive.

I have argued for many years that exercise in its most excessive form can be just as destructive as any other form of addictive behavior for the individual. It wasn't until 1997 that I had my first published paper on exercise addiction (Griffiths, 1997). It was (and still is) one of the few case study accounts providing a detailed account of an individual that I argued was genuinely addicted to exercise based on my 'components model of addiction' (Griffiths, 1996a, 1996b, 2005) and is among my most highly cited papers.

It wasn't until seven years later in 2004 that I published my second paper on exercise addiction. This paper was (in retrospect) pivotal in my career and maybe Attila's too. This was the first paper of many that Attila and

I coauthored, and it outlined the development of our new screening instrument – the Exercise Addiction Inventory (EAI) – which we developed with Annabel Terry when we were colleagues at Nottingham Trent University (Terry et al., 2004; Griffiths et al., 2005) and which was based on the aforementioned components model of addiction.

It was also the first time I had codeveloped a psychometric screening instrument, and since then I have codeveloped dozens more. For that alone, I am forever in Attila's debt. Since then, our first paper on the EAI has become our most highly cited paper in the exercise addiction field (close to 500 citations on *Google Scholar* at the time of writing) and has been translated into many languages and has included multicountry empirical and psychometric comparisons (Griffiths et al., 2015) as well as being adapted into a youth version (Lichtenstein et al., 2018) and a revised version (Szabo et al., 2019).

Since 2004, I have published over 30 more papers and book chapters on exercise addiction, and 19 of these have been with Attila and Zsolt as coauthors. One of these was the very first epidemiological study using a nationally representative sample to assess the prevalence of exercise addiction (Mónok et al., 2012), which all of us are still very proud of. Attila and Zsolt are both prolific scholars and wonderful research collaborators, and I am thankful to have worked with both of them for many years both inside and outside of the exercise addiction field.

Exercise is multifaceted and many factors may come into play in various ways and at different levels. They may be biological, social, or psychological. No single level of analysis is sufficient to explain exercise behavior. Individuals are self-determining agents. Examining exercise and problem exercise as a biopsychosocial behavior makes it evident that individual differences and broader contextual factors must all be considered. Moreover, it indicates that a variety of treatments, from a variety of standpoints, could be beneficial simultaneously. A narrow focus upon one theoretical perspective cannot be justified in understanding problematic exercise nor in treating it. This book provides an excellent 'one-stop shop' for the casual or interested reader to learn about some of these perspectives.

I very much hope that this book will become the first port of call for anyone working in the exercise addiction field. I wish Attila and Zsolt every success with the book and hope that readers will find it a stimulating and educational read as much as I did. I also hope that you, the reader, will feed back your own experiences and thoughts to the authors directly about the issues raised.

Dr. Mark Griffiths
Distinguished Professor of Behavioural Addiction
International Gaming Research Unit
Psychology Department
Nottingham Trent University
United Kingdom
November 2021

References

Brown, R. I. F. (1993). Some contributions of the study of gambling to the study of other addictions. In W. R. Eadington & J. Cornelius (Eds.), *Gambling behavior and problem gambling* (pp. 341–372). Reno, NV: University of Nevada Press.

Griffiths, M. D. (1996a). Behavioural addictions: An issue for everybody? *Journal of Workplace Learning, 8*(3), 19–25.

Griffiths, M. D. (1996b). Nicotine, tobacco and addiction. *Nature, 384*, 18.

Griffiths, M. D. (1997). Exercise addiction: A case study. *Addiction Research, 5*, 161–168.

Griffiths, M. D. (2005). A 'components' model of addiction within a biopsychosocial framework. *Journal of Substance Use, 10*, 191–197.

Griffiths, M. D., Szabo, A., & Terry, A. (2005). The exercise addiction inventory: A quick and easy screening tool for health practitioners. *British Journal of Sports Medicine, 39*, 30–31.

Griffiths, M. D., Urbán, R., Demetrovics, Z., Lichtenstein, M. B., de la Vega, R., Kun, B., Ruíz-Barquín, R., Youngman, J., & Szabo, A. (2015). A cross-cultural re-evaluation of the Exercise Addiction Inventory (EAI) in five countries. *Sports Medicine Open, 1*, 5.

Lichtenstein, M. B., Griffiths, M. D., Hemmingsen, S. D., Bojesen, A. B., & Støving, R. K. (2018). Exercise addiction in adolescents and emerging adults – Validation of a youth version of the Exercise Addiction Inventory. *Journal of Behavioral Addictions, 7*, 117–125.

Mónok, K., Berczik, K., Urbán, R., Szabó, A., Griffiths, M. D., Farkas, J., Magi, A., Eisinger, A., Kurimay, T., Kökönyei, G., Kun, B., Paksi, B., & Demetrovics, Z. (2012). Psychometric properties and concurrent validity of two exercise addiction measures: A population wide study in Hungary. *Psychology of Sport and Exercise, 13*, 739–746.

Szabo, A., Pinto, A., Griffiths, M. D., Kovacsik, R., & Demetrovics, Z. (2019). The psychometric evaluation of the revised Exercise Addiction Inventory: Improved psychometric properties by changing item response rating. *Journal of Behavioral Addictions, 8*, 157–161.

Terry, A., Szabo, A., & Griffiths, M. D. (2004). The Exercise Addiction Inventory: A new brief screening tool. *Addiction Research and Theory, 12*, 489–499.

Acknowledgments

We thank Professor Mark Griffiths for his thorough review of the book that helped us substantially in improving our first original draft. His comments and suggestions were extremely useful. We also thank Professor Griffiths for writing the Foreword to this book. Our work was supported by the Hungarian National Research, Development and Innovation Office (KKP126835).

1 Sports and exercise for healthy living

1.1 The need for physical activity today

The information age has changed the human way of life and fostered a significant decrease in work-related physical activity. Consequently, the evolutionary adaptation unfolding over millions of years to prepare the ancestors for a physically active lifestyle such as hunting, fishing, fighting, escaping predators, or building a shelter has suddenly been challenged by the fast-evolving information technology-driven transformations in people's lifestyles. These changes render contemporary living increasingly sedentary (Freese et al., 2018). A sedentary lifestyle characterized by prolonged sitting and physical inactivity is associated with many health risks (Blair, 2007). For example, low levels of physical activity were associated with increased incidence of all-cause mortality, various forms of cancer, type 2 diabetes mellitus, dyslipidemia, hypertension, immune deficiency, metabolic syndrome, neurological disorders, osteoporosis, obesity, oxidative stress, and sarcopenia (Knight, 2012).

Sitting, associated with most modern occupations, is the most hazardous component of physical inactivity. There is substantial evidence for the ill effect of prolonged sitting. For example, long hours of sitting could trigger premature aging and chronic diseases, including type 2 diabetes, substantial weight gain, cardiovascular disease, blood clots, cell death, inflammation, osteoporosis, and many other ailments (Lurati et al., 2017). Moreover, even increased leisure-time physical activity cannot compensate for the ill effects of prolonged sitting (Patel et al., 2010). Indeed, a large Canadian study showed that there appears to be a dose–response relationship between the length of sitting and all-cause mortality as well as cardiovascular disease, which is *independent* of the leisure-time physical activity (Katzmarzyk et al., 2009). The authors of the study have suggested that 'in addition to the promotion of moderate-to-vigorous physical activity and a healthy weight, physicians should discourage sitting for extended periods' (p. 998). Therefore, both sitting and physical inactivity may *independently* contribute to morbidity and mortality.

DOI: 10.4324/9781003173595-1

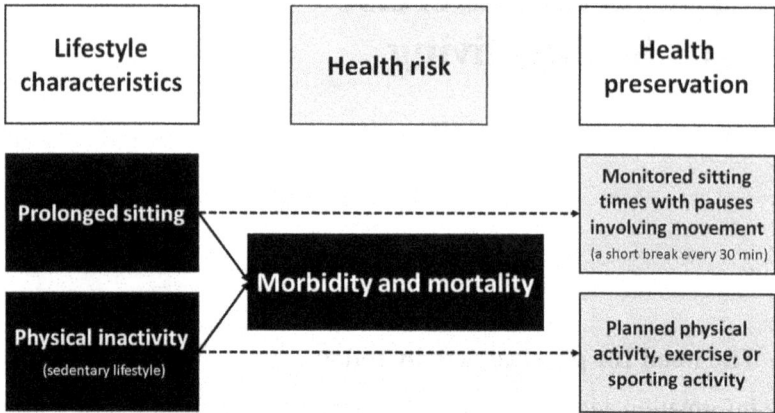

Figure 1.1 The ill effects of prolonged sitting and sedentary lifestyle on health and their behavioral means of prevention.

Shorter bouts of daily exercise episodes can counteract the ill effects of extended sitting. Sitting episodes should be interrupted by frequent brief pauses involving movement that raises the heart rate and favors blood circulation. Preset reminders from smart device applications could be helpful. The well-planned active pauses could buffer some ill effects of the sedentary lifestyle. Additionally, regular physical activity – planned exercise or sporting activity – should be incorporated into people's daily lives (Bushman & American College of Sports Medicine, 2017). Figure 1.1 illustrates this general principle.

1.2 The role of regular physical activity in health

Scholars agree that in addition to physical work, household activities, and active commuting, only regularly *planned* sports and exercise could compensate for the lost physical activity that was part of the earlier survival activities (Péronnet & Szabo, 1993). This scholastic point penetrates the mass media too (Berry et al. 2020). Consequently, most people realize and agree with the need to incorporate sports and exercise into their lifestyle. However, still, a large proportion of the world's population is not sufficiently active (Guthold et al., 2018).

Physical activity is conceptualized as *all forms* of movement which require energy expenditure to sustain work performed by the skeletal muscles. Primary examples are sports and exercise (Caspersen et al., 1985). While all movements are physical activities based on this definition, they may be categorized as planned and unplanned forms that serve different goals. Unplanned but necessary-for-living movements such as buying groceries, washing dishes, climbing the stairs, shoveling snow, or merely walking to work all help in mundane survival activities. Yet sports and exercise are *planned* physical activities aimed at benefiting people's health while mastering physical skills. These movements have a relatively stable pattern and volume, characterized by frequency, duration, and intensity. In addition to purposeful and planned skill practices, sports also involve 'rules' and 'contest,' making them more mastery-oriented compared to freely planned or self-organized forms of exercise, which are most often health-oriented (de la Vega et al., 2020; Szabo et al., 2019).

Research confirms that regular physical activity has numerous health benefits (Malm et al., 2019; Reiner et al., 2013). A literature review, including studies only with moderate and strong evidence (Powell et al., 2019), showed that regular physical activity in adults is related to lower risk of various cancers, lower risk of cardiovascular and all-cause mortality, reduced risk of weight gain, better cognitive function, improved quality of life, and improved sleep. Other studies connected habitual exercise with ameliorated cellular glucose uptake, glucose transport, and metabolism (Forsig & Richter, 2009), delayed cell aging (Forsig & Richter, 2009), suppression of cancer growth and apoptosis (Ambrose & Golightly, 2015), prevention of blood clots and increased calcium absorption (Charoenphandhu, 2007), and facilitation of bone formation, osteoblast formation, and osteoblastic cell growth (Cheng et al., 2020). Exercise also increases skeletal muscle interleukin 6, which plays a role in muscle repair after exercise and lipolysis (Meckel et al., 2009). The many health benefits of regular exercise, documented by *strong* or at least moderate research evidence, are summarized in Table 1.1.

Table 1.1 Health effects of regular physical activity. (Reproduced with permission from 'US Department of Health and Human Services (2018). *Physical Activity Guidelines for Americans*, 2nd edition. Washington, DC: US Department of Health and Human Services. [Table 2.1; Health Benefits Associated with Regular Physical Activity, p. 32]).' For the original source see: https://health.gov/sites/default/files/2019-09/Physical_Activity_Guidelines_2nd_edition.pdf.

Children and adolescents
- Improved bone (ages 3 through 17 years)
- Improved weight status (ages 3 through 17 years)
- Improved cardiorespiratory and muscular fitness (ages 6 through 17 years)
- Improved cardiometabolic health (ages 6 through 17 years)
- Improved cognition (ages 6 through 13 years) *
- Reduced risk of depression (ages 6 through 13 years)

Adults and older adults
- Lower risk of all-cause mortality
- Lower risk of cardiovascular disease mortality

(*Continued*)

Table 1.1 (Continued)

- Lower risk of cardiovascular disease (including heart disease and stroke)
- Lower risk of hypertension
- Lower risk of type 2 diabetes
- Lower risk of adverse blood lipid profile
- Lower risk of cancers of the bladder, breast, colon, endometrium, esophagus, kidney, lung, and stomach
- Improved cognition
- Reduced risk of dementia (including Alzheimer's disease)
- Improved quality of life
- Reduced anxiety
- Reduced risk of depression
- Improved sleep
- Slowed or reduced weight gain
- Weight loss, particularly when combined with reduced calorie intake
- Prevention of weight regain following initial weight loss
- Improved bone health
- Improved physical function
- Lower risk of falls (older adults)
- Lower risk of fall-related injuries (older adults)

Note: The Advisory Committee rated the evidence of health benefits of physical activity as strong, moderate, limited, or grade not assignable. Only outcomes with strong or moderate evidence of effect are included in this table. *See Table 1.3 for additional components of cognition and mental health.

1.3 The mental benefits of exercise

1.3.1 Acute effects of exercise

Regular sports and exercise participation are also linked to mental well-being (Biddle et al., 2019; Kekäläinen et al., 2019). For example, exercise relieves anxiety and aids in dealing with stress (Lucibello et al., 2019; Kim et al., 2019), one of the several motives for its practice. However, a single exercise session's *immediate* mental benefits are the primary incentive for regular exercise engagement. Such benefits occur after short workouts and usually manifest as improvement in feeling states, such as more positive affect and mood, or in anxiolytic effects. Research has demonstrated that exercise-induced affective changes were reported even after three minutes of exercise (Szabo et al., 2013). Studies have shown that many different exercises could yield positive psychological changes (Anderson & Brice, 2011; Dasilva et al., 2011). Table 1.2 presents some examples from research carried out in the last two decades on the acute mental benefits of *various forms* of exercise.

Table 1.2 Acute mental/psychological benefits of different forms of exercise.

Authors/year	Type of exercise	Duration of exercise	Main outcome
Crush et al., 2018	Treadmill running at moderate intensity	10, 20, 30, and 45 minutes	Regardless of duration, mood states improved significantly
Edwards & Loprinzi, 2018	Walking and meditation	10 minutes	Mood states have improved in both. Meditation had a larger mood-improving effect
Focht et al., 2015	Weight training	45 minutes	Feeling states improved
Glackin, & Beale, 2017	Outdoor cycling	Semistructured interviews	Outdoor cycling served to enhance the participants' sense of well-being and in doing so helped them cope with the mental challenges associated with their lives
Hoffman & Hoffman, 2008	Running on a treadmill (self-paced)	20 minutes	Vigor increased while fatigue decreased
Kovácsik & Szabo, 2019	Cheerleading	2 hours	Core- and positive affect increased while negative affect decreased
Li & Yin, 2008	Shadowboxing	1 hour	Tension, depression, and fatigue decreased while ego and vigor increased
Petruzzello et al., 2009; Rendi et al., 2008	Cycling (stationary)	20 minutes	Total mood disturbance and state anxiety decreased. In Rendi et al., positive engagement, tranquility, and revitalization increased
Rehor et al., 2001	Circuit training, weight training and racquetball	45 minutes	Mood states improved more after circuit training and weight training than after racquetball
Rokka et al., 2010	Dance aerobics	1 hour	Energy increased while tension, depression, aggressiveness, and confusion decreased

(*Continued*)

Table 1.2 (Continued)

Authors/year	Type of exercise	Duration of exercise	Main outcome
Sławińska et al., 2018	CrossFit	60 minutes	Mood stats have improved
Stark et al., 2011	Nordic walking	60 minutes	Calmness, activation, and mood improved whereas thoughtfulness, weakness, depression, and arousal decreased
Szabo et al., 2013	Warm-up, very light exercises	3 minutes	Perceived well-being has improved
Szabo et al., 2015	Spinning	35 minutes	Positive affect increased while negative affect decreased
Szabo et al., 2016	Bikram Yoga	90 minutes	Negative effect and anxiety decreased while positive affect increased
Szabo, 2003a, 2003b	Running outdoors and in the laboratory (self-paced)	20 minutes	Mood improved and anxiety decreased
Tolnai et al., 2016	Pilates	60 minutes	Negative affect and anxiety decreased while positive affect increased
Toskovic, 2001	Taekwondo	75 minutes	Tension, depression, anger, fatigue, and confusion decreased while vigor increased
Valentine & Evans, 2001	Swimming	30 minutes	Tense arousal decreased while hedonic tone and energetic arousal increased
Wang et al., 2010	Tai Chi	Various durations (review)	Stress, anxiety, depression, and mood disturbance decreased while self-esteem increased

Note: The table is not exhaustive. Its purpose is to provide some examples of the wide range of exercise forms and exercise durations that yield immediate psychological benefits.

1.3.2 Chronic effects of exercise

Regular exercise also benefits one's psychological health on the long term. Given that the acute effects of physical exercise are most evident in improved affect or mood and decreased stress or anxiety, it is not surprising that these cumulative effects, with regular exercise, yield long-term benefits primarily for depression and anxiety disorders. Gogulla et al.'s (2012) review showed that most research reports suggest that regular physical activity triggers a noticeable reduction of depression and fear of falling in healthy elderly. The review also concluded that high-intensity aerobic or anaerobic exercise might be the most effective in reducing depression. In contrast, Tai Chi and multimodal training may be more effective in alleviating the fear of falling.

A later meta-analysis found that exercise training also improves depressive symptoms in individuals with multiple sclerosis (Ensari et al., 2014). Furthermore, another review presented evidence for the antidepressant effects of aerobic exercise training if that is performed at least three times a week, at moderate intensity, and for a minimum of nine weeks (Stanton & Reaburn, 2014). Finally, a review by Herring et al. (2010) showed that exercise significantly reduces anxiety symptoms in patients with chronic illness compared to no treatment control conditions. The review also noted that the exercise interventions with the largest anxiolytic effect lasted no longer than 12 weeks, employed exercise sessions lasting at least 30 minutes, and assessed persistent anxiety lasting for more than one week.

Several other reviews also provide evidence for the long-term beneficial effects of various exercises. For example, a systematic review on the efficacy of Pilates training concluded that apart from physiological benefits, this form of exercise also improved the participants' mood and quality of life (Bullo et al., 2015). Another review supports the beneficial effect of resistance exercise training on the cognitive function of healthy older adults (Chang et al., 2012). Recently, two systematic reviews concluded that yoga improves mental health (Hendriks et al., 2017) and is effective for stress management (Wang & Szabo, 2020). Table 1.3 summarizes the evidence gathered by the United States Department of Health and Human Services on the benefits of exercise for mental health. The table only includes research outcomes with *strong or moderate evidence* for the beneficial effect of both acute and chronic (habitual) exercise.

1.4 Models explaining the positive psychological effects of exercise

1.4.1 Physiological models

The training volume has been implicated in most explanations for the positive effects of exercise. One relatively often-cited theory is the *endorphin hypothesis* (Steinberg & Sykes, 1985), which suggests that exercise performed for a prolonged time and with a certain intensity produces endorphins, an endogenous opiate similar to morphine. These molecules have mood- or affect-regulating properties and are responsible for the '*feeling good*' experience after exercise. Recent evidence on brain positron emission tomography (PET) showed that high-intensity exercise induces opioid release,

Table 1.3 The benefits of physical activity for mental health. (Reproduced with permission from 'US Department of Health and Human Services. (2018). *Physical Activity Guidelines for Americans, 2nd edition.* Washington, DC: US Department of Health and Human Services. [Table 2.3; The Benefits of Physical Activity for Brain Health, p. 40].)'

Outcome	Population	Benefit	Acute	Habitual
Cognition	Children aged 6 to 13 years	Improved cognition (performance on academic achievement test, executive function, processing speed, memory)	x	x
	Adults	Reduced risk of dementia (including Alzheimer's disease)		x
	Adults older than 50 years	Improved cognition (executive function, attention, memory, crystallized intelligence*, processing speed)		x
Quality of life	Adults	Improved quality of life		x
Depressed mood and depression	Children 6 to 17 years and adults	Reduced risk of depression Reduced depressed mood		x
Anxiety	Adults	Reduced short-term feelings of anxiety (state anxiety)	x	
	Adults	Reduced long-term feelings and signs of anxiety (trait anxiety) for people with and without anxiety disorders		x
Sleep	Adults	Improved sleep outcomes (increased sleep efficiency, sleep quality, deep sleep, reduced daytime sleepiness, frequency of use of medication to aid sleep)		x
	Adults	Improved sleep outcomes that increase with duration of an acute episode	x	

Source: https://health.gov/sites/default/files/2019-09/Physical_Activity_Guidelines_2nd_edition.pdf

Note: The Advisory Committee rated the evidence of health benefits of physical activity as strong, moderate, limited, or grade not assignable. Only outcomes with strong or moderate evidence of effect are included in this table. *Crystallized intelligence is the ability to retrieve and use information that has been acquired over time. It is different from fluid intelligence, which is the ability to store and manipulate new information.

which does not occur in response to moderate exercise (Saanijoki et al., 2017).

Another model for the mental benefits of sports and exercise is the *thermogenic hypothesis* (Koltyn, 1997). It is based on the premise that increased core body temperature induces physical (somatic) relaxation, decreases anxiety, and triggers a general feeling good subjective state. This hypothesis is still controversial because several studies failed to support it (Wininger & Green, 2011). However, *in situ* research in Bikram (hot) yoga (Szabo et al., 2016), performed at 40 degrees Celsius showed that after 90 minutes of workout, state anxiety and negative affect decreased, whereas positive affect increased in 53 participants. Still, the thermogenic hypothesis begs for more research in general and specific exercise settings.

Another physiological model explaining the role of exercise in mental health is the *monoamine hypothesis* (Dunn & Dishman, 1991; Lin & Kuo, 2013). It purports that physical exercise augments specific neurotransmitter (monoamine) activity in the brain, including serotonin, dopamine, and norepinephrine. Research shows that exercise induces increased monoamine levels in human plasma and urine (Motta, 2019). Neuroimaging evidence for increased exercise-induced dopaminergic activity in humans also exists in patients with Parkinson's disease (Sacheli et al., 2019). Still, the role of brain monoamines in regularly exercising healthy humans requires further empirical support.

1.4.2 Psychological models

A popular psychological model explaining exercise's mental benefits is the distraction hypothesis (Mikkelsen et al., 2017). It purports that beyond physiological changes produced by exercise, attentional 'time out' from some everyday problems, challenges, or stress could result in mood-elevating effects. Distracting oneself from unpleasant or worrying thoughts is a temporary relief that could cumulate and even have long-term benefits for coping with anxiety or depression. There is tentative research support for the distraction hypothesis (Crouzevialle & Butera, 2017; Szabo, 2003b; Szabo et al., 2005), but there is also contrary evidence. For very brief exercises, like those lasting three to ten minutes (see Table 1.2), the time-off or distraction is relatively short to expect an affect-improving effect. Yet, mood improvements were reported after such brief exercise episodes too. Empirical research also showed that regular exercisers report experiencing affective benefits after a single exercise session while non-exercisers do not (Hoffman & Hoffman, 2008). Exercisers may anticipate positive feelings after the exercise due to past positive experiences, whereas non-exercisers may not have such expectations in lack of past positive experiences. Therefore, in Hoffman and Hoffman's study, expected or conditioned response to exercise could be a more plausible explanation for exercise's mental benefits than distraction because both groups have had an equal amount of time.

The expectation-based placebo mechanism was also a posited model for exercise's psychological benefits (Szabo, 2013). The refreshing feelings after exercise workouts, along with the voluminous media information about the benefits of exercise, could shape the individual's expectations and mind-frame related to exercise. Indeed, research has shown that expectancy mediates the psychological effect of exercise. For example, in a study by Anderson and Brice (2011), exercise improved participants' mood after only 10 minutes. This positive effect was amplified by a biased recall of the pre-exercise mood. The authors concluded that exercisers' expectations regarding the benefits of exercise mediate the mood effects reported after exercise, thereby supporting the placebo explanation for the mental benefits of exercise.

Another related model is the self-efficacy or mastery hypothesis, which states that the physiological effects of completing an important-to-the-self and effortful task, such as a workout, trigger feelings of mastery and self-efficacy, which then yield positive mood states (Mikkelsen et al., 2017). Indeed, the positive feelings of mastery and self-efficacy may occur even after very short exercise. Therefore, distraction, anticipation, and mastery, along with some of the physiological effects of exercise, such as arousal, all could *jointly* contribute to the positive mental benefits of exercise even after very brief exercise sessions.

1.5 Exercise is Medicine

Knowing about the many physical and psychological benefits of physical activity and being concerned about the contemporary increasingly sedentary life, in 2007, the American College of Sports Medicine (ACSM) has started the Exercise is Medicine® (EIM) initiative (Thompson et al., 2020). It aims to make physical activity part of both prevention and treatment of various morbidities. Exercise is Medicine is a worldwide health initiative pursuing the mission to monitor and promote physical activity, a regular part of clinical practice and health care. Furthermore, EIM strives to connect the health-care systems with evidence-based physical activity resources for all people worldwide. EIM motivates doctors and health-care professionals to use planned physical activity when devising health-oriented treatment plans and to refer individuals to evidence-based exercise programs and qualified exercise professionals. During the past years, there have been significant developments in the influence-shaping ambitions of the EIM. An EIM global network comprising regional centers that coordinate the EIM partnerships in several nations worldwide has been established. The World Congress on 'Exercise is Medicine' was incorporated into the ACSM annual meeting to serve as an outlet for sharing knowledge and new research findings and establishing collaboration networks across the United States and worldwide. Finally, EIM created a solid on-campus network that is expanding continuously, and it is present in 275 higher education campuses around the world (Thompson et al., 2020). Overall, EIM is a key player in fighting the ill effects of sitting and sedentary lifestyle.

For most people, exercise is a pleasant and refreshing activity. It is a passion for most committed individuals. However, people exercise for many different reasons. For example, stress relief-motivated exercise is *therapeutic* by its nature (Szabo et al., 2019). Exercising individuals experiencing chronic or reoccurring stress may use exercise as a means of coping (Egorov & Szabo, 2013). For these people, exercise becomes *obligatory*, a must-do activity, to function well in their daily lives (Szabo, 2010). If exercise is not possible for some reason, obligatory exercisers experience severe withdrawal symptoms, such as anxiety, nervousness, irritability, negative affect, and other unpleasant emotions (Griffiths, 2005; Szabo, 2010). The presence of these symptoms in some individuals points toward an addictive aspect of sports and exercise behavior that forms the bulk of the discussion in this book.

1.6 Key points

1. Evolution prepared humans for movement.
2. In general, the modern human lifestyle is sedentary.
3. Sports and exercise buffer the ill effects of sedentary life.
4. Sports and exercise have proven mental health benefits.
5. Sports and exercise have positive health implications.

1.7 References

Ambrose, K., & Golightly, Y. (2015). Physical exercise as non-pharmacological treatment of chronic pain: Why and when. *Best Practice & Research Clinical Rheumatology, 29*, 120–130. doi:10.1016/j.berh.2015.04.022

Anderson, R. J., & Brice, S. (2011). The mood-enhancing benefits of exercise: Memory biases augment the effect. *Psychology of Sport and Exercise, 12*(2), 79–82. doi:10.1016/j.psychsport.2010.08.003

Berry, T. R., Yun, L., Faulkner, G., Rhodes, R. E., Chulak-Bozzer, T., Latimer-Cheung, A., . . . Tremblay, M. (2020). Implicit and explicit evaluations of a mass media physical activity campaign: Does everything get better? *Psychology of Sport and Exercise, 49*, 101684. doi:10.1016/j.psychsport.2020.101684

Biddle, S. J. H., Ciaccioni, S., Thomas, G., & Vergeer, I. (2019). Physical activity and mental health in children and adolescents: An updated review of reviews and an analysis of causality. *Psychology of Sport and Exercise, 42*, 146–155. doi:10.1016/j.psychsport.2018.08.011

Blair, S. N. (2007). Physical inactivity: A major public health problem. *Nutrition Bulletin, 32*(2), 113–117. doi:10.1111/j.1467-3010.2007.00632.x

Bullo, V., Bergamin, M., Gobbo, S., Sieverdes, J. C., Zaccaria, M., Neunhaeuserer, D., & Ermolao, A. (2015). The effects of Pilates exercise training on physical fitness and wellbeing in the elderly: A systematic review for future exercise prescription. *Preventive Medicine, 75*, 1–11. doi:10.1016/j.ypmed.2015.03.002

Bushman, B., & American College of Sports Medicine. (2017). *ACSM's complete guide to fitness & health* (2nd ed.). Champaign, IL: Human Kinetics.

Caspersen, C. J., Powell, K. E., & Christenson, G. M. (1985). Physical activity, exercise, and physical fitness: Definitions and distinctions for health-related research. *Public Health Reports, 100*(2), 126–131. PMID: 3920711

Chang, Y. K., Pan, C. Y., Chen, F. T., Tsai, C. L., & Huang, C. C. (2012). Effect of resistance-exercise training on cognitive function in healthy older adults: A review. *Journal of Aging and Physical Activity, 20*(4), 497–517. doi:10.1123/japa.20.4.497

Charoenphandhu, N. (2007). Physical activity and exercise affect intestinal calcium absorption: A perspective review. *Journal of Sports Science and Technology, 7*(1, 2), 171–181. Retrieved from: http://ftp.narattsys.com/press/JSST2007.pdf

Cheng, L., Khalaf, A. T., Lin, T., Ran, L., Shi, Z., Wan, J., . . . Zou, L. (2020). Exercise promotes the osteoinduction of HA/β-TCP biomaterials via the Wnt Signaling Pathway. *Metabolites, 10*(3), 90. doi:10.3390/metabo10030090

Crouzevialle, M., & Butera, F. (2017). Performance goals and task performance: Integrative considerations on the distraction hypothesis. *European Psychologist, 22*(2), 73–82. doi:10.1027/1016-9040/a000281

Crush, E. A., Frith, E., & Loprinzi, P. D. (2018). Experimental effects of acute exercise duration and exercise recovery on mood state. *Journal of Affective Disorders, 229*, 282–287. doi:10.1016/j.jad.2017.12.092

Dasilva, S. G., Guidetti, L., Buzzachera, C. F., Elsangedy, H. M., Krinski, K., De Campos, W., . . . Baldari, C. (2011). Psychophysiological responses to self-paced treadmill and overground exercise. *Medicine & Science in Sports & Exercise, 43*(6), 1114–1124. doi:10.1249/mss.0b013e318205874c

de la Vega, R., Almendros, L. J., Barquín, R. R., Boros, S., Demetrovics, Z., & Szabo, A. (2020). Exercise addiction during the COVID-19 pandemic: An international study confirming the need for considering passion and perfectionism. *International Journal of Mental Health and Addiction.* (Online first). doi:10.1007/s11469-020-00433-7

Dunn, A. L., & Dishman, R. K. (1991). Exercise and the neurobiology of depression. *Exercise and Sport Sciences Reviews, 19*(1), 41–98. doi:10.1249/00003677-199101000-00002

Edwards, M. K., & Loprinzi, P. D. (2018). Experimental effects of brief, single bouts of walking and meditation on mood profile in young adults. *Health Promotion Perspectives, 8*(3), 171–178. doi:10.15171/hpp.2018.23

Egorov, A. Y., & Szabo, A. (2013). The exercise paradox: An interactional model for a clearer conceptualization of exercise addiction. *Journal of Behavioral Addictions, 2*(4), 199–208. doi:10.1556/jba.2.2013.4.2

Ensari, I., Motl, R. W., & Pilutti, L. A. (2014). Exercise training improves depressive symptoms in people with multiple sclerosis: Results of a meta-analysis. *Journal of Psychosomatic Research, 76*(6), 465–471. doi:10.1016/j.jpsychores.2014.03.014

Focht, B. C., Garver, M. J., Cotter, J. A., Devor, S. T., Lucas, A. R., & Fairman, C. M. (2015). Affective responses to acute resistance exercise performed at self-selected and imposed loads in trained women. *Journal of Strength and Conditioning Research, 29*(11), 3067–3074. doi:10.1519/jsc.0000000000000985

Forsig, C., & Richter, E. (2009). Improved insulin sensitivity after exercise: Focus on insulin signaling. *Obesity, 17*, s15–s20. doi:10.1038/oby.2009.383

Freese, J., Klement, R. J., Ruiz-Núñez, B., Schwarz, S., & Lötzerich, H. (2018). The sedentary (r)evolution: Have we lost our metabolic flexibility? *F1000Research, 6*, 1787. doi:10.12688/f1000research.12724.2

Glackin, O. F., & Beale, J. T. (2017). "The world is best experienced at 18 mph". The psychological wellbeing effects of cycling in the countryside: An Interpretative phenomenological analysis. *Qualitative Research in Sport, Exercise and Health, 10*(1), 32–46. doi:10.1080/2159676x.2017.1360381

Gogulla, S., Lemke, N., & Hauer, K. (2012). Effects of physical activity and physical training on the psychological status of older persons with and without cognitive impairment. *Zeitschrift fur Gerontologie und Geriatrie, 45*(4), 279–289.

Griffiths, M. (2005). A "components" model of addiction within a biopsychosocial framework. *Journal of Substance Use, 10*(4), 191–197. doi:10.1080/14659890500114359

Guthold, R., Stevens, G. A., Riley, L. M., & Bull, F. C. (2018). Worldwide trends in insufficient physical activity from 2001 to 2016: A pooled analysis of 358 population-based surveys with 1·9 million participants. *The Lancet Global Health, 6*(10), e1077–e1086. doi:10.1016/s2214-109x(18)30357-7

Hendriks, T., de Jong, J., & Cramer, H. (2017). The effects of yoga on positive mental health among healthy adults: A systematic review and meta-analysis. *The Journal of Alternative and Complementary Medicine, 23*(7), 505–517. doi:10.1089/acm.2016.0334

Herring, M. P. O'Connor, P. J., & Dishman, R. K. (2010). The effect of exercise training on anxiety symptoms among patients. *Archives of Internal Medicine, 170*(4), 321–331. doi:10.1001/archinternmed.2009.530

Hoffman, M. D., & Hoffman, D. R. (2008). Exercisers achieve greater acute exercise-induced mood enhancement than non-exercisers. *Archives of Physical Medicine & Rehabilitation, 89*(2), 358–363. doi:10.1016/j.apmr.2007.09.026

Katzmarzyk, P. T., Church, T. S., Craig, C. L., & Bouchard, C. (2009). Sitting time and mortality from all causes, cardiovascular disease, and cancer. *Medicine & Science in Sports & Exercise, 41*(5), 998–1005. doi:10.1249/mss.0b013e3181930355

Kekäläinen, T., Freund, A. M., Sipilä, S., & Kokko, K. (2019). Cross-sectional and longitudinal associations between leisure time physical activity, mental wellbeing and subjective health in middle adulthood. *Applied Research in Quality of Life, 15*(4), 1099–1116. doi:10.1007/s11482-019-09721-4

Kim, H. J., Oh, S. Y., Lee, D. W., Kwon, J., & Park, E.-C. (2019). The effects of intense physical activity on stress in adolescents: Findings from Korea Youth Risk Behavior web-based survey (2015–2017). *International Journal of Environmental Research and Public Health, 16*(10), 1870. doi:10.3390/ijerph16101870

Knight, J. A. (2012). Physical inactivity: Associated diseases and disorders. *Annals of Clinical & Laboratory Science, 42*(3), 320–337. PMID: 22964623

Koltyn, K. F. (1997). The thermogenic hypothesis. In W. P. Morgan (Ed.), *Physical activity and mental health* (pp. 213–226). Washington, DC: Taylor and Francis.

Kovácsik, R., & Szabo, A. (2019). Dynamics of the affective states during and after cheerleading training in female athletes. *Polish Psychological Bulletin, 50*(1), 29–35. doi:10.24425/ppb.2019.12601

Li, G., & Yin, J. C. (2008). The effects of shadowboxing on mood and beta-Ep in still condition of female college students. *Journal of Beijing Sport University, 31*(3), 357–362.

Lin, T. W., & Kuo, Y. M. (2013). Exercise benefits brain function: The monoamine connection. *Brain Sciences, 3*(4), 39–53. doi:10.3390/brainsci3010039

Lucibello, K., Parker, J., & Heisz, J. (2019). Examining a training effect on the state anxiety response to an acute bout of exercise in low and high anxious individuals. *Journal of Affective Disorders, 247*, 29–35. doi:10.1016/j.jad.2018.12.063

Lurati, A. R. (2017). Health issues and injury risks associated with prolonged sitting and sedentary lifestyles. *Workplace Health & Safety, 66*(6), 285–290. doi:10.1177/2165079917737558

Malm, C., Jakobsson, J., & Isaksson, A. (2019). Physical activity and sports – real health benefits: A review with insight into the public health of Sweden. *Sports, 7*(5), 127. doi:10.3390/sports7050127

Meckel, Y., Eliakim, A., Seraev, M., Zaldivar, F., Cooper, D., Sagiv, D., & Nemet, D. (2009). The effect of a brief sprint interval exercise on growth factors and inflammatory mediators. *Journal of Strength & Conditioning Research, 23*, 225–230. doi:10.1519/JSC.0b013e3181876a9a

Mikkelsen, K., Stojanovska, L., Polenakovic, M., Bosevski, M., & Apostolopoulos, V. (2017). Exercise and mental health. *Maturitas, 106*, 48–56. doi:10.1016/j.maturitas.2017.09.003

Motta, R. (2019). The role of exercise in reducing PTSD and negative emotional states. In S. G. Taukeni (Ed.), *Psychology of health – biopsychosocial approach* (pp. 69–80). London, UK: IntechOpen Limited. doi:10.5772/intechopen.81012

Patel, A. V., Bernstein, L., Deka, A., Feigelson, H. S., Campbell, P. T., Gapstur, S. M., . . . Thun, M. J. (2010). Leisure time spent sitting in relation to total mortality in a prospective cohort of US adults. *American Journal of Epidemiology, 172*(4), 419–429. doi:10.1093/aje/kwq155

Péronnet, F., & Szabo, A. (1993). Sympathetic response to acute psychosocial stressors in humans: Linkage to physical exercise and training. In P. Seraganian (Ed.), *Exercise psychology: The influence of physical exercise on psychological processes* (pp. 172–217). New York, NY: Wiley.

Petruzzello, S. J., Snook, E. M., Gliottoni, R. C., & Motl, R. W. (2009). Anxiety and mood changes associated with acute cycling in persons with multiple sclerosis. *Anxiety, Stress & Coping, 22*(3), 297–307. doi:10.1080/10615800802441245

Powell, K. E., King, A. C., Buchner, D. M., Campbell, W. W., DiPietro, L., Erickson, K. I., . . . Whitt-Glover, M. C. (2019). The scientific foundation for the physical activity. *Journal of Physical Activity and Health, 16*, 1–11. doi:10.1123/jpah.2018-0618

Rehor, P. R., Stewart, C., Dunnagan, T., & Cooley, D. (2001). Alteration of mood state after a single bout of noncompetitive and competitive exercise programs. *Perceptual and Motor Skills, 93*(1), 249–256. doi:10.2466/pms.2001.93.1.249

Reiner, M., Niermann, C., Jekauc, D., & Woll, A. (2013). Long-term health benefits of physical activity – a systematic review of longitudinal studies. *BMC Public Health, 13*(1). doi:10.1186/1471-2458-13-813

Rendi, M., Szabo, A., Szabó, T., Velenczei, A., & Kovács, Á. (2008). Acute psychological benefits of aerobic exercise: A field study into the effects of exercise characteristics. *Psychology, Health & Medicine, 13*(2), 180–184.

Rokka, S., Mavridis, G., & Kouli, O. (2010). The impact of exercise intensity on mood state of participants in dance aerobics programs. *Physical Culture & Tourism, 17*(3), 241–245.

Saanijoki, T., Tuominen, L., Tuulari, J. J., Nummenmaa, L., Arponen, E., Kalliokoski, K., Hirvonen, J. (2017). Opioid release after high-intensity interval training in healthy human subjects. *Neuropsychopharmacology, 43*(2), 246–254. doi:10.1038/npp.2017.148

Sacheli, M. A., Neva, J. L., Lakhani, B., Murray, D. K., Vafai, N., Shahinfard, E., . . . Stoessl, A. J. (2019). Exercise increases caudate dopamine release and ventral striatal activation in Parkinson's disease. *Movement Disorders, 34*(12), 1891–1900. doi:10.1002/mds.27865

Sławińska, M., Stolarski, M., & Jankowski, K. S. (2018). Effects of chronotype and time of day on mood responses to CrossFit training. *Chronobiology International, 36*(2), 237–249. doi:10.1080/07420528.2018.1531016

Stanton, R., & Reaburn, P. (2014). Exercise and the treatment of depression: A review of the exercise program variables. *Journal of Science and Medicine in Sport, 17*(2), 177–182. doi:10.1016/j.jsams.2013.03.010

Stark, R., Schöny, W., & Kopp, M. (2011). [Acute effects of a single bout of moderate exercise on psychological well-being in patients with affective disorder during hospital treatment]. *Neuropsychiatrie: Klinik, Diagnostik, Therapie und Rehabilitation: Organ der Gesellschaft Osterreichischer Nervenarzte und Psychiater, 26*(4), 166–170. doi:10.1007/s40211-012-0033-7

Steinberg, H., & Sykes, E. A. (1985). Introduction to symposium on endorphins and behavioural processes: Review of literature on endorphins and exercise. *Pharmacology Biochemistry and Behavior, 23*(5), 857–862. doi:10.1016/0091-3057(85)90083-8

Szabo, A. (2003a). Acute psychological benefits of exercise performed at self-selected workloads: Implications for theory and practice. *Journal of Sports Science and Medicine, 2*(3), 77–87. PMID: 24627659

Szabo, A. (2003b). The acute effects of humor and exercise on mood and anxiety. *Journal of Leisure Research, 35*(2), 152–162. doi:10.1080/00222216.2003.11949988

Szabo, A. (2010). *Addiction to exercise: A symptom or a disorder?* New York, NY: Nova Science Publishers.

Szabo, A. (2013). Acute psychological benefits of exercise: Reconsideration of the placebo effect. *Journal of Mental Health, 22*(5), 449–455. doi:10.3109/09638237.2012.734657

Szabo, A., Ainsworth, S. E., & Danks, P. K. (2005). Experimental comparison of the psychological benefits of aerobic exercise, humor, and music. *Humor, 18*(3). doi:10.1515/humr.2005.18.3.235

Szabo, A., Boros, S., & Bősze, J. P. (2019). Are there differences in life-satisfaction, optimism, pessimism and perceived stress between therapeutic and mastery exercisers? A preliminary investigation. *Baltic Journal of Sport and Health Sciences, 3*(114). doi:10.33607/bjshs.v3i114.807

Szabo, A., Gaspar, Z., & Abraham, J. (2013). Acute effects of light exercise on subjectively experienced wellbeing: Benefits in only three minutes. *Baltic Journal of Health and Physical Activity, 5*(4). doi:10.2478/bjha-2013-0024

Szabo, A., Gáspár, Z., Kiss, N., & Radványi, A. (2015). Effect of spinning workouts on affect. *Journal of Mental Health, 24*(3), 145–149. doi:10.3109/09638237.2015.1019053

Szabo, A., Nikházy, L., Tihanyi, B., & Boros, S. (2016). An in-situ investigation of the acute effects of Bikram yoga on positive- and negative affect, and state-anxiety in context of perceived stress. *Journal of Mental Health, 26*(2), 156–160. doi:10.1080/09638237.2016.1222059

Thompson, W. R., Sallis, R., Joy, E., Jaworski, C. A., Stuhr, R. M., & Trilk, J. L. (2020). Exercise is medicine. *American Journal of Lifestyle Medicine, 14*(5), 511–523. doi:10.1177/1559827620912192

Tolnai, N., Szabó, Z., Köteles, F., & Szabo, A. (2016). Physical and psychological benefits of once-a-week Pilates exercises in young sedentary women: A 10-week longitudinal study. *Physiology & Behavior, 163*, 211–218. doi:10.1016/j. physbeh.2016.05.025

Toskovic, N. N. (2001). Alterations in selected measures of mood with a single bout of dynamic Taekwondo exercise in college-age students. *Perceptual and Motor Skills, 92*(3c), 1031–1038. doi:10.2466/pms.2001.92.3c.1031

US Department of Health and Human Services. (2018). *Physical activity guidelines for Americans* (2nd ed.). Washington, DC: US Department of Health and Human Services.

Valentine, E., & Evans, C. (2001). The effects of solo singing, choral singing and swimming on mood and physiological indices. *British Journal of Medical Psychology, 74*(1), 115–120. doi:10.1348/000711201160849

Wang, C., Bannuru, R., Ramel, J., Kupelnick, B., Scott, T., & Schmid, C. H. (2010). Tai Chi on psychological wellbeing: Systematic review and meta-analysis. *BMC Complementary and Alternative Medicine, 10*(23), 1–16. doi:10.1186/1472-6882-10-23

Wang, F., & Szabo, A. (2020). Effects of yoga on stress among healthy adults: A systematic review. *Alternative Therapies in Health & Medicine, 26*(4), 58–64.

Wininger, S. R., & Green, J. M. (2011). Effects of hot vs. cold environment on psychological outcomes during cycling. *Athletic Insight, 2*(3), 179–186.

2 Passion

Definitions and conceptualization

2.1 Passion

There are several definitions for passion, ranging from simple to complex conceptualizations. The online edition of the *Dictionary of Psychology* of the American Psychological Association (2021) defines *passion* as 1) 'an intense, driving, or overwhelming feeling or conviction. Passion is often contrasted with emotion, in that passion affects a person unwillingly'; 2) 'intense sexual desire,' and 3) 'a strong enthusiasm for or devotion to an activity, object, concept, or the like.' These sets of terminologies all attempt to describe passion as feeling or emotion. However, passion itself perhaps cannot be felt as a distinct feeling state. Still, the feelings *resulting from passion* could have a strong impact on the person. Examples are love, political ideology, religious or moral convictions, or activities like fishing, hunting, doing research, running, playing cards, collecting butterflies or stamps, etc. These feelings might include, among several others, affinity and dedication (Fernández-Carrasco et al., 2019), desire (Yitshaki & Kropp, 2016), attachment (Paquette et al., 2020; Wang et al., 2021), salience (Rao & Tobias Neely, 2019; Reynaud et al., 2010), cognitive distortion (Schellenberg & Bailis, 2018), fantasy (Orosz et al., 2018), love (D'Acquisto, 2019; Paquette et al., 2020), and need of sacrifice (Bélanger et al., 2014). The collection of such feelings and emotions may be interpreted as passion. In our view, passion is a behavioral manifestation, which is *overtly observable* and reflects the presence of a solid and persistent motivational incentive (Sigmundsson et al., 2020) for a relationship (i.e., love), ideology (i.e., religious), object (i.e., stamp/coin collection), or action (i.e., gardening).

Observing passion makes it hard to distinguish it from commitment. However, by understanding the emotions of the individual, the intensity and nature of passion become evident. Commitment is the onset of a passionate relationship. Then passion emerges at various levels and could unfold to include compulsion, obsession, and may occasionally even turn into addiction (Lichtenstein et al., 2020). Like passion, commitment and addiction are behavioral manifestations of the individual's feelings and affective states generated by emotions. The fine line between passion

DOI: 10.4324/9781003173595-2

and addiction is *self-harm*. Addiction involves self-harm (Blasco-Fontecilla et al., 2016; Szabo et al., 2015). Therefore, there is continuity from a healthy-balanced involvement in an ideology, activity, or social relationship to a self-destructive symbiosis. This continuity represents the path from passion to addiction. Indeed, when one is exposed to mental or physical danger in a romantic partnership and still stays in the self-harming relationship, the behavior is connotated as addictive (Earp et al., 2017; Frascella et al., 2010). Addiction could also be noticed when a person indulges in an adopted behavior, such as sport or exercise, to the extent that the behavior becomes self-harming (repeated injuries, personal losses, etc.; Szabo et al., 2015).

In both Plato's and Spinoza's views, passion involves *losing control* and even rational thought (Vallerand & Verner-Filion, 2020), and, etymologically, the word means *suffering* (Hacker, 2018). In this view, passion leads to irrational beliefs that control people and make them slaves of the objects of their passion. What is the difference, then, between passion characterized by suffering and addiction? The answer is *self-harm*. One can suffer without apparent self-harm, but the suffering (i.e., compulsive and obsessive uncontrolled passion) is the path to self-harm. Indeed Descartes, as an adversary to Stoic philosophy, borrowed from the Stoics the view of *acceleration disorder* concerning passion that persistently *controls* the individual and passion that has an instant impact (Descartes [translated by Stephen H. Voss], 1989). Consequently, there is a *time* (duration) and *impact* (intensity) component of passion, which could be evolutionary or revolutionary (surfacing suddenly and having an intense, immediate impact; Egorov & Szabo, 2013). Consequently, passion can be conceptualized on a spectrum ranging from health (harmony) to dysfunction (obsession prone to turn into addiction) as proposed by the dual model of passion (Vallerand et al., 2003), presented later.

Most people adopt an activity for pleasure and fun. Although they could develop a passionate relationship with their chosen activity, generally, they remain in control and experience pleasures stemming from the involvement. Joy and satisfaction are the intrinsic rewards linked to autonomy and control that significantly motivate the activity's persuasion, thereby strengthening the individuals' commitment. This symbiosis with the chosen activity reflects the healthy passion, enhancing the individual's well-being (Moè, 2016). In some cases, however, involvement becomes obligatory because if it is not undertaken, the person experiences negative feelings (i.e., withdrawal effects). Then the activity starts to control the person, and the passionate relationship switches from autonomous into obligatory. This shift reflects the transformation of passion, from healthy (enjoyment) to dysfunctional (suffering) passion that could turn into an addiction. However, there must be a trigger for this transformation to occur, specific to the individual experience. Therefore, the behavioral manifestation of passion could be either positive or negative (Vallerand, 2012) but could also turn from positive into negative, with a trigger between the two, which could be explained by a tripartite model of passion (Lichtenstein et al., 2020) described later.

2.2 Passion and flow

Research attention dedicated to the passion for sports and exercise started around the late 1990s. While passion was most often associated with love and its erotic manifestations (i.e., Davies, 2003; Luhmann, 1986), there was little or no research on passion toward an activity (Vallerand, 2008). But how can one isolate passion from flow? First, flow is total absorption into a beloved activity, characterized by euphoric feelings, merging of awareness with the action, intrinsic motivation, and the inability to perceive the elapse of time (Csikszentmihalyi, 1990). There are commonalities and differences between passion and flow. Flow is an affective and cognitive state of mind, while passion is a feeling-based motivational construct bridging feeling states and personality traits (Philippe et al., 2009). In our view, motivational constructs are inseparable from affective and cognitive states, so in this regard, passion is relatively like flow. The difference is in passion's *chronic* (persistently present) nature versus the periodical *acute* (momentary) flow experience.

On the one hand, passion for a beloved activity persists continuously and surfaces in cognitive and affective forms (i.e., longing for it when remembering a pleasant moment) even when the person is not engaged in the activity. On the other hand, the flow experience is only momentary. It can be experienced when people engage in their passionate activity. Its occurrence is the *optimal* human experience (Csikszentmihalyi, 1990), manifesting as joy and happiness. The euphoric feeling associated with a flow experience is the intrinsic reward for the passionate activity. It is also the motivational fuel of the action. This link explains the strong correlation between passion and flow (Carpentier et al., 2012; Curran et al., 2015).

2.3 Dualistic model for passion

Vallerand and his coworkers (Vallerand et al., 2003) developed a dualistic model for passion based on the self-determination theory (Deci & Ryan, 2000). They postulated that, over a lifetime, people get involved in different activities for satisfying their personal needs for 1) *autonomy*, interpreted as an inner eagerness to experience self-initiative; 2) *competence*, viewed as the inner desire to master a given situation; and 3) *relatedness*, conceptualized as the inner ambition to connect with other people. The authors separate survival activities from leisure activities. From among the latter, experienced through trial and error, people will adopt and commit to those concrete activities that could fulfill their desire for autonomy, competence, and relatedness. Vallerand et al. (2003) conceptualize passion as a strong affinity toward an activity that the individual loves, values, and invests effort and time in it. Love and value distinguish this activity from others toward which the individual exhibits interest or even intrinsic motivation but are of lesser significance (Mageau et al., 2009).

People may show an affinity for their beloved activity in both autonomous and controlled ways, which determines the nature of their passion, being *harmonious* or *obsessive*, through behavioral regulation. For example, people could love and value their chosen activity (i.e., a sport) for *autonomous reasons* underpinned by the activity's inherent satisfaction or *controlled reasons* related to its compensatory function (Mageau et al., 2009; Vallerand et al., 2003). While the segregation of the two reasons may be impractical, an activity done for autonomous reasons primarily reflects *harmonious passion*. Alternately, activities practiced for controlled reasons mirror *obsessive passion* (Mageau et al., 2009). Consequently, harmonious passion results from autonomous internalization that triggers a strong but controlled drive to be part of the activity that the person freely adopts. It is congruent with the aspects of the self in which it becomes integrated (Mageau et al., 2009).

Harmonious passion emerges when the person flexibly engages in the autonomously internalized activity. This behavior is directly related to positive affect while being inversely associated with negative affect (Vallerand et al., 2003; Vallerand & Miquelon, 2007). However, obsessive passion may emerge in the lack of fulfillment of one's intrinsic needs, resulting in the internalization of intra- or interpersonal pressures or both. It appears when a person internalizes the activity in a controlled way, when the participation is rigidly controlled, which is associated with negative affect (Stenseng et al., 2011; Vallerand et al., 2003; Vallerand & Miquelon, 2007). Additionally, activity contingencies such as self-esteem and escape from problems (i.e., stress) are critical for the obsessively passionate person. The attachment to or reliance on these contingencies makes it difficult for one to stop or even interrupt the passionate activity. Therefore, self-pressures may arise from contingencies linked to the activity and loss of control over the activity or social pressure (Mageau et al., 2009). Vallerand et al. (2003) proposed that undertaking an activity with obsessive passion may also reflect compensation for perceived lack of low self-worth that motivates the indulging into the activity for ego nourishment. Obsessively passionate people feel obliged to pursue their passionate activity. Therefore, while they like, or even love, their chosen activity, they feel an urge to engage in it because of internal contingencies.

2.4 A tripartite model of passion

A recent study found that passion might have three dimensions (Lichtenstein et al., 2020). While this study's results stem from a culturally heterogeneous exercising sample, the third dimension of passion shown by the authors to be represented by *discovery* is worth further consideration. The common-sense prerequisite for discovery is interest and curiosity, which are inner psychological *needs* to investigate and explore for the sake of *discovering* something (Fitzgerald, 1999). Therefore, this need's fulfillment comes via investigation (i.e., searching, and self-directed learning) and exploration (experiencing or trying out things). For example, trying out a new sport for its personally appealing features (internal motivation) or peer, physical activity teacher, or parental pressure (external motivation) could lead to the *discovery* of the potential for the satisfaction of the desire for autonomy, competence, and relatedness, as postulated in the self-determination theory. Alternately, it can lead to disappointment and disengagement. The discovery of the positive experience is associated with positive affect and will increase commitment to the activity (Harter, 1981). Through a repeated cycle of personally rewarding sessions, the person might develop a harmonious passion for the new sport. However, a disappointment with the novel experience (whether initiated by inner or outer motivation) will generate negative affect and lead to no further interest in the activity as predicted by the competence motivation theory (Harter, 1981).

In an autonomously internalized passionate activity, being in harmony with the chosen sport or exercise also involves the continuous discovery of personal growth, new skills, more efficient techniques, better performance, bodily changes, and rewarding social feedback. These slight but continuously surfacing changes and associated feelings could reflect a passion for discovery. In Lichtenstein et al.'s (2020) work, items reflecting *discovery* passion were: 1) 'The new things that I discover with this activity allow me to appreciate it even more,' 2) 'This activity reflects the qualities I like about myself,' and 3) 'This activity allows me to live a variety of experiences.' All these items reflect the affinity for novelty and discovery. Although the second item may appear unrelated to novelty or discovery, the *liked qualities* emerging as novelty resulting from engagement in the activity reflect the *discovery* of a better and more positive self. Perhaps a good example of *discovery passion* is the scientist passionate about academic research which is in harmony with the work. To maintain this harmony, rewarding experiences, in the form of discoveries (i.e., fulfilling the research's aim), is essential. In this regard, according to Lichtenstein et al. (2020), there could be a continuum ranging from commitment to addiction, to a given activity, with the three forms of passion between them, in a hierarchical order (see Figure 2.1). However, as we discuss in the last chapter, this relationship is probably more complex.

The tripartite model for passion (Lichtenstein et al., 2020) does not attempt to fully separate harmonious passion and obsessive passion into two distinct categories. Instead, it proposes that passion exists on a continuum, ranging from harmony to obsession, with inner rewarding novelty and discovery between the two. Passion toward an activity can only develop following the commitment to the respective activity. Therefore, commitment is a prerequisite for passion. Committed engagement in the chosen activity leads to harmonious passion, which results from autonomous internalization and

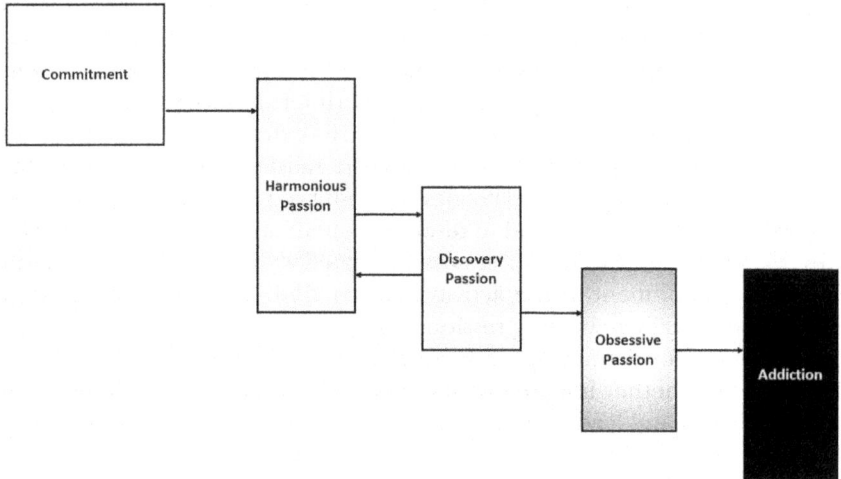

Figure 2.1 The continuum from the commitment to an activity to addiction, encompassing three forms of passion in a hierarchical order.

integration with the freely adopted activity (Mageau et al., 2009). It manifests in many positive feelings, such as affinity, intense desire, commitment, prioritization, joy, and love. Flow is likely to occur during the performance of the activity. Flow is a very pleasant, or even gratifying, 'optimal' human experience (Csikszentmihalyi, 1990), posited to explain the link between harmonious passion and well-being (Carpentier et al., 2012).

The new satisfying experiences stemming from improved skill, mastery, enjoyment, flow state, and increasingly closer association with the adopted activity continuously provide rewarding feelings in the form of novel discoveries about the relationship between the person and the chosen activity. For example, in sports, people discover that they can do better today than yesterday. They feel increasingly greater control, have more confidence, enjoy a particular session more than before, feel flow more often, and identify with their sport more closely. These are rewarding discoveries of growth and self-discovery of a perceived better self, resulting from the chosen activity. They also generate expectancies of discoveries, which in turn can act as motivational incentives in sport and exercise.

In some instances, a person can get *hooked* to these rewarding feelings as they may provide the most or the only satisfying life experience. For example, the discovery that a sport or exercise helps relieve stress could lead to adopting the activity for coping with stress (Egorov & Szabo, 2013). Through this novel discovery, the harmoniously performed activity is practiced for controlled reasons (instead of feeling like exercising for a positive reward, one *must* exercise to avoid stress) that reflect obsessive passion (Mageau et al., 2009). Indeed, the person becomes dependent on the chosen activity (i.e., a sport or exercise) at this stage. Dependence ranges from very low to very high, eventually culminating in addiction (Szabo et al., 2018). The relationship with the tripartite model of passion is that this model posits that the three forms of passion, *harmonious, discovery*, and *obsessive* passion, are positioned between commitment, characterized by very *low dependence*, and addiction, characterized by a very *high dependence* level.

2.5 Passion as a single action-motivating energy

Lawrie (1980) presented the concept of passion as a form of energy specific to the person's desire. The craving to fulfill the desire mobilizes this energy via emotions, feelings, and thoughts. Only in the presence of this energy does passion become evident. If the energy fueling the satisfaction of the desire is thwarted, a powerful emotional response occurs, and the person becomes unable to contain the passion. Is such frustrated passion identical to negative, or the *obsessive*, passion in Vallerand et al.'s (2003) dual model of passion? Can the obstruction of desire reflect the *discovery* (i.e., a new challenge, change, transformation) posited by the tripartite model? Lawrie (1980) suggested that various manifestations could characterize *one* passion. Accordingly, passion reflects how the feelings and emotions of the person generate behavioral expression toward another person, ideology, object, or action. Then, passion mirrors the affinity to a beloved activity (or event, object, or ideology). It is a mirror that reflects control or lack of it, and perhaps more closely enjoyment and harmony (harmonious passion), or slavery to a strong habit and suffering, potentially leading to self-harm (obsessive passion), bridged by a change in the relationship with the passionate activity, representing the trigger (discovery passion), when undergoing change or transformation.

Consequently, in line with Lawrie, passion is the behavioral manifestation of the desire-driven motivational energy generated by emotion-driven feelings that deeply connect the person with another person, animal or plant, an event, object(s), or activity. Passion is, therefore, a yearning-derived motivational energy that could trigger positive reinforcement (harmonious passion) when the reward surfaces as gain to the individual (satisfaction, enjoyment, fun, feeling of competence, etc.). Alternately, it is the fuel for negative reinforcement (obsessive passion) when the reward appears as salvation (avoidance of something negative such as stress, weight gain, risk of morbidity, etc.). Indeed, as Lawrie (1980) implies, it is the *same* energy the individual connects in different ways (harmoniously or obsessively). The type of connection can be a function of complex personal and situational factors, and, therefore, it is idiographic (Egorov & Szabo, 2013) and suggests a dynamic nature for passion.

Nevertheless, a transition from commitment to addiction may rarely occur. In many cases, either one type of passion, harmonious or obsessive, predominates the individual's relationship with a person, plant, or animal, an event, object(s), or activity, or both forms may be present. As Lawrie (1980) suggests, if both are energy, they could add up, and the *absolute passion* (i.e., peak motivating power) emerges as the sum of harmonious, discovery, and obsessive passion. In this case, there is no transition but coexistence. For example, romantic love and athletic excellence comprise the features of both obsessive and harmonious passion. The desire to be close to and be intimate with the loved person is autonomous and reflects *harmonious* characteristics of romantic love. The inner urge to think about her, call her, know what she is doing at this moment, asking for forgiveness, and external need of conforming and adapting (the person's lifestyle, family, needs, and emotions) are controlling characteristics of romantic love, which can be associated with obsessive passion (Mageau et al., 2009). A similar coexistence of harmonious and obsessive passion can also be observed in elite athletes. A passionate athlete can be expected to score high on both obsessive and harmonious passion measures (Szabo, 2018). However, athletes are unlikely to become addicted to their sport because through self-harm that would also hurt their performance and sporting career.

2.6 Key points

1. Passion is a complex inner motivating combination of feelings and emotions.
2. Passion can be harmonious, obsessive, or both depending on one's level of involvement.
3. There might be another motivating passion embracing change, novelty, and discovery.
4. Both positive and negative reinforcement could fuel all manifestations of passion.
5. Passion forms can also reflect a dynamic and symbiotic combination of feelings.

2.7 References

American Psychological Association (2021). *APA dictionary of psychology*. Retrieved from: https://dictionary.apa.org/passion
Bélanger, J. J., Caouette, J., Sharvit, K., & Dugas, M. (2014). The psychology of martyrdom: Making the ultimate sacrifice in the name of a cause. *Journal of Personality and Social Psychology, 107*(3), 494–515. doi:10.1037/a0036855
Blasco-Fontecilla, H., Fernández-Fernández, R., Colino, L., Fajardo, L., Perteguer-Barrio, R., & de Leon, J. (2016). The addictive model of self-harming (non-suicidal and suicidal) behavior. *Frontiers in Psychiatry, 7.* doi:10.3389/fpsyt.2016.00008
Carpentier, J., Mageau, G. A., & Vallerand, R. J. (2012). Ruminations and flow: Why do people with a more harmonious passion experience higher well-being? *Journal of Happiness Studies, 13*(3), 501–518. doi:10.1007/s10902-011-9276-4

Csikszentmihalyi, M. (1990). *Flow: The psychology of optimal experience.* New York, NY: Harper & Row.

Curran, T., Hill, A. P., Appleton, P. R., Vallerand, R. J., & Standage, M. (2015). The psychology of passion: A meta-analytical review of a decade of research on intrapersonal outcomes. *Motivation and Emotion, 39*(5), 631–655. doi:10.1007/s11031-015-9503-0

D'Acquisto, F. (2019). Quisquis amat valeat! (Whoever loves, may he be well) Why love and passion are important for the well-being of the immune system. *Frontiers in Education, 4*, 1–7. doi:10.3389/feduc.2019.00062

Davies, J. M. (2003). Falling in love with love oedipal and postoedipal manifestations of idealization, mourning, and erotic masochism. *Psychoanalytic Dialogues, 13*(1), 1–27. doi:10.1080/10481881309348718

Deci, E. L., & Ryan, R. M. (2000). The "what" and "why" of goal pursuits: Human needs and the self-determination of behavior. *Psychological Inquiry, 11*, 227–268. doi:10.1207/s15327965pli1104_02

Descartes, R. ([translated by Stephen H. Voss], 1989). *Passions of the soul.* Cambridge, MA: Hackett Publishing.

Earp, B. D., Wudarczyk, O. A., Foddy, B., & Savulescu, J. (2017). Addicted to love: What is love addiction and when should it be treated? *Philosophy, Psychiatry, & Psychology, 24*(1), 77–92. doi:10.1353/ppp.2017.0011

Egorov, A. Y., & Szabo, A. (2013). The exercise paradox: An interactional model for a clearer conceptualization of exercise addiction. *Journal of Behavioral Addictions, 2*(4), 199–208. doi:10.1556/jba.2.2013.4.2

Fernández-Carrasco, F. J., González-Mey, U., Rodríguez-Díaz, L., Vázquez-Lara, J. M., Gómez-Salgado, J., & Parrón-Carreño, T. (2019). Significance of affection changes during pregnancy: Intimacy, passion, and commitment. *International Journal of Environmental Research and Public Health, 16*(13), 2254. doi:10.3390/ijerph16132254

Fitzgerald, F. T. (1999). Curiosity. *Annals of Internal Medicine, 130*(1), 70–72. doi:10.7326/0003-4819-130-1-199901050-00015

Frascella, J., Potenza, M. N., Brown, L. L., & Childress, A. R. (2010). Shared brain vulnerabilities open the way for non-substance addictions: Carving addiction at a new joint? *Annals of the New York Academy of Sciences, 1187*(1), 294–315.

Hacker, P. M. S. (2018). *The passions: A study of human nature.* Oxford, UK: Wiley Blackwell. doi:10.1111/j.1749-6632.2009.05420.x

Harter, S. (1981). A model of mastery motivation in children: Individual differences and developmental change. In W. A. Collins (Ed.), *Aspects of the development of competence: The Minnesota symposia on child psychology* (Vol. 14, pp. 215–255). Hillsdale, NJ: Lawrence Erlbaum Associates.

Lawrie, R. (1980). Passion. *Philosophy and Phenomenological Research, 41*(1/2), 106–126.

Lichtenstein, M. B., Jensen, E. S., Larsen, P. V., Omdahl, M. K., & Szabo, A. (2020). Passion for exercise has three dimensions: Psychometric evaluation of the Passion Scale in a Danish fitness sample. *Translational Sports Medicine, 3*(6), 638–648. doi:10.1002/tsm2.173

Luhmann, N. (1986). *Love as passion: The codification of intimacy.* Cambridge, MA: Harvard University Press.

Mageau, G. A., Vallerand, R. J., Charest, J., Salvy, S. J., Lacaille, N., Bouffard, T., & Koestner, R. (2009). On the development of harmonious and obsessive passion: The role of autonomy support, activity specialization, and identification with the activity. *Journal of Personality, 77*(3), 601–646. doi:10.1111/j.1467-6494.2009.00559.x

Moè, A. (2016). Harmonious passion and its relationship with teacher well-being. *Teaching and Teacher Education, 59*, 431–437. doi:10.1016/j.tate.2016.07.017

Orosz, G., Zsila, Á., Vallerand, R. J., & Böthe, B. (2018). On the determinants and outcomes of passion for playing Pokémon Go. *Frontiers in Psychology, 9.* doi:10.3389/fpsyg.2018.00316

Paquette, V., Rapaport, M., St-Louis, A. C., & Vallerand, R. J. (2020). Why are you passionately in love? Attachment styles as determinants of romantic passion and conflict resolution strategies. *Motivation and Emotion, 44*(4), 621–639. doi:10.1007/s11031-020-09821-x

Philippe, F. L., Vallerand, R. J., Andrianarisoa, J., & Brunel, P. (2009). Passion in referees: Examining their affective and cognitive experiences in sport situations. *Journal of Sport and Exercise Psychology, 31*(1), 77–96. doi:10.1123/jsep.31.1.77

Rao, A. H., & Tobias Neely, M. (2019). What's love got to do with it? Passion and inequality in white-collar work. *Sociology Compass, 13*(12), 1–14, e12744. doi:10.1111/soc4.12744

Reynaud, M., Karila, L., Blecha, L., & Benyamina, A. (2010). Is love passion an addictive disorder? *The American Journal of Drug and Alcohol Abuse, 36*(5), 261–267. doi:10.3109/00952990.2010.495183

Schellenberg, B. J. I., & Bailis, D. S. (2018). When decisions are clouded by passion: A look at casino patrons. *Motivation Science, 4*(3), 274–279. doi:10.1037/mot0000086

Sigmundsson, H., Haga, M., & Hermundsdottir, F. (2020). The passion scale: Aspects of reliability and validity of a new 8-item scale assessing passion. *New Ideas in Psychology, 56*, e100745. doi:10.1016/j.newideapsych.2019.06.001

Stenseng, F., Rise, J., & Kraft, P. (2011). The dark side of leisure: Obsessive passion and its covariates and outcomes. *Leisure Studies, 30*(1), 49–62. doi:10.1080/02614361003716982

Szabo, A. (2018). Addiction, passion, or confusion? New theoretical insights on exercise addiction research from the case study of a female body builder. *Europe's Journal of Psychology, 14*(2), 296–316. doi:10.5964/ejop.v14i2.1545

Szabo, A., Demetrovics, Z., & Griffiths, M. D. (2018.). Morbid exercise behavior: Addiction or psychological escape? In H. Budde & M. Wegner (Eds.), *The exercise effect on mental health: Neurobiological mechanisms* (pp. 277–311). New York, NY: Routledge. doi:10.4324/9781315113906-11

Szabo, A., Griffiths, M. D., Marcos, R. D. L. V., Mervó, B., & Demetrovics, Z. (2015). Focus: Addiction: Methodological and conceptual limitations in exercise addiction research. *The Yale Journal of Biology and Medicine, 88*(3), 303–308. PMCID: PMC4553651

Vallerand, R. J. (2008). On the psychology of passion: In search of what makes people's lives most worth living. *Canadian Psychology/Psychologie Canadienne, 49*(1), 1–13. doi:10.1037/0708-5591.49.1.1

Vallerand, R. J. (2012). The role of passion in sustainable psychological well-being. *Psychology of Well-Being: Theory, Research and Practice, 2*(1), 1. doi:10.1186/2211-1522-2-1

Vallerand, R. J., Blanchard, C., Mageau, G. A., Koestner, R., Ratelle, C., Léonard, M., . . . Marsolais, J. (2003). Les passions de l'ame: On obsessive and harmonious passion. *Journal of Personality and Social Psychology, 85*(4), 756–767. doi:10.1037/0022-3514.85.4.756

Vallerand, R. J., & Miquelon, P. (2007). Passion for sport in athletes. In D. Laval-lee & S. Jowett (Eds.), *Social psychology in sport* (pp. 249–262). Champaign, IL: Human Kinetics.

Vallerand, R. J., & Verner-Filion, J. (2020). Theory and research in passion for sport and exercise. In G. Tenenbaum & R. C. Eklund (Eds.), *Handbook of sport psychology* (4th ed., pp. 206–229). New York, NY: John Wiley & Sons, Inc.

Wang, T., Thai, T. D.-H., Ly, P. T. M., & Chi, T. P. (2021). Turning social endorse-ment into brand passion. *Journal of Business Research, 126,* 429–439. doi:10.1016/j.jbusres.2021.01.011

Yitshaki, R., & Kropp, F. (2016). Motivations and opportunity recognition of social entrepreneurs. *Journal of Small Business Management, 54*(2), 546–565. doi:10.1111/jsbm.12157

3 Passion in athletes and leisure exercisers

3.1 Passion in sports

Athletes must be highly motivated and passionate about their chosen sport to succeed in competitions (Gustafsson et al., 2011). Most successful athletes have an 'inner fire burning' for their sport with which they identify (Mallett & Hanrahan, 2004). This fire is the passion for the chosen sport; it is internalized and may become an important, or the most important, aspect of the athletes' identity (Vallerand et al., 2008a). The athletic identity reflects the degree to which athletes identify themselves with their sport (Giannone et al., 2017). This relationship with the beloved sport can be harmonious and obsessive, as discussed in the previous chapter. The form of passion is impacted by, and impacts, affective states or emotions, of which the individual is aware (Paul et al., 2020). Therefore, affect is a strong determinant of passion and its form.

Affect refers to subjective feeling states having a valence (pleasant or unpleasant, positive or negative; Russell, 2009). Therefore, the measurement of affect is aimed at gauging the intensity of positive and negative feeling states. A distinction can be made between affect and mood. The *Diagnostic and Statistical Manual of Mental Disorders* (*DSM-4*; American Psychiatric Association, 2000) defines affect as reflections of behaviors due to subjective emotional states and mood as a persisting, more general, emotion. In accord with Manjunatha et al. (2009), the mood might be perceived as a persisting emotional climate, in contrast to affect, which mirrors the changing (i.e., momentary) emotional weather.

Consequently, mood mirrors enduring emotions, while affect is the momentary valence (positive or negative) of those emotions (Williams & Tappen, 2007), significantly influenced by the situation. Still, the interdependence between the two prognosticates how affective valence influences mood. Indeed, repeated events that generate negative affect will eventually result in a persisting negative mood. However, not only the frequency of the affective valence is crucial in shaping one's mood but also its intensity (Diener et al., 1985). For example, a traumatic or an exhilarating event generates a strong effect that immediately impacts mood, while less intense

DOI: 10.4324/9781003173595-3

events shape the person's mood through their frequency of occurrence. Research in athletes has primarily focused on the relationship between affect and passion.

3.2 Passion in athletes

3.2.1 Affect

A longitudinal study with 205 male football players (Vallerand et al., 2003, Study 2) showed that harmonious passion predicted the increase in positive affect while unrelated to negative affect. On the contrary, obsessive passion was associated with increased negative affect over the season while unrelated to positive affect, but the shared variance was relatively small (i.e., <10%). These results support the theoretical relationship predicting a direct relationship between positive affect and harmonious passion and negative affect and obsessive passion. Similar results emerged from a study examining 210 competitive basketball players (Vallerand et al., 2006, Study 2). In this study, harmonious passion was positively and significantly correlated (shared variance = 12.96%) with positive affect, but it was not connected to negative affect. However, obsessive passion was positively and significantly correlated with negative affect (shared variance = 9.61%) but not with positive affect.

Another research examining 94 female and 164 male competing athletes from various sports (Gustafsson et al., 2011) also demonstrated that harmonious passion was positively related to positive affect (shared variance = 15.21%), while obsessive passion was positively associated with negative affect (shared variance = 5.29%). Furthermore, obsessively passionate athletes scored significantly higher on negative affect than harmoniously passionate athletes. Conversely, the latter scored significantly higher on positive affect than obsessively passionate athletes. Similar findings emerged from research with soccer referees (Philippe et al., 2009). These studies support a direct (positive) relationship between harmonious passion and positive affect and obsessive passion and negative affect.

A possible explanation for these findings, connecting affect and passion, could be that harmonious passion stems from the autonomous internalization of the beloved activity in the person's identity with no rigidly associated contingencies. Consequently, it is likely to generate a desire to experience (yearning for the objecft of passion) what is occurring at the very moment (Philippe et al., 2009). This openness to the (a) new experience and the situation permits the integration of the activity and promotes pleasant feelings or positive affect. On the contrary, obsessive passion stems from controlled internalization (Vallerand et al., 2003) of the action in the person's identity. It is associated with rigid contingencies and related expectations attached to it. Therefore, the individual's self-evaluation depends on participation and the extent of excelling in the passionate activity (Ashley et al.,

2020). Imperfect (personally judged as not satisfying) action-result hurts the ego and generates an emotional threat, or negative self-evaluation and negative affect, which hampers the experience of positive affect (Philippe et al., 2009). However, there is also research evidence showing that obsessive passion does not hamper positive affect when the reason for being passionate is fulfilled (Vallerand et al., 2008b).

3.2.2 Burnout

Raedeke et al. (2002) defined burnout in sport, or in athletic context, as 'a withdrawal from [sport] noted by a reduced sense of accomplishment, devaluation/resentment of sport, and physical/psychological exhaustion' (p. 181). Passion represents a double-edged sword concerning burnout. While obsessive passion could lead to burnout, harmonious passion may be a shield against it (Vallerand et al., 2010). Indeed, differences were reported between harmonious and obsessive passion concerning their relationship with burnout. According to Vallerand et al. (2010), obsessive passion appears to be positively associated with burnout, whereas harmonious passion seems to be negatively related to burnout in *occupational* settings (Carbonneau et al., 2008; Vallerand et al., 2010). In sports, research with 149 young soccer players (Curran et al., 2011) showed an inverse relationship between harmonious passion and athletic burnout mediated by increased levels of self-determined motivation. This finding hints toward the adaptive role of harmonious passion for athletes. However, this research did not disclose an association between obsessive passion and athlete burnout.

Another study of 173 young soccer players (Curran et al., 2013) assessing passion for sport, psychological need satisfaction, and athlete burnout found that psychological need satisfaction mediated the relationship between harmonious passion and athlete burnout. In accord with Vallerand et al. (2010), these findings support an inverse relationship between harmonious passion and burnout. On the contrary, like in Curran et al.'s earlier study (2011), obsessive passion was unrelated to burnout in these athletes.

A study with university volleyball players (Schellenberg et al., 2013) examined the relationship between harmonious and obsessive passion and coping skills. It tested whether coping mediated the relationship between passion, risk of burnout, and goal attainment, from the start to the end of an athletic season. The results indicated that the two forms of passion were indirectly associated with the risk of burnout and goal attainment through coping. Harmonious passion was positively associated with task-oriented coping, which was positively related to the change in goal attainment. Obsessive passion was related to disengagement-oriented coping, while the latter was positively linked to burnout and negatively to goal attainment changes. This study provided evidence for the association between passion and coping that could be instrumental in athletic burnout.

A study by Kent and her colleagues (2018) investigated whether psychological need satisfaction mediates the relationship between passion and athletes' burnout. They tested 120 competitive athletes participating in 21 different sports. Their results indicated that both harmonious and obsessive passion were significantly related to the sport devaluation dimension of athletic burnout but not to exhaustion and sense of accomplishment. The psychological need for autonomy was the only significant mediating variable in the relationship between passion and the sport devaluation component of burnout.

In a more recent study, Lopes and Vallerand (2020) tested the role of harmonious and obsessive passion in various, mainly individual, athletes' perceptions of burnout. Two correlational studies involved different athletes with a mixed level of athletic skills. In the first study, the authors found that obsessive passion was positively related to the perception of burnout, while harmonious passion exhibited an inverse relationship with it. These results were supported in another study of 316 individual athletes. Additionally, the authors found support for the mediating role of conflict and need satisfaction in the relationships between the two forms of passion and the athletes' perceptions of burnout. They also reported, as a novel finding, in accord with Vallerand et al. (2010), that harmonious passion for a second activity was negatively related to the perceptions of burnout. In contrast, obsessive passion for a second activity was positively associated with it. These results, however, are new and await replication and critical evaluation.

Further support for a direct relationship between obsessive passion and burnout and an inverse relationship between harmonious passion and burnout comes from Gustafsson et al. (2011) and Martin and Horn (2013). In the first study, 258 Swedish national-level athletes from 21 different sports were tested. Athletes' harmonious passion was inversely associated with the risk of athletic burnout, while obsessive passion was positively related only to the exhaustion component of athletic burnout. In the other study, 186 female adolescent athletes were examined to determine whether harmonious and obsessive passion and athletic identity could predict burnout (Martin & Horn, 2013). Like Gustafsson et al., the findings showed that athletes' harmonious passion negatively predicted athletic burnout. In contrast, obsessive passion was positively linked again only to the exhaustion component of athletic burnout. Therefore, these studies provided partial support for the positive relationship between athletic burnout and obsessive passion, while they both showed the potentially protective role of harmonious passion in athletic burnout.

Most studies investigating the relationship between passion and athletic burnout suggest a varying association level between the two. Still, other factors appear to mediate the relationship to a variable extent. Moreover, obsessive passion seems to bear a weaker relationship with athletic burnout. Indeed, an investigation based on responses from 356 young Norwegian elite athletes participating in various sports (Moen et al., 2016a) yielded a moderate negative correlation between harmonious passion and athletic burnout and a statistically still significant but weak negative correlation between obsessive passion and burnout. However, in predicting burnout, obsessive passion was statistically no longer significant in the regression equation. Another report by Moen and his colleagues (2016b) examined whether passion, perceived performance, stress, and worry predict athletic burnout in 318 young elite athletes participating in various sports. The results showed that all dependent measures, *except obsessive passion*, were related to burnout. In contrast, a study with 267 athletes from various sports in Turkey reported that obsessive passion, perfectionism subdimensions of perceived parental pressure, and concern over mistakes predicted the sport devaluation component of athletic burnout (Demirci & Çepikkurt, 2018).

Considering the heterogeneity of the examined samples in various studies and the different mediating variables studied, the link between passion and burnout appears somewhat tentative. A relatively recent mini literature review (Bicalho & Da Costa, 2018) showed that all three included studies reported a negative relationship between harmonious passion and burnout in elite athletes. Two studies showed a positive relationship between obsessive passion and personal accomplishment and all three established a positive link between obsessive passion and exhaustion dimension of burnout. Obsessive passion was negatively associated with the sport devaluation dimension of burnout in two of the studies. The authors concluded that harmonious passion is negatively related to burnout. In contrast, obsessive passion is positively connected to the dimensions of reduced self-accomplishment and exhaustion while being negatively associated with the devaluation dimension of athletic burnout in elite athletes. Despite the small number of studies included in this review, the findings agree with the extant research, suggesting a consistent negative relationship between harmonious passion and athletic burnout. In contrast, the relationship between obsessive passion and athletic burnout appears weaker and often positive. Consequently, harmonious passion may have a protective role in athletic burnout, while obsessive passion could represent a risk factor. However, these relationships may not be direct, and substantially more research should be conducted to unveil the contribution of various mediating factors to this relationship.

3.2.3 Coach–athlete relationship

A positive relationship between athletes and their coaches appears to foster the passion for a chosen sport. A study with 200 male handball players in Turkey (Güllü, 2019) showed a positive link between the coach–athlete relationship and sports passion. In this study, both harmonious passion and obsessive passion were weakly positively correlated with the coach–athlete relationship scores. An earlier report, presenting the results of two studies (Lafrenière et al., 2008), showed that harmonious passion positively predicted the quality of the coach–athlete relationship in 157 athletes involved in various team sports. In contrast, obsessive passion was mainly unrelated to this relationship. However, like in Güllü's (2019) study, all correlations were positive. In the second study reported by Lafrenière et al., only harmonious passion predicted the coach–athlete relationship's quality in 106 coaches from various team and individual sports. Positive emotions fully mediated the observed effects. Furthermore, the quality of the coach–athlete relationship emerged as a positive predictor of coaches' well-being. Surely, being in an occupational harmonious relationship promotes well-being (Liu et al., 2021).

In a later study of 103 coach–athlete dyads, Lafrenière et al. (2011) found that harmonious passion for coaching was a positive predictor of the athletes' autonomy-support. In contrast, obsessive passion for coaching was a predictor of controlling behaviors. Furthermore, autonomy-support from the coaches' part predicted high-quality coach–athlete relationships, as subjectively perceived by the athletes, which positively predicted athletes' general happiness. A more recent study of 278 athletes involved in various individual sports at different levels of competition (Güllü et al., 2020) reported that athletes participating at a higher level of competition (national level) exhibited more obsessive passion than those participating in lower levels of competition. The authors also noticed a statistically significant positive relationship between coach–athlete (all dimensions) and harmonious and obsessive passion. Therefore, a positive relationship between the coach–athlete relationship and passion, especially harmonious passion, seems to be supported in the limited literature on the topic. Obsessive passion also appears to be linked to the coach–athlete relationship, perhaps at the higher levels of competition.

3.2.4 Performance

Only a few studies have tested the relationship between sports performance and passion. Both harmonious passion and obsessive passion could positively influence performance through the motivational energy of passion. However, the relationship, like the passion-burnout relationship, is often mediated by other factors rather than being a direct one. For example, a series of three studies with team athletes tested whether harmonious passion, less than obsessive passion, influences the last-minute sport performance via integrated temporal positivity comprising 1) positive past, 2) positive present, 3) positive future, and 4) negative past (Sverdlik et al., 2019). The researchers found that harmonious passion for the chosen sport led to the positive appraisal of the past, present, and future, facilitating the crucial last-minute performance on the field. In contrast, obsessive passion for the sport yielded a less positive appraisal of the temporal perspectives and a more negative evaluation of the past, which harmed the last-minute performance. The bivariate correlations (direct association) between harmonious/obsessive passion and the last-minute performance, however, were relatively weak.

Two studies, one with 184 basketball players and another with 67 synchronized swimmers and water-polo players, examined whether harmonious and obsessive passions could predict performance via deliberate practice (Vallerand et al., 2008a). The first study showed that both harmonious and obsessive passion predicted deliberate practice in basketball, which then predicted performance. In the second study, harmonious passion predicted mastery goals, which predicted performance via deliberate practice while obsessive passion inversely predicted performance via performance-avoidance goals. However, the direct correlations between harmonious/obsessive passion and performance were relatively weak. Comparably, in a study of 645 Chinese high school athletes (Li, 2010), mastery approach goals, which were predicted by both harmonious and obsessive passion, predicted sports performance. In Li's study, the two forms of passion also directly predicted sports performance, despite a low correlation between them. However, the direct effect vanished when achievement and mastery (approach and avoidance goals) were entered into the equation. These findings suggest that the direct influence of passion on performance is only minimal. Still, passion affects performance by facilitating mastery goals, especially mastery approach goals, positively affecting performance.

Indeed, the reported correlations between passion, both obsessive and harmonious passion, and perceived performance are usually weak. Moen et al. (2016b), for example, reported statistically significant positive correlations between perceived performance and both harmonious and obsessive passion but they explained less than 10% of the variance, supporting the contention that the direct effect of passion on performance is weak. Similarly, weak correlations (explaining <10% of the variance) were observed between harmonious and obsessive passion and performance, as *perceived* by soccer coaches, and harmonious and obsessive passion and *objective* performance, as based on the number of games played in ice hockey (Verner-Filion et al., 2017). However, this study, matching the results of most other related studies in the field, also disclosed an indirect link between harmonious passion and performance mediated by need satisfaction (in soccer and hockey) and achievement goals (in hockey), and obsessive passion and performance mediated by deliberate practice (in both soccer and hockey).

Overall, it appears that, in accord with the conceptualization of passion in Chapter 2, there is an energy mobilization that stems from high affinity, love, and dedication to the sports activity, often to the extent of symbiotic unity with the beloved sport. The source of this energy could be harmonious or obsessive or both. Indeed, the conceptualization of passion on a single spectrum may be inadequate. Often athletes score high on both harmonious and obsessive passion (Szabo, 2018). Such observation makes sense when the controlling and rigid aspects of competitive sports are considered. These characteristics of competitive sports stem from the required self-discipline to adhere to the strict and highly demanding training regimen that controls the athlete's life in striving for successful performance.

High harmonious passion reflects autonomously internalized activity, pride in success, and the joy of good performance. Consequently, competitive athletes can be expected to report high scores on both obsessive and harmonious passion, one reflecting a surrender to conformity (e.g., 'I have to do it . . . I must train. . ., No pain, no gain. . .,' etc.). On the one hand, high obsessive passion could mirror the self-set and coach-*imposed* pressures that are not mere choices but perceived obligations the athlete needs to succumb to succeed. Therefore, they are 'controlled' internalizations that stem from intra- and interpersonal pressures (Vallerand, 2012). On the other hand, high scores of harmonious passion reflect the pleasant and rewarding *binding* (enjoyed, beloved, integrated) aspects of the sporting behavior. They involve dedication, aspiration, and commitment mediated by the positive reinforcement of regular training, reflecting the energy fueling the internal motivation. However, it is more than internal motivation because dedicated athletes identify with what they are doing (Vallerand, 2012), which is part of their identity. The greater this part is, the higher the passion; obsessive passion surfaces with conformity and self-imposed pressure to achieve her goal while harmonious passion arises with pride, enjoyment, and satisfaction (Figure 3.1).

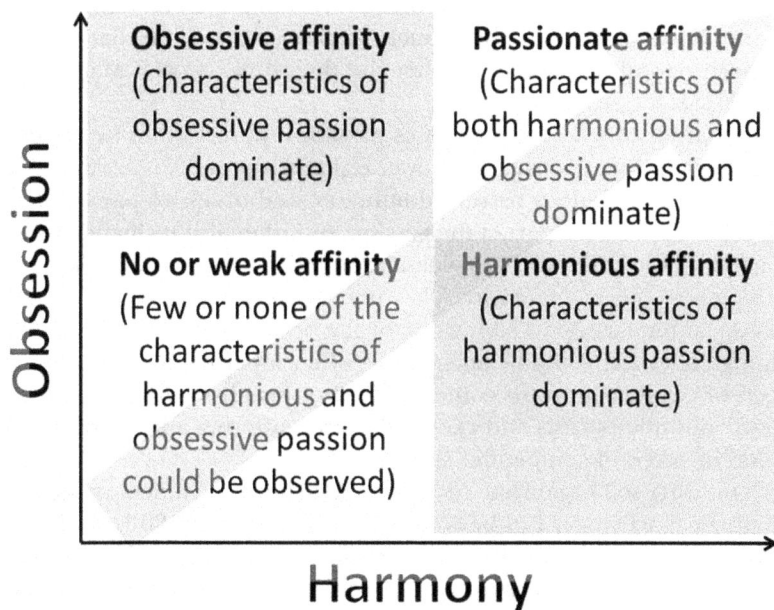

Figure 3.1 Two dimensions of passion: Diagram of harmonious and obsessive passion in athletes.

3.3 Passion as energy in athletes

A two-dimensional view of passion posits that total passion is observable when both the harmonious and obsessive characteristics of passion dominate the person's relationship with the beloved sport. If we accept that passion is a form of energy (Lawrie, 1980), then, as mentioned in Chapter 2, harmonious and obsessive passion could add up to yield total or absolute passion as a form of maximum desire-driven energy. This energy emerges in the top right quadrant in Figure 3.1, and it is in full accord with the classical views of passion encompassing *joy* and *suffering*. Like in Christian religions, for example, the suffering and death of Jesus Christ also involve his joy of going to Heaven, to the Father, and disciples' joy for Christ (He is going to the Father) and the salvation of humanity. 'You heard Me say, 'I am going away, and I am coming back to you.' If you loved Me, you would rejoice [in Christ's Passion] that I am going to the Father, because the Father is greater than I' (Bible, John 14:28).

Similarly, in sport achievement, there is the *joy* of excelling, feeling great, and winning, which are accompanied by *suffering* from the daily long hours of training, sacrifice in personal needs and relationships, forced adaptation to training schedules, environment, travel, coach, and teammates, and so on. The following quote from Michael Jordan illustrates the pain and gain or the suffering and joy involved in passion: 'I've failed over and over again. And that is why I succeed.' True passion is such motivational energy that one feels that the passion is worth dying for: 'I've done everything you can imagine. It just depends on how much I can push myself on that exact day. But there's no quit in me, I'd rather die than quit' (Coach Mag, December 8, 2015).

Total passion is when the object of passion is perceived to be worth the life of the passionate person. The lower right quadrant of Figure 3.1 reflects a case when harmonious passion dominates, and obsessive passion is relatively low. This case is a part of the passion, or rather affinity manifested in a balanced relationship with the pleasant or joyful aspect of the relationship with a person, object, or activity. A harmonious relationship with a friend or a spouse, a usual run on a sunny day, or the occasional admiration of one's painting collection could be an example of harmonious affinity for various objects of passion. In sports contests, whether healthy or not, the 'no pain, no gain' attitude persists and exemplifies the suffering and joy of the elite athletes involved in competitive sports.

In contrast, self-organized recreational exercises (noncompetitive leisure physical activities) can be void of pain or suffering. Still, as discussed in Chapter 2 in the context of the tripartite model, the beloved activity may start to control the passionate person. In this case, there could be two possible outcomes. One is when the controlled aspects of obsession with the activity remain balanced with the harmonious elements, in which case a total passion is observable (upper right quadrant in Figure 3.1). This scenario is total, or true, passion: ' . . . when individuals are passionate for an activity, they tend to strongly endorse items from both (harmonious and obsessive) subscales. . .' (Guérin et al., 2013, p. 9, parenthesis added).

The other scenario is when obsessive characteristics of the passionate relationship tend to dominate. In this situation, with a concomitant loss in harmonious affinity, there is a shift from the harmonious to obsessive affinity, which starts to characterize the person's relationship to the object of passion (upper-left quadrant in Figure 3.1). Perhaps more rarely, a similar shift from obsessive toward harmonious passion may also occur. Based on the tripartite model of passion, presented in Chapter 2, the transition from a harmonious to an obsessive passion – via the loss of internal control and progressively increasing internal (self) pressure – could lead to addiction (refer to Figure 2.1). Finally, in the lower-left quadrant of Figure 3.1, low levels of both harmonious and obsessive affinity may reflect the lack of significant desire and elevated motivation toward a possible object of passion. It is important to note that there is large intraindividual and interindividual variability in the two dimensions of passion. For example, one person may be fully passionate about golf while having an obsessive passion for red wine and a harmonious passion for mountain biking. Another order may prevail in another person.

3.4 Passion in recreational exercisers

Recreational exercisers, unlike athletes, have autonomy and control over their preferred exercise(s); these characteristics of leisure exercises foster a harmonious relationship between individuals and their physical activities. Several studies examined passion in recreational exercisers. For example, Guérin et al. (2013) studied 63 women in a 14-day experience sampling study assessing affect and physical activity. Results indicated that 60 participants were passionate, and the mean scores of harmonious passion were 2.68 times higher than scores of obsessive passion. The harmonious and obsessive passion levels moderated the association between activity engagement and positive affect; obsessively passionate participants felt significantly worse on days when they were inactive. The results also indicated that vitality was inversely associated with obsessive passion while directly related to harmonious passion. As expected, this study provides support for greater harmonious passion than obsessive passion in recreational exercise.

3.4.1 Team versus individual exercise

A study with recreational university athletes compared harmonious and obsessive passion between the team and individual exercisers (Kovacsik et al., 2020). The study results showed that team exercisers scored significantly higher on harmonious passion, but not obsessive, passion, than individual exercisers. The findings agree with the results obtained by Vallerand et al. (2003, Study 1). Furthermore, these results replicated earlier findings reported by de la Vega et al. (2016) in terms of harmonious passion. However, in the latter study, obsessive passion was also greater in the team exercisers than in individual exercisers, probably due to a mixed sample studied by De La Vega et al. comprising competitive and noncompetitive exercisers.

An explanation for greater harmonious passion in team exercisers in contrast to individual exercisers is that in addition to the physical and psychological aspects of exercise activity found in individual activities, team workouts have social components that could influence harmonious passion. Such components are collective motivation, shared success, and successful cooperation, all of which could be associated with greater harmonious passion in team versus individual sports. Furthermore, socialization, which is more characteristic in the team than individual sports (Devecioglu et al., 2012), might also contribute to greater harmonious passion in the former than the latter group. Overall, team sports provide a greater opportunity for enjoyment, fun, and shared experience via their social aspects, which could foster greater harmonious affinity than individual exercises.

3.4.2 Gender and cultural differences

Several studies examined whether there are differences between men and women exercisers in passion. A cross-sectional research with 516 adult Greek exercisers showed no difference in passion between men and women (Parastatidou et al., 2012). Similarly, another cross-sectional investigation with 480 Canadian university students participating in various individual exercisers found no difference in passion between men and women (Paradis et al., 2013). Also, there was no gender difference in passion among 313 Spanish exercisers (de la Vega et al., 2016). In contrast, another study found that women exercising at lower intensities reported greater obsessive and harmonious passion than men exercising at similar exercise intensities (Kovacsik et al., 2019).

Cultural differences in passion were reported in a study comparing 1002 Hungarian and Spanish exercisers (Szabo et al., 2018). In this study, Hungarian women scored significantly higher on harmonious and obsessive passion than their Spanish counterparts, but Hungarian men only scored higher on obsessive passion when compared to Spanish men. These findings suggest that gender differences are likely to exist at a cultural level. In addition, more gender differences emerged in a study of 1255 Danish fitness exercisers in obsessive but not harmonious passion, with men scoring higher than women (Lichtenstein et al., 2020). Overall, research on gender, physical activity, and passion is still meager. It is possible that the form and volume of exercise, along with cultural factors, could both influence passion in different ways. Therefore, substantially more research is needed in this area.

3.5 Key differences in passion between athletes and leisure exercisers

As discussed earlier in this chapter, competing athletes may exhibit (and most do, i.e., Szabo, 2018) total or absolute passion and report high levels of both harmonious and obsessive passion. In contrast, by maintaining complete control over their exercise, leisure exercisers are more likely to show greater harmonious than obsessive passion, as evidenced in the literature. Still, there could be a unidirectional shift (via discovery passion) from harmonious to obsessive passion leading to addiction. Both passions are (desire-motivated) forms of mental energy that add up and culminate in a mental state, often equating the passionate activity with life's worth.

3.6 Key points

1. Passion in sports and exercise may not be categorical but rather two-dimensional.
2. Harmonious passion appears to have a protective role in athletic burnout.
3. Positive affect is associated with harmonious passion while negative affect is more closely related to obsessive passion.
4. Passion has a small and primarily indirect effect on athletic performance.
5. Total passion can be described as high harmonious and obsessive passion, seen in competitive athletes and, therefore, supporting a two-dimensional view of passion.

3.7 References

American Psychiatric Association (2000). *Diagnostic and statistical manual of mental disorders* (4th ed., Text Revision). Washington, DC: Author.

Ashley, S. L., Brown, A., & Crocker, J. (2020). Contingencies of self-worth. In V. Zeigler-Hill & T. K. Shackelford (Eds.), *Encyclopedia of personality and individual differences* (pp. 885–888). Cham, Switzerland: Springer Nature Switzerland AG. doi:10.1007/978-3-319-24612-3_300542

Bicalho, C. C. F., & Da Costa, V. T. (2018). Burnout in elite athletes: A systematic review. *Cuadernos de Psicología del Deporte, 18*(1), 89–102.

Carbonneau, N., Vallerand, R. J., Fernet, C., & Guay, F. (2008). The role of passion for teaching in intrapersonal and interpersonal outcomes. *Journal of Educational Psychology, 100*(4), 977–987. doi:10.1037/a0012545

Coach Mag (2015, December 8). *Tony Bellew: "I'd rather die than quit!"*. Retrieved from: www.coachmag.co.uk/people/4984/tony-bellew-id-rather-die-than-quit

Curran, T., Appleton, P. R., Hill, A. P., & Hall, H. K. (2011). Passion and burnout in elite junior soccer players: The mediating role of self-determined motivation. *Psychology of Sport and Exercise, 12*(6), 655–661. doi:10.1016/j.psychsport.2011.06.004

Curran, T., Appleton, P. R., Hill, A. P., & Hall, H. K. (2013). The mediating role of psychological need satisfaction in relationships between types of passion for sport and athlete burnout. *Journal of Sports Sciences*, *31*(6), 597–606. doi:10.1080/0264 0414.2012.742956

de la Vega, R., Parastatidou, I. S., Ruíz-Barquín, R., & Szabo, A. (2016). Exercise addiction in athletes and leisure exercisers: The moderating role of passion. *Journal of Behavioral Addictions*, *5*(2), 325–331. doi:10.1556/2006.5.2016.043

Demirci, E., & Çepikkurt, F. (2018). Examination of the relationship between passion, perfectionism and burnout in athletes. *Universal Journal of Educational Research*, *6*(6), 1252–1259. doi:10.13189/ujer.2018.060616

Devecioglu, S., Sahan, H., Yildiz, M., Tekin, M., & Sim, H. (2012). Examination of socialization levels of university students engaging in individual and team sports. *Procedia – Social and Behavioral Sciences*, *46*, 326–330. doi:10.1016/j. sbspro.2012.05.115

Diener, E., Larsen, R. J., Levine, S., & Emmons, R. A. (1985). Intensity and frequency: Dimensions underlying positive and negative affect. *Journal of Personality and Social Psychology*, *48*(5), 1253–1265. doi:.1037/0022-3514.48.5.1253

Giannone, Z. A., Haney, C. J., Kealy, D., & Ogrodniczuk, J. S. (2017). Athletic identity and psychiatric symptoms following retirement from varsity sports. *International Journal of Social Psychiatry*, *63*(7), 598–601. doi:10.1177/0020764017724184

Guérin, E., Fortier, M. S., & Williams, T. (2013). "I just NEED to move . . .": Examining women's passion for physical activity and its relationship with daily affect and vitality. *Psychology of Well-Being: Theory, Research and Practice*, *3*(1), 4. doi:10.1186/2211-1522-3-4

Güllü, S. (2019). The effect of the coach-athlete relationship on passion for sports: The case of male handball players in super league. *Journal of Education and Training Studies*, *7*(1), 38–47. doi:10.11114/jets.v7i1.3724

Güllü, S., Keskin, B., Ates, O., & Hanbay, E. (2020). Coach-athlete relationship and sport passion in individual sports. *Acta Kinesiologica*, *14*(1), 9–15.

Gustafsson, H., Hassmén, P., & Hassmén, N. (2011). Are athletes burning out with passion? *European Journal of Sport Science*, *11*(6), 387–395. doi:10.1080/17461391 .2010.536573

Kent, S., Kingston, K., & Paradis, K. F. (2018). The relationship between passion, basic psychological needs satisfaction and athlete burnout: Examining direct and indirect effects. *Journal of Clinical Sport Psychology*, *12*(1), 75–96. doi:10.1123/ jcsp.2017-0030

Kovacsik, R., Griffiths, M. D., Pontes, H. M., Soós, I., de la Vega, R., Ruíz-Barquín, R., . . . Szabo, A. (2019). The role of passion in exercise addiction, exercise volume, and exercise Intensity in long-term exercisers. *International Journal of Mental Health and Addiction*, *17*(6), 1389–1400. doi:10.1007/s11469-018-9880-1

Kovacsik, R., Soós, I., de la Vega, R., Ruíz-Barquín, R., & Szabo, A. (2020). Passion and exercise addiction: Healthier profiles in team than in individual sports. *International Journal of Sport and Exercise Psychology*, *18*(2), 176–186. doi:10.1080/1612 197X.2018.1486873

Lafrenière, M.-A. K., Jowett, S., Vallerand, R. J., & Carbonneau, N. (2011). Passion for coaching and the quality of the coach–athlete relationship: The mediating role of coaching behaviors. *Psychology of Sport and Exercise*, *12*(2), 144–152. doi:10.1016/j.psychsport.2010.08.002

Lafrenière, M.-A. K., Jowett, S., Vallerand, R. J., Donahue, E. G., & Lorimer, R. (2008). Passion in sport: On the quality of the coach–athlete relationship. *Journal of Sport and Exercise Psychology*, *30*(5), 541–560. doi:10.1123/jsep.30.5.541

Lawrie, R. (1980). Passion. *Philosophy and Phenomenological Research*, *41*(1/2), 106–126.

Li, C. H. (2010). Predicting subjective vitality and performance in sports: The role of passion and achievement goals. *Perceptual and Motor Skills*, *110*(3), 1029–1047. doi:10.2466/05.06.07.14.PMS.110.C.1029-1047

Lichtenstein, M. B., Jensen, E. S., Larsen, P. V., Omdahl, M. K., & Szabo, A. (2020). Passion for exercise has three dimensions: Psychometric evaluation of The Passion Scale in a Danish fitness sample. *Translational Sports Medicine*, *3*(6), 638–648. doi:10.1002/tsm2.173

Liu, Y., Zemke, R., Liang, L., & Gray, J. M. (2021). Occupational harmony: Embracing the complexity of occupational balance. *Journal of Occupational Science*, 1–15. (Online first). doi:10.1080/14427591.2021.1881592

Lopes, M., & Vallerand, R. J. (2020). The role of passion, need satisfaction, and conflict in athletes' perceptions of burnout. *Psychology of Sport and Exercise*, *48*, 101674. doi:10.1016/j.psychsport.2020.101674

Mallett, C. J., & Hanrahan, S. J. (2004). Elite athletes: Why does the "fire" burn so brightly? *Psychology of Sport and Exercise*, *5*(2), 183–200. doi:10.1016/s1469-0292(02)00043-2

Manjunatha, N., Khess, C. R., & Ram, D. (2009). The conceptualization of terms: 'Mood' and 'affect' in academic trainees of mental health. *Indian Journal of Psychiatry*, *51*(4), 285–288. doi:10.4103/0019-5545.58295

Martin, E. M., & Horn, T. S. (2013). The role of athletic identity and passion in predicting burnout in adolescent female athletes. *The Sport Psychologist*, *27*(4), 338–348. doi:10.1123/tsp.27.4.338

Moen, F., Myhre, K., Sandbakk, Ø., & Moen, F. (2016a). Psychological determinants of burnout, illness and injury among elite junior athletes. *The Sport Journal*, *19*, 1–14.

Moen, F., Myhre, K., & Stiles, T. C. (2016b). An exploration about how passion, perceived performance, stress and worries uniquely influence athlete burnout. *Journal of Physical Education and Sports Management*, *3*(1), 88–107. doi:10.15640/jpesm.v3n1a7

Paradis, K. F., Cooke, L. M., Martin, L. J., & Hall, C. R. (2013). Too much of a good thing? Examining the relationship between passion for exercise and exercise dependence. *Psychology of Sport and Exercise*, *14*(4), 493–500. doi:10.1016/j.psychsport.2013.02.003

Parastatidou, I. S., Doganis, G., Theodorakis, Y., & Vlachopoulos, S. P. (2012). Exercising with passion: Initial validation of the Passion Scale in exercise. *Measurement in Physical Education and Exercise Science*, *16*(2), 119–134. doi:10.1080/1091367x.2012.657561

Paul, E. S., Sher, S., Tamietto, M., Winkielman, P., & Mendl, M. T. (2020). Towards a comparative science of emotion: Affect and consciousness in humans and animals. *Neuroscience & Biobehavioral Reviews*, *108*, 749–770. doi:10.1016/j.neubiorev.2019.11.014

Philippe, F. L., Vallerand, R. J., Andrianarisoa, J., & Brunel, P. (2009). Passion in referees: Examining their affective and cognitive experiences in sport situations. *Journal of Sport and Exercise Psychology*, *31*(1), 77–96. doi:10.1123/jsep.31.1.77

Raedeke, T. D., Lunney, K., & Venables, K. (2002). Understanding athlete burnout: Coach perspectives. *Journal of Sport Behavior*, *25*, 181–206.

Russell, J. A. (2009). Emotion, core affect, and psychological construction. *Cognition and Emotion*, *23*(7), 1259–1283. doi:10.1080/02699930902809375

Schellenberg, B. J. I., Gaudreau, P., & Crocker, P. R. E. (2013). Passion and coping: Relationships with changes in burnout and goal attainment in collegiate volleyball players. *Journal of Sport and Exercise Psychology*, *35*(3), 270–280. doi:10.1123/jsep.35.3.270

Sverdlik, A., Vallerand, R. J., St-Louis, A., Tion, M. S., & Porlier, G. (2019). Making the final shot: The role of passion and integrated temporal positivity in last-second sport performance. *Journal of Sport and Exercise Psychology*, *41*(6), 356–367. doi:10.1123/jsep.2019-0058

Szabo, A. (2018). Addiction, passion, or confusion? New theoretical insights on exercise addiction research from the case study of a female body builder. *Europe's Journal of Psychology*, *14*(2), 296–316. doi:10.5964/ejop.v14i2.1545

Szabo, A., Griffiths, M. D., Demetrovics, Z., Vega, R., Ruíz-Barquín, R., Soós, I., & Kovacsik, R. (2018). Obsessive and harmonious passion in physically active Spanish and Hungarian men and women: A brief report on cultural and gender differences. *International Journal of Psychology*, *54*(5), 598–603. doi:10.1002/ijop.12517

Vallerand, R. J. (2012). From motivation to passion: In search of the motivational processes involved in a meaningful life. *Canadian Psychology/Psychologie Canadienne*, *53*(1), 42–52. doi:10.1037/a0026377

Vallerand, R. J., Blanchard, C., Mageau, G. A., Koestner, R., Ratelle, C., Léonard, M., . . . Marsolais, J. (2003). Les passions de l'ame: On obsessive and harmonious passion. *Journal of Personality and Social Psychology*, *85*(4), 756–767. doi:10.1037/0022-3514.85.4.756

Vallerand, R. J., Mageau, G. A., Elliot, A. J., Dumais, A., Demers, M.-A., & Rousseau, F. (2008a). Passion and performance attainment in sport. *Psychology of Sport and Exercise*, *9*(3), 373–392. doi:10.1016/j.psychsport.2007.05.003

Vallerand, R. J., Ntoumanis, N., Philippe, F. L., Lavigne, G. L., Carbonneau, N., Bonneville, A., . . . Maliha, G. (2008b). On passion and sports fans: A look at football. *Journal of Sports Sciences*, *26*(12), 1279–1293. doi:10.1080/02640410802123185

Vallerand, R. J., Paquet, Y., Philippe, F. L., & Charest, J. (2010). On the role of passion for work in burnout: A process model. *Journal of Personality*, *78*(1), 289–312. doi:10.1111/j.1467-6494.2009.00616.x

Vallerand, R. J., Rousseau, F. L., Grouzet, F. M. E., Dumais, A., Grenier, S., & Blanchard, C. M. (2006). Passion in sport: A look at determinants and affective experiences. *Journal of Sport and Exercise Psychology*, *28*(4), 454–478. doi:10.1123/jsep.28.4.454

Verner-Filion, J., Vallerand, R. J., Amiot, C. E., & Mocanu, I. (2017). The two roads from passion to sport performance and psychological well-being: The mediating role of need satisfaction, deliberate practice, and achievement goals. *Psychology of Sport and Exercise*, *30*, 19–29. doi:10.1016/j.psychsport.2017.01.009

Williams, C. L., & Tappen, R. M. (2007). Effect of exercise on mood in nursing home residents with Alzheimer's disease. *American Journal of Alzheimer's Disease & Other Dementias*, *22*(5), 389–397. doi:10.1177/1533317507305588

4 Runner's high

A path from healthy to dysfunctional exercise?

4.1 Healthy and unhealthy exercise

What is dysfunctional exercise? If regular physical activity is good for health, how can it be dysfunctional? This question is valid and begs for an answer before discussing morbidity in relationship to exercise behavior. Perhaps the most common thought about dysfunctional exercise pertains to uncontrolled indulgence in long and heavy workouts. Overexercising is an objective manifestation of an exercise motive that could be healthy or unhealthy. A healthy exercise motive could be, for example, training for a competition while maintaining control over the training regimen.

In contrast, unhealthy exercise motives could often be related to *another* psychological problem. For example, setting an exercise-related goal that exceeds the person's capabilities may be a mental problem because the people involved cannot accept their physical/mental limits. In nonathletic settings, overexercising could be associated with stress, trauma, other psychological issues (Egorov & Szabo, 2013), or eating disorders (i.e., Dumitru et al., 2018). The former is referred to as *primary exercise dependence or addiction*, whereas the latter is termed *secondary exercise dependence or addiction*. (In parenthesis, we should highlight that dependence and addiction, although erroneously often used as synonyms in the literature, are not the same, and we will elaborate on the difference in a later chapter.) Therefore, *dysfunctional exercise* most often connotates an *uncontrolled dependence or addiction* to exercise. In dysfunctional exercise, the behavior is geared toward achieving an objective that is usually *unrelated to exercise*, such as dealing with stress (Szabo, 2010), body image (Mącik & Kowalska-Dąbrowska, 2015), body dysmorphia (Nogueira et al., 2018), and weight loss, or management of various eating disorders (Freimuth et al., 2011).

However, high-intensity exercise, which externally appears to be excessive, seldom indicates dysfunction because most exercisers have a healthy motive for their exercise. For example, progressively increased endurance and strength permit longer and more intensive exercise workouts for the sake of enjoyment, fun, and other pleasant mental states experienced after exercise. One of these pleasant states is the *runner's high*, experienced by

DOI: 10.4324/9781003173595-4

many hard-exercising individuals while maintaining complete control over their exercise regimen. Therefore, a dysfunctional exercise refers to cases in which people use exercise as *a means* to achieve a non-exercise-related objective or set unrealistic performance goals, which are incongruent with their physical capabilities, resulting in the loss of control and self-harm (Egorov & Szabo, 2013). However, most exercise workouts are healthy and beneficial for the exercising person and psychologically uplifting even into an altered state of consciousness (Kasos et al., 2021). The runners' high feeling is an example of such a mental state.

4.2 Runners' high: too much of a good thing?

For many years now, marathon or long-distance runners, joggers, and other athletes have reported a subjective feeling state characterized by the euphoria that also buffered the fatigue and pain resulting from physical exertion. This euphoria is analogous to the sensation of 'flying'; it is characterized by automatic and effortless movements (flow), and it is connoted as 'the zone' (Goldberg, 1988). However, the evidence for the existence of the runner's high is incongruent. The question is whether a biochemical or psychophysiological explanation for the runner's high exists, or is it an anecdotal terminology conceptualized and popularized by runners? Most regular exercisers experience deprivation feelings or withdrawal symptoms when they cannot exercise for an unexpected reason. Their symptoms might include guilt, irritability, anxiety, and other unpleasant sensations (Szabo, 1995). Research showed that the human body produces its opiate-like peptides, called endorphins, which have a chemical structure similar to morphine. These peptides could cause dependence (Farrell et al., 1982) and, consequently, may be the biochemical source of the withdrawal symptoms. In general, endorphins are responsible for pain and pleasure responses in the central nervous system. Morphine and other exogenous (taken externally) opiates bind to the endogenous (within the body) opioids or endorphin receptors. Since the analgesic and euphoric effects of morphine are well documented in the literature, similar effects resulting from endogenous (internally produced) endorphins are expectable (Sforzo, 1988).

Studies were conducted to examine the effects of aerobic fitness levels, gender, and exercise intensity on endogenous opioid – mainly β-endorphin – production during cycling, running on a treadmill, participating in aerobic dance, and running marathons. Biddle and Mutrie (1991) summarized research findings showing that aerobic exercise could cause a fivefold increase in β-endorphin levels compared to pre-exercise baseline levels. Furthermore, the fitness levels of the research participants appear to be irrelevant as both trained and untrained individuals experience an increase in β-endorphin levels. However, the metabolism of β-endorphins seems to be more efficient in well-trained than in less-trained athletes (Goldfarb & Jamurtas, 1997).

Goldfarb et al. (1998) examined whether men and women differ in β-endorphin production during exercise. Their results failed to reveal gender differences in β-endorphin response to exercise training. Other studies have demonstrated that both exercise intensity and duration are mediators of β-endorphin concentrations. For example, the exercise needs to be performed at above 60% of the individual's maximal aerobic capacity (Goldfarb & Jamurtas, 1997) and for at least three minutes (Kjaer & Dela, 1996) to detect changes in endogenous opioids.

The researchers have further explored these findings by looking at the correlation between the exercise-induced increase in β-endorphin levels and mood changes using the Profile Of Mood States (POMS) inventory (Farrell et al., 1982). The POMS was presented to all participants before and after the exercise session. Respondents gave numerical ratings to five negative mood categories (tension, depression, anger, fatigue, and confusion) and one positive category (vigor). Adding the five negative affect scores and then subtracting *vigor* yields a 'Total Mood Disturbance' (TMD) score. In Farrell's study, the TMD scores improved by 15 and 16 raw score units from the baseline after participants exercised at 60% and 80% VO_2 max. Quantitatively, mood improved around 50%, similar to clinical observations in which people's mood is elevated after exercise workouts. Using radioimmunoassay, Farrell et al. (1982) also observed a twofold to fivefold increase in peripheral plasma β-endorphin concentrations from pre- to postexercise.

However, Farrell et al.'s research was relatively inconclusive. First, they only studied six well-trained endurance athletes. The six participants showed significant individual differences in β-endorphin response to submaximal treadmill exercise. Second, the exercise-induced change in mood scores was not different between pre- and postexercise scores. Third, there was no significant relationship between mood measures obtained with the POMS inventory and plasma β-endorphin levels. Therefore, the obtained results could not prove that β-endorphins cause mood elevations. However, a more questionable issue, also recognized by Farrell et al., is that the β-endorphin measures in the experiment come from plasma, implying that the measured β-endorphin came from the peripheral circulation. Because of their chemical makeup, β-endorphins cannot cross the Blood–Brain Barrier (BBB).

Consequently, plasma β-endorphin fluctuations do not reflect the β-endorphin changes in the brain. Some researchers have speculated that endogenous opiates in the plasma may act centrally and, therefore, can be used to trace the central nervous system's activity (Biddle & Mutrie, 1991). At this time, the model concerning plasma β-endorphins transport to the brain could only rely on the circumstantial evidence that met-enkephalin and dynorphin, two opioids manifesting modification mechanisms, could transport them across the BBB (Sforzo, 1988). Unfortunately, at this time, direct measurement of changes in brain β-endorphins levels involves cutting open the skull and doing radioimmunoassay on brain slices, which is impossible in research with humans.

To solve this problem, scholars proposed that naloxone could help test whether β-endorphins play a role in central nervous system-mediated affective responses to exercise (Markoff et al., 1982). Given that naloxone is a potent opioid receptor antagonist, it competes with β-endorphins to bind to the opioid receptors. Therefore, injection of naloxone in humans should neutralize the euphoric and analgesic effects of the runners' high feeling if β-endorphins perpetrate such effects indeed. Markoff et al.'s (1982) findings showed that naloxone did not reverse the exercise-induced positive changes in mood. Consequently, they concluded that endorphins are not involved in the affective response to exercise, and therefore the opioid theory of runners' high may be invalid.

Using positron emission tomography (PET), a more recent study provided promising evidence for adaptation in the opioid receptors during exercise. Saanijoki et al. (2014) found that cycling exercise – performed between the aerobic and anaerobic threshold for 60 minutes – triggered an increase in the availability of μ-opioid receptors in the anterior cingulate cortex, prefrontal and temporal cortex of young, healthy recreational exercisers. Relatedly, earlier animal studies with rats, suggestive of an increased opioid release, have shown a rise in opioid receptor binding following physical exercise (Sforzo et al., 1986).

Later, Saanijoki et al. (2018) examined the effects of a single bout of exercise on the cerebral μ-opioid receptors in healthy male leisure exercisers, using PET along with a μ-opioid receptor-selective radioligand. The μ-opioid receptor binding was determined in three experimental conditions: 1) after 60 minutes of moderate-intensity aerobic exercise, 2) after high-intensity cycling interval training, and 3) in a control session after rest. Affect was measured repeatedly throughout the experiment. The high-intensity cycling interval training resulted in significantly reduced μ-opioid receptor binding. This finding was selectively characteristic of the frontolimbic area involved in pain, reward, and emotional regulation (thalamus, insula, orbitofrontal cortex, hippocampus, and anterior cingulate cortex). The decreased receptor binding also correlated with increased negative emotionality. Moderate-intensity exercise did not change μ-opioid receptor binding, but an increased euphoria correlated with decreased receptor binding.

Therefore, Saanijoki et al. (2018) unveiled the role of μ-opioid receptors in mediating affective responses *in high-intensity exercise* but not in moderate workouts. Moreover, although the reduction in μ-opioid receptor availability implies increased opioid release during high-intensity exercise, instead of yielding euphoria, the very intense exercise resulted in more negative affect, exhaustion, irritation, and energy loss. These findings are in discord with earlier work, also using PET with a nonselective binding ligand, which supported the opioid theory of the runner's high (Boecker et al., 2008) by showing that euphoria has significantly increased following a two-hour session of endurance running. The difference between the two studies might be ascribed to several factors. Two of the most important are selective versus nonselective ligand use and the different types of exercises, such as high-intensity interval training (anaerobic) versus prolonged running (aerobic). It is noteworthy that the runner's high (as the term suggests) was most often reported in runners. Still, apart from the type of exercise, individual differences could play a significant role as well. Nevertheless, future empirical studies should examine the differences in the brain opioid dynamics in response to aerobic and anaerobic exercises and, perhaps the emotional states associated with the exercise bout (i.e., artificial laboratory settings versus green space exercise).

4.3 Positive effects of exercise without opioids

Mounting evidence suggests that β-endorphins are not necessary for euphoria experienced by exercisers. Earlier, Harte et al. (1995) noted that although exercise produces both positive emotions and a rise in β-endorphin levels, these simultaneous changes are not necessarily connected. Indeed, some physically undemanding activities like watching humor or listening to music produce mood elevations identical to exercise (Szabo, 2006; Szabo et al., 2005) while accompanying surges in β-endorphins could not be observed after either humor (Berk et al., 1989) or music (McKinney et al., 1997). Similarly, Harte et al. (1995) found that both running and meditation resulted in significant positive changes in mood. Furthermore, in addition to taking mood measures, Harte et al. (1995) also measured plasma β-endorphin levels of the participants. As expected, the individuals in the meditation group did not show an increase in β-endorphin levels despite reporting elevated mood states. Such results present a dilemma for research that directly links mood improvement and β-endorphin levels after exercise.

Reversing the examination of increased mood and increased β-endorphin level relationship, early experiments were conducted in which β-endorphin was directly injected into the participants' bloodstream. On the one hand, as summarized by Biddle and Mutrie (1991), the results of these studies failed to evoke any mood changes in healthy participants. However, on the other hand, β-endorphin injections positively affected clinically depressed patients (Biddle & Mutrie, 1991).

The lack of β-endorphin release during meditation and the lack of mood alteration after β-endorphin injection call attention to other factors that could influence β-endorphin levels. Researchers have realized that the peripheral opioid system requires further investigation to consolidate peripheral β-endorphin data with the central nervous effects. Taylor et al. (1994) proposed that exercise-induced acidosis is the actual trigger of β-endorphin secretion in the bloodstream. Their results showed that the blood pH level strongly correlated with the β-endorphin levels (acidic conditions raise the β-endorphin concentration, and buffering the blood attenuates this response). The explanation behind such observations is that acidosis increases respiration and stimulates a feedback inhibition mechanism through β-endorphins. The latter interacts with the neurons responsible for respiratory control, and β-endorphin, therefore, serves to prevent hyperventilation (Taylor et al., 1994).

How is then this physiological mechanism connected to brain-mediated emotional responses? Sforzo (1988) noted that since opioids have inhibitory functions in the brain, another neural pathway must be involved if a system is activated through opioids. Therefore, instead of trying to establish how peripheral levels of the β-endorphin act on the brain, researchers could develop an alternate physiological model demonstrating how the emotional effects of opioids may be activated through the inhibition of peripheral sympathetic activity (Sforzo, 1988).

While the 'runner's high' phenomenon lacks empirical evidence and β-endorphins have a questionable role, studies have shown that peripheral β-endorphins affect centrally mediated behavior. For example, electroacupuncture used to treat morphine addiction by diminishing cravings and relieving withdrawal symptoms, caused β-endorphin levels to rise (McLachlan et al., 1994). Since exercise also increases β-endorphin levels in the plasma, McLachlan et al. (1994) investigated whether exercise could lower exogenous opiate intake. Rats were fed morphine and methadone for several days and then randomly divided into an exercise and a no-exercise group. The voluntary exogenous opiate intake was recorded to determine whether exercise would affect the consumption of opiates in the exercising rats. The results showed that while opiate consumption has increased in both groups, exercising rats did not consume as much as non-exercising animals, and the difference was statistically significant (McLachlan et al., 1994). These findings suggested that exercise decreases craving.

In conclusion, the relationship between β-endorphins and the runner's high is an elegant explanation without sufficient empirical support. It is likely that the intense positive emotional experience, to which athletes, runners, and scientists refer as 'runner's high,' is evoked by several mechanisms acting jointly. For example, a study carried out about 15 years ago by the first author of this book showed that while exercise and humor were equally effective in decreasing negative moods and increasing positive mood states, the effects of exercise lasted longer than that of humor (Szabo, 2006). These results may serve as evidence for the involvement of more than one mechanism in mood alteration after physically active and inactive, or relatively passive, interventions. But the critical point emerging from research reviewed in this section is that it is doubtful that exercise results in massive quantities of endogenous opiates, which could trigger dysfunctional exercise behavior, such as addiction.

4.4 Endocannabinoids and runner's high

Scholars proposed the endocannabinoid hypothesis as an alternative to the opioid/endorphin hypothesis to explain the runner's high phenomenon (Dietrich & McDaniel, 2004). This model relies on empirical research evidence showing that exercise increases serum concentrations of endocannabinoids (Heyman et al., 2012; Sparling et al., 2003). For example, Sparling et al. (2003) tested trained male university students who either ran on a treadmill or cycled on a stationary bike for 50 minutes at moderate exercise intensity. Blood samples were drawn before and after the exercise. The collected samples were tested for two plasma endocannabinoids, namely anandamide and 2-arachidonoylglycerol. The results showed that exercise increased anandamide but not 2-arachidonoylglycerol levels. The authors interpreted the findings in terms of a new mechanism explaining exercise-induced analgesia and possibly other adaptations to exercise.

In a later work, Heyman et al. (2012) tested 11 healthy cyclists to examine the effects of a 90-minute intense exercise on anandamide and 2-arachidonoylglycerol and their relationship with Brain-Derived Neurotrophic Factor (BDNF). Similar to the results obtained by Sparling et al. (2003), anandamide levels have increased during and after exercise while 2-arachidonoylglycerol levels did not change. The BDNF levels also increased significantly during exercise but then decreased in the postexercise recovery period. There was a strong positive correlation between anandamide and BDNF levels after exercise and the recovery period. The authors proposed that increased anandamide during exercise might have triggered a rise in the peripheral BDNF levels and that increased anandamide levels during the recovery period may delay the recovery of BDNF levels. Evidence suggests that BDNF mediates the positive effects of exercise on affective states (Szuhany et al., 2015). Therefore, this work showed an indirect, mediator effect of an endocannabinoid in exercise's mood-enhancing effects.

Both studies (i.e., Heyman et al., 2012; Sparling et al., 2003) tested trained participants who exercised at high and moderate levels of exercise intensity. A laboratory investigation by Raichlen and his colleagues (2013) measured the circulating levels of anandamide and 2-arachidonylglycerol in ten healthy recreational runners before and after 30 minutes of treadmill running at four different exercise intensities (<50%, 70%, 80%, and 90% of the age-adjusted Maximal Heart Rate [MHR]) on different test days. Similar to earlier research findings (Heyman et al., 2012; Sparling et al., 2003), their results showed that anandamide but not 2-arachidonylglycerol levels have risen after exercise. However, the increase was statistically significant only after 70% and 80% MHR moderate exercise intensity. Indeed, very low (<50% MHR) and very high (90% MHR) intensity exercise did not affect or tended to decrease the circulating endocannabinoid levels

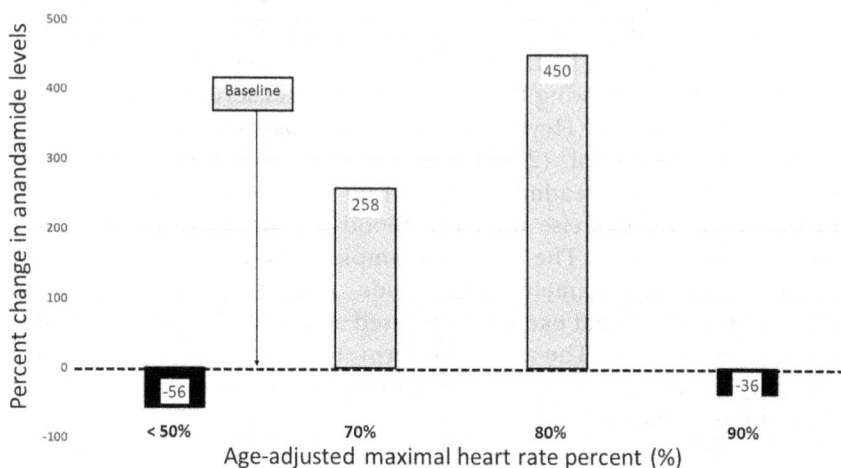

Figure 4.1 Approximate changes in anandamide levels after exercise at different intensities. Increases (grey bars) were statistically significant. The current authors created the figure, and the percent changes were estimated from figure 1 of Raichlen et al. (2013).

(Figure 4.1). These findings agree with the results reported by Sparling and his colleagues (2003), who also employed a moderate-intensity exercise protocol but seem to disagree with results of Heyman et al., who found an increase in anandamide levels after high-intensity exercise. Noteworthy is mentioning the difference in the training status of the participants in the two studies: one study tested trained cyclists, whereas the other examined recreational runners. Training status, reflecting adaptation to high-intensity exercise, could make a difference in endocannabinoid response to vigorous exercise. Consequently, the right-most column in Figure 4.1 may look different in trained athletes.

A laboratory investigation assessing anandamide and 2-arachidonoylglycerol levels and mood before and after prescribed and preferred exercise in three groups (one exercising less than 60 minutes per week, another exercising between 150 and 299 minutes per week, and another exercising more than 300 minutes per week) found no group differences in endocannabinoid response to moderate exercise (Brellenthin et al., 2017). However, both preferred and prescribed exercises triggered an increase in circulating anandamide and 2-arachidonoylglycerol levels. The increase in anandamide levels was more significant in the prescribed condition. Similarly, both preferred and prescribed exercise have induced positive mood changes compared to baseline values. Still, the changes in state anxiety,

TMD, and confusion were more significant in the preferred than in the prescribed condition. Changes in 2-arachidonoylglycerol levels inversely correlated with changes in depression, tension, and TMD scores in the preferred exercise condition, and changes in anandamide levels were positively correlated with vigor in the prescribed condition. Therefore, this study divulges a relationship between changes in the levels of circulating endocannabinoids and various mood states as a result of exercise. Furthermore, the study also demonstrates that prescribed and preferred exercise have different relationships with the changes in the circulating endocannabinoids.

In contrast to opioids, endocannabinoids can easily pass through the BBB to exert their effects on the central nervous system (Dietrich & McDaniel, 2004). The movement of endocannabinoids across biological membranes is facilitated by transporter proteins (Fu et al., 2012). In vitro research has shown that some endocannabinoids modulate human BBB permeability themselves. However, while anandamide decreased BBB permeability, 2-arachidonoylglycerol had no effect on permeability (Hind et al., 2015). Exercise intervention studies (Brellenthin et al., 2017; Heyman et al., 2012; Raichlen et al., 2013; Sparling et al., 2003) suggest that moderate exercise augments blood anandamide levels, which based on in vitro research (Hind et al., 2015) might decrease the permeability of the BBB, making it potentially more difficult for some molecules to reach the central nervous system.

A cross-species study (Raichlen et al., 2012) assessed circulating endocannabinoids in humans, dogs, and ferrets pre- and post-treadmill exercise. The findings indicated that humans and dogs manifested a significant increase in circulating endocannabinoids as a result of high-intensity exercise. The results also showed that endocannabinoid signaling did not increase significantly after low-intensity walking in these species, and endocannabinoid signaling did not increase in ferrets, regardless of the exercise intensity. Raichlen et al.'s (2012) results presented evidence for the exercise-induced increase in endocannabinoids and the cross-species variation in mammalian neurotransmitter signaling. The authors conjectured that the neurobiological reward, an example being the runner's high experience, for endurance forms of exercise could explain why humans along with other cursorial (long-distance running) mammals engage in aerobic exercise, despite the high energy costs of these activities and risk of injury, and why non-cursorial mammals, such as ferrets, avoid this form of movement. At this point, it should be mentioned that increased levels of endocannabinoids alone cannot be associated with dysfunctional exercise. While such changes may be connected to the euphoric feeling of runner's high, similar to opioids, they do not seem to be connected with maladaptive behavioral manifestations to date. The runner's high, a pleasant internal reward, is unlikely to be the path to dysfunctional exercise.

4.5 Key points

1. Currently, the runner's high phenomenon has limited empirical support.
2. There is limited knowledge about the brain's opioid response to exercise.
3. There is a link between exercise intensity and circulating anandamide levels.
4. Preferred and prescribed activities impact the anandamide levels differently.
5. Temporal neurochemical changes in the brain do not point to morbid exercise.

4.6 References

Berk, L. S., Tan, S. A., Fry, W. F., Napier, B. J., Lee, J. W., Hubbard, R. W., . . . Eby, W. C. (1989). Neuroendocrine and stress hormone changes during mirthful laughter. *The American Journal of the Medical Sciences, 298*(6), 390–396. doi:10.1097/00000441-198912000-00006

Biddle, S. J. H., & Mutrie, N. (1991). *Psychology of physical activity and exercise.* London: Springer-Verlag London Ltd.

Boecker, H., Sprenger, T., Spilker, M. E., Henriksen, G., Koppenhoefer, M., Wagner, K. J., . . . & Tolle, T. R. (2008). The runner's high: Opioidergic mechanisms in the human brain. *Cerebral Cortex, 18*(11), 2523–2531. doi:10.1093/cercor/bhn013

Brellenthin, A. G., Crombie, K. M., Hillard, C. J., & Koltyn, K. F. (2017). Endocannabinoid and mood responses to exercise in adults with varying activity levels. *Medicine & Science in Sports & Exercise, 49*(8), 1688–1696. doi:10.1249/mss.0000000000001276

Dietrich, A., & McDaniel, W. F. (2004). Endocannabinoids and exercise. *British Journal of Sports Medicine, 38*(5), 536–541. doi:10.1136/bjsm.2004.011718

Dumitru, D. C., Dumitru, T., & Maher, A. J. (2018). A systematic review of exercise addiction: Examining gender differences. *Journal of Physical Education and Sport, 18*(3), 1738–1747. doi:10.7752/jpes.2018.03253

Egorov, A. Y., & Szabo, A. (2013). The exercise paradox: An interactional model for a clearer conceptualization of exercise addiction. *Journal of Behavioral Addictions, 2*(4), 199–208. doi:10.1556/JBA.2.2013.4.2

Farrell, P. A., Gates, W. K., Maksud, M. G., & Morgan, W. P. (1982). Increase in plasma beta-endorphin/beta-lipotropin immunoreactivity after treadmill running in humans. *Journal of Applied Physiology: Respiratory, Environmental and Exercise Physiology, 52*(5), 1245–1249. doi:10.1152/jappl.1982.52.5.1245

Freimuth, M., Moniz, S., & Kim, S. R. (2011). Clarifying exercise addiction: Differential diagnosis, co-occurring disorders, and phases of addiction. *International Journal of Environmental Research and Public Health, 8*(10), 4069–4081. doi:10.3390/ijerph8104069

Fu, J., Bottegoni, G., Sasso, O., Bertorelli, R., Rocchia, W., Masetti, M., . . . Piomelli, D. (2012). A catalytically silent FAAH-1 variant drives anandamide transport in neurons. *Nature Neuroscience, 15*(1), 64–69. doi:10.1038/nn.2986

Goldberg, A. S. (1988). The *sports mind: A workbook of mental skills for athletes*. Northampton, MA: Competitive Advantage.

Goldfarb, A. H., & Jamurtas, A. Z. (1997). β-Endorphin response to exercise. *Sports Medicine, 24*(1), 8–16. doi:10.2165/00007256-199724010-00002

Goldfarb, A. H., Jamurtas, A. Z., Kamimori, G. H., Hegde, S., Otterstetter, R., & Brown, D. A. (1998). Gender effect on beta-endorphin response to exercise. *Medicine and Science in Sports and Exercise, 30*(12), 1672–1676. doi:10.1097/00005768-199812000-00003

Harte, J. L., Eifert, G. H., & Smith, R. (1995). The effects of running and meditation on beta-endorphin, corticotropin-releasing hormone and cortisol in plasma, and on mood. *Biological Psychology, 40*(3), 251–265. doi:10.1016/0301-0511(95)05118-T

Heyman, E., Gamelin, F.-X., Goekint, M., Piscitelli, F., Roelands, B., Leclair, E., . . . Meeusen, R. (2012). Intense exercise increases circulating endocannabinoid and BDNF levels in humans – Possible implications for reward and depression. *Psychoneuroendocrinology, 37*(6), 844–851. doi:10.1016/j.psyneuen.2011.09.017

Hind, W. H., Tufarelli, C., Neophytou, M., Anderson, S. I., England, T. J., & O'Sullivan, S. E. (2015). Endocannabinoids modulate human blood-brain barrier permeability in vitro. *British Journal of Pharmacology, 172*(12), 3015–3027. doi:10.1111/bph.13106

Kasos, E., Kasos, K., Józsa, E., Varga, K., Bányai, E., Költő, A., & Szabo, A. (2021). Altered states of consciousness during exercise, active-alert hypnosis and everyday waking state. *International Journal of Clinical and Experimental Hypnosis*. (In press)

Kjaer, M., & Dela, F. (1996). Endocrine response to exercise. In L. Hoffman-Goetz (Ed.), *Exercise and immune function* (pp. 6–8). Boca Raton, FL: CRC Press.

Mącik, D., & Kowalska-Dąbrowska, M. (2015). The risk of muscle dysmorphia and the perception of change in retrospective, current and ideal self-image – preliminary study. *Health Psychology Report, 1*, 24–34. doi:10.5114/hpr.2015.47087

Markoff, R. A., Ryan, P., & Young, T. (1982). Endorphins and mood changes in long-distance running. *Medicine & Science in Sports & Exercise, 14*(1), 11–15. doi:10.1249/00005768-198214010-00002

McKinney, C. H., Tims, F. C., Kumar, A. M., & Kumar, M. (1997). The effect of selected classical music and spontaneous imagery on plasma β-endorphin. *Journal of Behavioral Medicine, 20*(1), 85–99. doi:10.1023/A:1025543330939

McLachlan, C. D., Hay, M., & Coleman, G. J. (1994). The effects of exercise on the oral consumption of morphine and methadone in rats. *Pharmacology Biochemistry and Behavior, 48*(2), 563–568. doi:10.1016/0091-3057(94)90572-X

Nogueira, A., Molinero, O., Salguero, A., & Márquez, S. (2018). Exercise addiction in practitioners of endurance sports: A literature review. *Frontiers in Psychology, 9*. doi:10.3389/fpsyg.2018.01484

Raichlen, D. A., Foster, A. D., Gerdeman, G. L., Seillier, A., & Giuffrida, A. (2012). Wired to run: Exercise-induced endocannabinoid signaling in humans and cursorial mammals with implications for the 'runner's high'. *Journal of Experimental Biology, 215*(8), 1331–1336. doi:10.1242/jeb.063677

Raichlen, D. A., Foster, A. D., Seillier, A., Giuffrida, A., & Gerdeman, G. L. (2013). Exercise-induced endocannabinoid signaling is modulated by intensity. *European Journal of Applied Physiology, 113*(4), 869–875. doi:10.1007/s00421-012-2495-5

Saanijoki, T., Tuominen, L., Nummenmaa, L., Arponen, E., Kalliokoski, K., & Hirvonen, J. (2014). Physical exercise activates the μ-opioid system in human brain. *Journal of Nuclear Medicine, 55*(suppl. 1), p. 1909.

Saanijoki, T., Tuominen, L., Tuulari, J. J., Nummenmaa, L., Arponen, E., Kallioko-ski, K., & Hirvonen, J. (2018). Opioid release after high-intensity interval training in healthy human subjects. *Neuropsychopharmacology, 43*(2), 246–254. doi:10.1038/npp.2017.148

Sforzo, G. A. (1988). Opioids and exercise. *Sports Medicine, 7*(2), 109–124. doi:10.2165/00007256-198907020-00003

Sforzo, G. A., Seeger, T. F., Pert, C. B., Pert, A., & Dotsen, C. O. (1986). In vivo opioid receptor occupation in the rat brain following exercise. *Medicine and Science in Sports and Exercise, 18*, 380–384. doi:10.1249/00005768-198608000-00003

Sparling, P. B., Giuffrida, A., Piomelli, D., Rosskopf, L., & Dietrich, A. (2003). Exercise activates the endocannabinoid system. *NeuroReport, 14*(17), 2209–2211. doi:10.1097/00001756-200312020-00015

Szabo, A. (1995). The impact of exercise deprivation on well-being of habitual exer-cisers. *The Australian Journal of Science and Medicine in Sport, 27*, 68–75.

Szabo, A. (2006). Comparison of the psychological effects of exercise and humor. In A. M. Lane (Ed.), *Mood and human performance: Conceptual, measurement, and applied issues* (pp. 201–216). New York, NY: Nova Science Publishers.

Szabo, A. (2010). *Addiction to exercise: A symptom or a disorder?* New York, NY: Nova Science Publishers.

Szabo, A., Ainsworth, S. E., & Danks, P. K. (2005). Experimental comparison of the psychological benefits of aerobic exercise, humor, and music. *Humor, 18*(3), 235–246. doi:10.1515/humr.2005.18.3.235

Szuhany, K. L., Bugatti, M., & Otto, M. W. (2015). A meta-analytic review of the effects of exercise on brain-derived neurotrophic factor. *Journal of Psychiatric Research, 60*, 56–64. doi:10.1016/j.jpsychires.2014.10.003

Taylor, D. V., Boyajian, J. G., James, N., Woods, D., Chicz-Demet, A., Wilson, A. F., & Sandman, C. A. (1994). Acidosis stimulates beta-endorphin release dur-ing exercise. *Journal of Applied Physiology, 77*(4), 1913–1918. doi:10.1152/jappl.1994.77.4.1913

5   Behavioral addictions
Overview and classifications

5.1 Brief historical perspective

For several decades, addiction research has traditionally focused on psychoactive substance dependence. This approach has naturally emerged from most handbooks and overviews of addiction. Many of these books almost exclusively (except for sometimes included chapters on pathological gambling) focused on substance dependence and discussed the characteristics of intoxication and dependence to specific psychoactive substances and their treatments. The psychoactive substances most often reviewed are alcohol, nicotine, and the so-called 'classic' leisure drugs such as heroin, cocaine, cannabis, amphetamines, LSD, etc. However, it is also essential to look at the changes that occurred during the past decades.

In this chapter's framework, we briefly present the non-substance-related, so-called behavioral addictions, with an expanded discussion on the place of *exercise addiction* within this category of dysfunctions. These disorders surfaced through their similarity to problematic gambling, initially conceptualized as an impulse control disorder and now as *gambling disorder* in the latest (fifth) edition of the *Diagnostic and Statistical Manual of Mental Disorders* (*DSM-5*; American Psychiatric Association, 2013). In *DSM-5*, the chapter on 'Substance-Related and Addictive Disorders' includes gambling disorder as the only nonsubstance-related addiction under the new (but almost a decade old) category of behavioral addictions. Accordingly, gambling disorder is classified within this category. This classification indicates that reliable research findings underpin that gambling disorder is akin to substance-related dysfunctions in its clinical manifestation, including behavioral tendencies, brain mechanisms, comorbidity, psychophysiology, and treatment.

Several other behavioral addictions were also considered for possible inclusion in the *DSM-5*. Specifically, sex, shopping, and exercise addiction were elaborated but not included in the manual because the working group concluded that 'at this time there is insufficient peer-reviewed evidence to establish the diagnostic criteria and course descriptions needed to identify these behaviors as mental health disorders' (p. 481; American Psychiatric

DOI: 10.4324/9781003173595-5

Association, 2013). However, since many people may suffer from such conditions, it is essential to continue researching and collecting scientific information on these behaviors to improve public health initiatives and treatment.

5.2 Behavioral addictions receiving research attention

There are several behavioral addictions currently researched. Table 5.1 presents a summary of these behaviors. Behavioral addictions are also often referred to as *addictive behaviors* (Yu & Sussman, 2020). However, the latter classification also denotes substance or chemical addictions (Schall et al., 2020). Apart from the gambling disorder, as discussed earlier, none of the behavioral addictions in Table 5.1 can be diagnosed on the basis of universally accepted diagnostic criteria such as the *DSM-5*. However, the International Classification of Diseases (ICD) latest version, the 11th revision, in addition to gambling disorder (6C50), also includes gaming disorders (6C51) (World Health Organization, 2019). Further, the ICD-11 has a category named 'Disorders due to addictive behaviors' including the subcategory of 'other specified disorders due to addictive behaviors,' which is described as:

> Disorders due to addictive behaviours are recognizable and clinically significant syndromes associated with distress or interference with personal functions that develop as a result of repetitive rewarding behaviours other than the use of dependence-producing substances. Disorders due to addictive behaviours include gambling disorder and gaming disorder, which may involve both online and offline behaviour.

Still, the diagnostic criteria for other addictive behaviors (than gambling or gaming disorder) fitting into this category are unspecified. There is, however, a proposal for a set of criteria that might differentiate some pathological behavioral addictions from other passionate, habitual, and rewarding behaviors (Brand et al., 2020).

Behavioral addictions include the category of gambling addictions that involve risk-taking or playing for the sake of winning, which is the reward in this form of addiction. Sex and relationship addictions include watching or reading pornography for the sake of self-gratification through masturbation and other paraphilias and sex-related addictive behaviors. Also, in this category, but somewhat different from pornography addiction, is sex addiction which includes having multiple sexual partners and taking risks for the sake of sexual gratification (such as not wearing a condom), spending a lot of money on prostitutes, and engaging in prostitution, or sexual perversions. Passionate love is also considered by some to be an addiction (Earp et al., 2017).

Technology-related addictions include Internet addiction, smartphone addiction, television addiction, online (Internet) gaming addiction, and social media addiction. In this category, the affected person is not addicted to the medium itself (i.e., the Internet) but a *specific activity* on the Internet (Griffiths & Szabo, 2014). Similarly, addiction to smartphones refers to an addiction to some *specific* applications that can be accessed with this type of device (Csibi et al., 2017). Further, television addiction describes the uncontrolled needs and urges to watch television for extended periods and not miss perceived as important and rewarding programs (Kubey, & Csikszentmihalyi, 2002). Online gaming disorder is like offline gaming disorder, and social media addiction involves the uncontrolled urge and craving to contact, know, and share information with others.

Eating addictions are in a distinct and obscured category because they may be classified as behavioral addictions but also as substance addiction (Hauck et al., 2020) since they involve the introduction of a substance (food) in the body that is similar to alcohol use, smoking, caffeine or leisure drugs. The distinguishing feature is that alcohol and other substances are *psychoactive* while food, in general, is not psychoactive and therefore is not a source of substance addiction. Eating addiction includes food addiction or addiction to specific foods like chocolate. The former could be described as an addictive pattern of eating that may manifest in habitual consumption of certain highly palatable, highly processed, and complex foods, usually containing large amounts of calories through their sugar and fat content (Hauck et al., 2020). Chocolate is only one example of a popular and *specific* food that can be highly addictive (Rajeswari, 2020), and unlike general foods, it appears to have a psychoactive effect (Nasser et al., 2011). However, according to Hauck et al. (2020), food addiction is not different from eating disorders and should be treated within this category of mental dysfunction.

5.3 Positive addictions that are 'never positive'

In the middle of Table 5.1, we treat the category of positive addictions with special attention because it includes addictions manifested in socially acceptable behaviors that usually are rewarded. However, too many of these behaviors culminating in obsession and compulsion can also be detrimental. Still, Glasser (1976) believed that too much of a good thing is better than little of a bad thing. He described six categories for positive addictions: 1) must be noncompetitive and needing about an hour a day; 2) easy, so no mental effort is required; 3) easy to be done alone, not dependent on people; 4) believed to be having some value (physical, mental, and spiritual); 5) believed that if persisted in, some improvement will result; and 6) involve no self-criticism. However, these criteria do not mirror addiction or dysfunctional behavior (Griffiths, 1996a), Glasser used them to identify

Table 5.1 Various general categories of currently studied behavioral addictions.

Gambling addictions	Sex and relationship addictions[1]	Positive addictions[2]	Technology-related addictions	Eating addictions
Gambling disorder	Pornography addiction	Work addiction	Internet addiction	Food addiction
	Sex addictions (many types, i.e., paraphilias, and voyeurism)	Exercise addiction	Smartphone addiction	Chocolate addiction (specific food addiction)
	Love or relationship addiction	Shopping addiction	Television addiction	
		Religious addiction	Online gaming addictions	
		Tanning addiction	Social media addiction	

Note: [1]This category could be distinct too (i.e., sex and relationship). [2]This category refers to socially accepted and healthy behaviors, but when abused, they are dysfunctional. In fact, in an addicted form, they are not positive at all.

positive addiction attempting to distinguish between excessive behaviors that are personally and socially rewarding from self-destructive behaviors like drug, tobacco, or alcohol abuse. Unfortunately, the 'positive' prefix with the term addiction resulted in the widespread and perhaps negligent use of the term in the academic literature. We state here clearly that addiction is *always negative* and dysfunctional, unlike passion or commitment.

A few years later, Morgan (1979) has recognized that the term *positive addiction* gives rise to a semantic problem because the *positive* prefix obscures maladaptive situations in which a transition occurs from healthy to pathological behavior. For example, in sports and exercise, high levels of commitment to the activity under some circumstances might shift into exercise addiction. Therefore, to highlight the morbid aspects of exaggerated and abused positive behaviors, he introduced *negative addiction* to Glasser's positive addiction as an antonym. Like other authors, we believe that *all addictions reflect a dysfunction and, consequently, are always negative* (Rozin & Stoess, 1993; Zou et al., 2017). Indeed, the term *addiction* by its definition implies pathological/disordered behavior.

Glasser's (1976) 'positive' notion referred to the benefits of commitment to a socially accepted and praised behavior compared to some 'unhealthy' or socially unaccepted or even condemned behaviors. Among positive addictions (Table 5.1), we mention work, exercise, shopping, religion, and tanning addictions. People who work hard may be responsible for their families and financial future, apart from having a high affinity for the job that they are doing. Work also could be a means of escape from ongoing and unresolved situations. Workaholism is a widely researched behavioral dysfunction (Avanzi et al., 2020). Then habitual exercisers work hard to take care of their health or appearance. Athletes are examples representing the pride of a nation. A subcategory of exercise addiction, dance addiction, has also been reported in the literature (Maráz et al., 2015a, 2015b; Targhetta et al., 2013). Paradoxically, these behaviors were also used to treat substance addictions (Colledge et al., 2018).

Extensive shopping mirrors affluence and social privilege to the outsider, putting the shopper in an enviable social position. On the contrary, shopping can be addictive (Kyrios et al., 2018; Maráz et al., 2015c; Müller et al., 2019; Weinstein et al., 2016). Further, even if some criticize or condemn, religious commitment often reflects a striving for goodness and a form of living based on a particular religion's moral and ethical values. However, some view religious addiction as a 'disease' (Taylor, 2002). Finally, tanning addiction also stems from a generally healthy behavior (relaxation, vitamin D) if done in moderation, but apparently, it can be addictive (Kourosh et al., 2010). In the academic literature, one can find numerous less investigated but potentially highly addictive behaviors such as hoarding, kleptomania, tattoo addiction, and even brand addiction (Cui et al., 2018), but the discussion and evaluation of these tentatively maladaptive behaviors are beyond the scope of this book. One note, however, should be added. We speak about addiction only in excessively practiced behaviors that *endanger and harm* the health and well-being of the person.

In this book's context, we are especially interested in sport and exercise as behaviors that can become addictive, among other similar addictions behind which an individual can easily hide due to the general *positive* connotation of the behavior. What makes these *positive* behaviors addictive? Like most addictive behaviors, they could provide a means of coping and *escape* from a problem or compensation for the emotional or physical *pain* caused by that problem. The escape occurs by momentary gratification obtained from the performance of the behavior (Goodman, 1990). They all share common symptoms, like substance addiction, that aid in their identification as a dysfunction. The symptom-based models will be presented later in this chapter, but we briefly look at exercise addiction before that.

5.4 Exercise addiction

The existence of exercise addiction is based on anecdotal and scholastic evidence presenting substantial loss and suffering due to uncontrolled exercise behavior (Juwono & Szabo, 2020). Most, if not all, nomothetic research can only assess the *risk* of exercise addiction because actual cases can only be identified through the idiographic examination of the affected person's antecedents, symptoms, and consequences. There is only a fine borderline between high commitment and addiction. Glasser's (1976) *positive addiction* in sport and exercise sciences and psychology may be interpreted as a synonym to high commitment or dedication to the activity (Carmack & Martens, 1979). However, when 'commitment' to exercise is considered a synonym to exercise addiction or to exercise dependence as termed by some scholars (i.e., Reche et al., 2018), a significant conceptual confusion emerges. For example, a while ago, Thornton and Scott (1995) thought that they could classify 77% of a sample of runners as moderately or highly addicted to running. Now, this figure is unrealistically high compared to the mere 3% to 5% being at risk of exercise addiction in a population-wide study (Mónok et al., 2012). Indeed, such a figure is vastly exaggerated. For example, if we take 20,000 runners participating in a marathon race, over 15,000 of them would be addicted to exercise. This prevalence would be greater than the prevalence of any known disease in the world. Like most other behavioral addictions, exercise addiction is identified through the symptoms also characteristic of substance addictions. Exercise addiction and its difference from commitment are treated in a separate chapter in this book.

5.5 Recognizing behavioral addictions

Behavioral addictions share common symptoms and underlying dysfunctional processes with substance addictions (Sussman et al., 2017). Earlier, Goodman (1990) proposed 14 signs, but out of 9, only a minimum of 5 should be present for the identification of the addictive behavior (Table 5.2). Later, Griffiths (1996b, 2005) presented the components model of addictions modified from Brown (Griffiths, 2005). These components are salience, mood modification, tolerance, withdrawal, conflict, and relapse. These six symptoms in the components model serve as the infrastructure for several instruments assessing various behavioral addictions, such as the Exercise Addiction Inventory (Terry et al., 2004) that gauges the risk of exercise addiction, the Smartphone Application-Based Addiction Scale (Csibi et al., 2017), and numerous other questionnaires.

Grüsser and Thalemann's (2006) list of symptoms of addictions is longer than those in the components model of addictions (Griffiths, 2005). However, the list incorporates most, if not all (directly or implicitly), of the six components of addiction proposed by Griffiths. Furthermore, there is a great overlap with Goodman's (1990) model. Any of the three models could help in appraising the *risk* of addiction. However, some of these symptoms overlap with nonaddictive characteristics associated with behaviors that could be addictive. For example, in Goodman's list, 'Pleasure or relief at the time of engaging in the behavior' could be linked to almost any habitual passionate activity. In Griffiths' list, *mood modification* appears to be a generally observable consequence of engaging in even very brief leisure activities, such as three minutes of exercise (Szabo et al., 2013). Finally, on Grüsser and Thalemann's list, the *function*, as a mood-regulatory incentive

Table 5.2 Three proposed sets of criteria for behavioral addictions. The shaded boxes indicate overlap with another model.

Goodman (1990)	Griffiths (2005)	Grüsser and Thalemann (2006)
Repeated failure to resist impulses to engage in a specified behavior	Salience (the behavior is the most important in the person's life)	The exaggerated behavior is exhibited over a long period of at least 12 months in an abused aberrant form, deviating from the norm in frequency and intensity
Increased tension immediately before the initiation of the behavior	Mood modification (altered mood as a result of the behavior)	Loss of control over the behavior (duration, frequency, intensity, risk) when the behavior started
Pleasure or relief at the time of engaging in the behavior	Conflict (intra- and interpersonal conflict because of too much attention and time devoted to the behavior)	Reward effect (e.g., the behavior is rewarding, process a desired and enjoyed feeling state)
Feeling of lack of control while engaging in the behavior	Withdrawal (negative mood, feeling bad, or guilty when the behavior is missed)	Development of tolerance (behavior performed longer, more often, and more intensively to achieve the desired effect; in unvaried form, intensity and frequency, the desired effect fails to appear)
At least five of the following:	Tolerance (increasingly more engagement is needed to achieve the same effects as before)	Behavior initially perceived as pleasant, positive, and rewarding is progressively considered to be an unpleasant obligation
1) Frequent preoccupation with the behavior or activity that leads to it	Relapse (unsuccessful attempt to cut down or to stop the behavior)	Irresistible urge or craving to engage in the behavior
2) Frequent engaging in the behavior to a greater extent or over a more extended period than intended		Function (the purpose of the behavior is to regulate the emotions or mood)

(Continued)

Table 5.2 (Continued)

Goodman (1990)	Griffiths (2005)	Grüsser and Thalemann (2006)
3) Repeated efforts to reduce, control, or stop the behavior		The expectancy of the effect (anticipation of pleasant feelings as a result of the behavior)
4) Significant time spent with activities necessary for the behavior, engaging in the behavior, or recovering from its effect(s)		Limited behavior patterns (does not wish to try out new things in life)
5) Frequent engaging in the behavior when expected to fulfill an occupational, academic, domestic, or social obligation		Mental preoccupation buildup (execution and follow-up activities linked to the behavior and the anticipated effects of possibly even more indulgence in the behavior)
6) Important social, occupational, or recreational activities reduced or given up because of the behavior		Irrational perception of different aspects of the behavior
7) Continuation of the behavior despite knowledge of having a persistent or recurrent social, financial, psychological, or physical problem that is caused or exacerbated by the behavior		Withdrawal symptoms (both psychological and physical)

(*Continued*)

Goodman (1990)	Griffiths (2005)	Grüsser and Thalemann (2006)
8) Tolerance or need to increase the intensity or frequency of the behavior to achieve the desired effect or diminished effect with continued behavior of the same intensity		Continued involvement in excessive behavior despite already experienced negative consequences (health-related, occupational, and social)
9) Restlessness or irritability if unable to engage in the behavior		Conditioned responses (resulting from the confrontation with internal and external stimuli related to the excessive behavior and mental preoccupation with it)
Some symptoms of the disturbance have persisted for at least one month or have occurred repeatedly over a longer period		Suffering, pain management (desire to alleviate perceived suffering)

behind the behavior, can be observed in many leisure and social activities (i.e., one goes for a walk to unwind). Therefore, the presence and severity of these symptoms reflect a certain level of predisposition or risk.

5.6 Etiology of behavioral addictions

Most behavioral addictions, including exercise addiction, have antecedents represented by the interaction of several personal and situational factors. For exercise addiction, we will present several models in Chapter 11 of this book. A more general explanation of the etiology of behavioral addictions is discussed below. This viewpoint is primarily based on a stress-coping model of addictions (Sussman, 2017). This orientation closely matches the interactional model for exercise addiction (Egorov & Szabo, 2013).

Behavioral addictions can very often be traced back to ongoing or chronic stress or a high-impact traumatic experience (Egorov & Szabo, 2013). Individuals search for a mode of escape from stress or a means of coping that alleviates pain and suffering associated with chronic stress, such as being bullied at work, or a trauma, such as losing a loved one. Personal values and attitudes play an essential role in determining how people will cope with stress and trauma. For example, a perfectionist, or socially highly conscious individual, will turn to positive or socially accepted coping methods, such as spending more and more time at work, exercising, shopping, or praying (Çakın et al., 2021). These behaviors are socially acceptable. Therefore, the suffering individual could hide behind them.

In contrast, some people may turn to drugs or alcohol, hoping that others will not notice the change. The difference between behavioral addictions and substance addiction is that the former requires time and energy-demanding action(s) to exert their effects. In contrast, the other only requires access to the substance that can yield an immediate impact. The desired results, regardless of the form of addiction, are always only temporary. Its dissipation leads to the urge to repeat the behavior. The longer time elapses between the dissipation of the effect and the repetition of the addictive behavior, the stronger is the urge and craving. However, the path from chronic stress or trauma to full-blown behavioral addiction is not instantaneous; instead, it is a sequential process (Figure 5.1).

As illustrated in Figure 5.1, the ongoing stress or sudden trauma, for which the individual is unprepared, triggers the search to resolve the problem or cope. Coping can be passive (the event or situation cannot be changed) or active (the situation is manageable). In passive coping, the stress or trauma causes mental discomfort and pain that begs for relief. Since the affected person cannot change the situation, temporary relief is sought through substance use (immediate effect of alcohol, drugs, etc.)

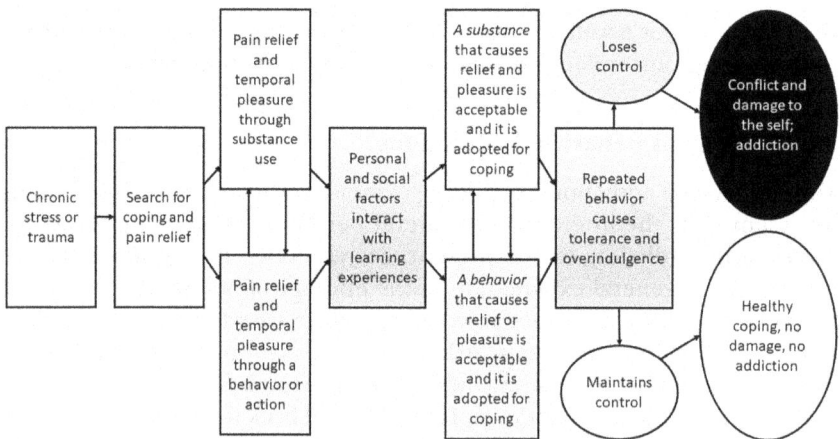

Figure 5.1 A stress-based model for the development of addictions, showing the path to behavioral addictions.

or specific behaviors that cause distraction and pleasure (delayed effect). The individual must have experience with the substance and behavior. For example, if one does not know about the joyous feelings after exercise, that person is unlikely to resort to exercise for coping. However, suppose a person usually winds down with a coffee or playing golf (earlier rewarding experience). At the time of stress, the adopted behavior is retrieved from the memory as a schematic cue for pleasure and feeling good. Subsequently, it is reproduced to relieve the discomfort caused by the stress. Therefore, the behavior slowly starts to control the individual. It must be done or else something will go wrong.

Therefore, the behavior becomes a means of coping with passive stress, represented by an uncontrollable life event. While substances usually have an *instant* effect in contrast to behaviors that produce a *delayed* effect, the latter may still be preferred if the self-image or social prestige is vital to the person who has a positive experience with the adopted behavior. Using an addictive substance and addictive behavior in coping may co-occur (Freimuth et al., 2008). Most often, one predominates (the one that causes the problem) and eventually leads to tolerance and overindulgence, resulting in intra- and interpersonal conflict and health problems, signaling the transfer into the addiction phase. In this phase, the affected person becomes dependent on the addictive behavior (or substance) to function normally. Not fulfilling the behavior (or having access to the addicted substance) causes deprivation feelings and withdrawal symptoms because the behavior controls the person, which is a characteristic of addictive behaviors. A behavioral addiction, based on an expert group's definition, is:

> A repeated behaviour leading to significant harm or distress. The behaviour is not reduced by the person and persists over a significant period of time. The harm or distress is of a functionally impairing nature.
> (Kardefelt-Winther et al., 2017, p. 1710)

5.7 Biological basis of behavioral addictions

There is a psychobiological similarity between substance and behavioral addictions. With its progression, addiction reshapes the brain's neurochemistry. Psychoactive substance addiction affects nearly all neurochemical pathways in the brain. For example, the dopaminergic system is linked to reward, craving, and relapse. Therefore, it is involved in all forms of addictions (Solinas et al., 2018). The dopaminergic pathways lie mainly in the limbic system, the brain's reward center (Fletcher et al., 2015). A chief component of the reward center is the mesolimbic dopamine system (Serafini et al., 2020). It comprises nerve cells originating from the ventral tegmental area, which innervate central regions that regulate executive, emotional, and motivational functions, including the prefrontal cortex, amygdala, and nucleus accumbens (Serafini et al., 2020). It was suggested that the dopamine pathway from the ventral tegmental area to the nucleus accumbens plays a vital role in maintaining the addiction (Nestler & Malenka, 2004).

In addition to dopamine, other neurotransmitters (i.e., serotonin, noradrenaline, and opioids) also play significant roles in substance and behavioral addictions. For example, while serotonin is associated with behavioral inhibition, dopamine mediates motivation, learning, and reward; both may have a critical function in the two forms of addictions (Grant et al., 2010). Indeed, neuroimaging studies support the existence of common neural pathways in substance use and behavioral addictions (Brewer & Potenza, 2008). Abnormal ventral medial prefrontal cortex function was observed in patients with substance addiction. It was also related to impulsive decision-making in risk-reward assessments and decreased response to gambling cues in pathological gamblers (Grant et al., 2010). As mentioned earlier, the dopaminergic mesolimbic pathway, leading from the ventral tegmental area to the nucleus accumbens, is involved in substance and behavioral addiction, as evidenced by neuroimaging studies (Grant et al., 2010). These biological similarities reveal a close relationship between chemical and behavioral addictions and support their continued scientific exploration.

5.8 Key points

1. Gambling disorder (6C50) and gaming disorder (6C51) are the only behavioral addictions recognized in the ICD-11.
2. Behavioral addictions reflect ordinarily normal behaviors abused by some people.
3. Symptom-based models aid in recognizing behavioral addictions.
4. Behavioral addictions often reflect means of coping with ongoing stress or trauma.
5. The dopaminergic mesolimbic pathway is involved in both substance and behavioral addictions.

5.9 References

American Psychiatric Association. (2013). *Diagnostic and statistical manual of mental disorders* (5th ed.). doi:10.1176/appi.books.9780890425596

Avanzi, L., Perinelli, E., Vignoli, M., Junker, N. M., & Balducci, C. (2020). Unravelling work drive: A comparison between workaholism and overcommitment. *International Journal of Environmental Research and Public Health, 17*(16), 5755. doi:10.3390/ijerph17165755

Brand, M., Rumpf, H.-Jü., Demetrovics, Z., MÜller, A., Stark, R., King, D. L., . . . Potenza, M. N. (2020). Which conditions should be considered as disorders in the International Classification of Diseases (ICD-11) designation of "other specified disorders due to addictive behaviors"? *Journal of Behavioral Addictions.* (Online first). doi:10.1556/2006.2020.00035

Brewer, J. A., & Potenza, M. N. (2008). The neurobiology and genetics of impulse control disorders: Relationships to drug addictions. *Biochemical Pharmacology*, 75(1), 63–75. doi:10.1016/j.bcp.2007.06.043

Brown, R. I. F. (1993). Some contributions of the study of gambling to the study of other addictions. In W. R. Eadington & J. A. Cornelius (Eds.), *Gambling behavior and problem gambling* (pp. 241–272). Reno: University of Nevada Press.

Çakın, G., Juwono, I. D., Potenza, M. N., & Szabo, A. (2021). Exercise addiction and perfectionism: A systematic review of the literature. *Current Addiction Reports*, 8(1), 144–155. doi:10.1007/s40429-021-00358-8

Carmack, M. A., & Martens, R. (1979). Measuring commitment to running: A survey of runners' attitudes and mental states. *Journal of Sport and Exercise Psychology*, 1(1), 25–42. doi:10.1123/jsp.1.1.25

Colledge, F., Gerber, M., Pühse, U., & Ludyga, S. (2018). Anaerobic exercise training in the therapy of substance use disorders: A systematic review. *Frontiers in Psychiatry*, 9. doi:10.3389/fpsyt.2018.00644

Csibi, S., Griffiths, M. D., Cook, B., Demetrovics, Z., & Szabo, A. (2017). The psychometric properties of the Smartphone Application-Based Addiction Scale (SABAS). *International Journal of Mental Health and Addiction*, 16(2), 393–403. doi:10.1007/s11469-017-9787-2

Cui, C. C., Mrad, M., & Hogg, M. K. (2018). Brand addiction: Exploring the concept and its definition through an experiential lens. *Journal of Business Research*, 87, 118–127. doi:10.1016/j.jbusres.2018.02.028

Earp, B. D., Wudarczyk, O. A., Foddy, B., & Savulescu, J. (2017). Addicted to love: What is love addiction and when should it be treated? *Philosophy, Psychiatry, & Psychology*, 24(1), 77–92. doi:10.1353/ppp.2017.0011

Egorov, A. Y., & Szabo, A. (2013). The exercise paradox: An interactional model for a clearer conceptualization of exercise addiction. *Journal of Behavioral Addictions*, 2(4), 199–208. doi:10.1556/jba.2.2013.4.2

Fletcher, G. J., Simpson, J. A., Campbell, L., & Overall, N. C. (2015). Pair-bonding, romantic love, and evolution: The curious case of Homo sapiens. *Perspectives on Psychological Science*, 10(1), 20–36. doi:10.1177/1745691614561683

Freimuth, M., Waddell, M., Stannard, J., Kelley, S., Kipper, A., Richardson, A., & Szuromi, I. (2008). Expanding the scope of dual diagnosis and co-Addictions: Behavioral addictions. *Journal of Groups in Addiction & Recovery*, 3(3–4), 137–160. doi:10.1080/15560350802424944

Glasser, W. (1976). *Positive addiction.* New York, NY: Harper and Row.

Goodman, A. (1990). Addiction: Definition and implications. *British Journal of Addiction*, 85(11), 1403–1408. doi:10.1111/j.1360-0443.1990.tb01620.x

Grant, J. E., Potenza, M. N., Weinstein, A., & Gorelick, D. A. (2010). Introduction to behavioral addictions. *The American Journal of Drug and Alcohol Abuse*, 36(5), 233–241. doi:10.3109/00952990.2010.491884

Griffiths, M. D. (1996a). Behavioural addiction: An issue for everybody? *Employee Counselling Today*, 8(3), 19–25. doi:10.1108/13665629610116872

Griffiths, M. D. (1996b). Nicotine, tobacco and addiction. *Nature*, 384, 18.

Griffiths, M. D. (2005). A "components" model of addiction within a biopsychosocial framework. *Journal of Substance Use*, 10(4), 191–197. doi:10.1080/146598 90500114359

Griffiths, M. D., & Szabo, A. (2014). Is excessive online usage a function of medium or activity? *Journal of Behavioral Addictions*, 3(1), 74–77. doi:10.1556/jba.2.2013.016

Grüsser, S. M., & Thalemann, C. N. (2006). *Verhaltenssucht Diagnostik, Therapie, Forschung*. Bern: Huber.

Hauck, C., Cook, B., & Ellrott, T. (2020). Food addiction, eating addiction and eating disorders. *Proceedings of the Nutrition Society, 79*(1), 103–112. doi:10.1017/s0029665119001162

Juwono, I. D., & Szabo, A. (2020). 100 cases of exercise addiction: More evidence for a widely researched but rarely identified dysfunction. *International Journal of Mental Health and Addiction*. (Online first). doi:10.1007/s11469-020-00264-6

Kardefelt-Winther, D., Heeren, A., Schimmenti, A., van Rooij, A., Maurage, P., Carras, M., . . . Billieux, J. (2017). How can we conceptualize behavioural addiction without pathologizing common behaviours? *Addiction, 112*(10), 1709–1715. doi:10.1111/add.13763

Kourosh, A. S., Harrington, C. R., & Adinoff, B. (2010). Tanning as a behavioral addiction. *The American Journal of Drug and Alcohol Abuse, 36*(5), 284–290. doi:10.3109/00952990.2010.491883

Kubey, R., & Csikszentmihalyi, M. (2002). Television addiction is no mere metaphor. *Scientific American, 286*(2), 74–80.

Kyrios, M., Trotzke, P., Lawrence, L., Fassnacht, D. B., Ali, K., Laskowski, N. M., & Müller, A. (2018). Behavioral neuroscience of buying-shopping disorder: A review. *Current Behavioral Neuroscience Reports, 5*(4), 263–270. doi:10.1007/s40473-018-0165-6

Maráz, A., Király, O., Urbán, R., Griffiths, M. D., & Demetrovics, Z. (2015a). Why do you dance? Development of the dance motivation inventory (DMI). *PLoS ONE 10*(3), e0122866. doi:10.1371/journal.pone.0122866

Maráz, A., Urbán, R., Griffiths, M. D., & Demetrovics, Z. (2015b). An empirical investigation of dance addiction. *PLOS ONE, 10*(5), e0125988. doi:10.1371/journal.pone.0125988

Maráz, A., van den Brink, W., & Demetrovics, Z. (2015c). Prevalence and construct validity of compulsive buying disorder in shopping mall visitors. *Psychiatry Research, 228*(3), 918–924. doi:10.1016/j.psychres.2015.04.012

Mónok, K., Berczik, K., Urbán, R., Szabo, A., Griffiths, M. D., Farkas, J., . . . Demetrovics, Z. (2012). Psychometric properties and concurrent validity of two exercise addiction measures: A population wide study. *Psychology of Sport and Exercise, 13*(6), 739–746. doi:10.1016/j.psychsport.2012.06.003

Morgan, W. P. (1979). Negative addiction in runners. *The Physician and Sports Medicine, 7*(2), 55–77. doi:10.1080/00913847.1979.11948436

Müller, A., Brand, M., Claes, L., Demetrovics, Z., de Zwaan, M., Fernández-Aranda, F., . . . Kyrios, M. (2019). Buying-shopping disorder – is there enough evidence to support its inclusion in ICD-11? *CNS Spectrums, 24*(4), 374–379. doi:10.1017/s1092852918001323

Nasser, J. A., Bradley, L. E., Leitzsch, J. B., Chohan, O., Fasulo, K., Haller, J., . . . Del Parigi, A. (2011). Psychoactive effects of tasting chocolate and desire for more chocolate. *Physiology & Behavior, 104*(1), 117–121. doi:10.1016/j.physbeh.2011.04.040

Nestler, E. J., & Malenka, R. C. (2004). The addicted brain. *Scientific American 290*(3), 78–85.

Rajeswari, P. (2020). Can chocolate be addictive? *Food and Agriculture Spectrum Journal, 1*(3). 1–8. Retrieved from: https://foodagrispectrum.org/index.php/fasj/article/view/71/28

Reche, C., De Francisco, C., Martínez-Rodríguez, A., & Ros-Martínez, A. (2018). Relationship among sociodemographic and sport variables, exercise dependence, and burnout: A preliminary study in athletes. *Anales de Psicología, 34*(2), 398. doi:10.6018/analesps.34.2.289861

Rozin, P., & Stoess, C. (1993). Is there a general tendency to become addicted? *Addictive Behaviors, 18*(1), 81–87. doi:10.1016/0306-4603(93)90011-w

Schall, T. A., Wright, W. J., & Dong, Y. (2020). Nucleus accumbens fast-spiking interneurons in motivational and addictive behaviors. *Molecular Psychiatry, 26*(1), 234–246. doi:10.1038/s41380-020-0683-y

Serafini, R. A., Pryce, K. D., & Zachariou, V. (2020). The mesolimbic dopamine system in chronic pain and associated affective comorbidities. *Biological Psychiatry, 87*(1), 64–73. doi:10.1016/j.biopsych.2019.10.018

Solinas, M., Belujon, P., Fernagut, P. O., Jaber, M., & Thiriet, N. (2018). Dopamine and addiction: What have we learned from 40 years of research. *Journal of Neural Transmission, 126*(4), 481–516. doi:10.1007/s00702-018-1957-2

Sussman, S. (2017). *Substance and behavioral addictions: Concepts, causes, and cures.* Cambridge, UK: Cambridge University Press.

Sussman, S., Rozgonjuk, D., & van den Eijnden, R. J. J. M. (2017). Substance and behavioral addictions may share a similar underlying process of dysregulation. *Addiction, 112*(10), 1717–1718. doi:10.1111/add.13825

Szabo, A., Gaspar, Z., & Abraham, J. (2013). Acute effects of light exercise on subjectively experienced well-being: Benefits in only three minutes. *Baltic Journal of Health and Physical Activity, 5*(4). doi:10.2478/bjha-2013-0024

Targhetta, R., Nalpas, B., & Perney, P. (2013). Argentine tango: Another behavioral addiction? *Journal of Behavioral Addictions, 2*(3), 179–186. doi:10.1556/jba.2.2013.007

Taylor, C. Z. (2002). Religious addiction: Obsession with spirituality. *Pastoral Psychology, 50*(4), 291–315.

Terry, A., Szabo, A., & Griffiths, M. (2004). The Exercise Addiction Inventory: A new brief screening tool. *Addiction Research & Theory, 12*(5), 489–499. doi:10.1080/16066350310001637363

Thornton, E. W., & Scott, S. E. (1995). Motivation in the committed runner: Correlations between self-report scales and behaviour. *Health Promotion International, 10*(3), 177–184. doi:10.1093/heapro/10.3.177

Weinstein, A., Maraz, A., Griffiths, M. D., Lejoyeux, M., & Demetrovics, Z. (2016). Compulsive buying – Features and characteristics of addiction. In V. R. Preedy (Ed.). *Neuropathology of drug addictions and substance misuse. Volume 3: General processes and mechanisms, prescription medications, caffeine and areca, polydrug misuse, emerging addictions and non-drug addictions* (pp. 993–1007). London: Academic Press.

World Health Organization. (2019). *International statistical classification of diseases and related health problems* (11th ed.). Retrieved from: https://icd.who.int/

Yu, S., & Sussman, S. (2020). Does smartphone addiction fall on a continuum of addictive behaviors? *International Journal of Environmental Research and Public Health, 17*(2), 422. doi:10.3390/ijerph17020422

Zou, Z., Wang, H., d' Oleire Uquillas, F., Wang, X., Ding, J., & Chen, H. (2017). Definition of substance and non-substance addiction. In Zhang, X., Shi, J., & Tao, R. (Eds.). *Substance and non-substance addiction* (pp. 21–41). Singapore: Springer. doi:10.1007/978-981-10-5562-1_2

6 Uncovering exercise addiction

A historical perspective

6.1 Too much or unhealthy exercise

Overexercising to the point where individuals *lose control* over their exercise routine and walk on the path of self-destruction is generally referred to as *exercise addiction* (Szabo, 2000, 2010). The same concept is also often described as *exercise dependence* by many scholars (e.g., Cockerill & Riddington, 1996; Hausenblas & Downs, 2002). Furthermore, some academics refer to the condition as *obligatory exercising* (e.g., Pasman & Thompson, 1988), probably emphasizing the behavior's external control and compulsive aspect. Indeed, in the public or mass media, the condition is frequently termed as *compulsive exercise* (Eberle, 2004), *obsessive exercise* (Boone, 1990), or *exercise abuse* (Davis, 2000). Other terms like excessive exercise or pathological exercise are also often used in the literature. It is important to note that all these synonymous words, theoretically, are intended to label the *same* psychological condition (Table 6.1). Recently, the term 'morbid exercise' was proposed to encompass all deviations from healthy exercise (Szabo et al., 2018). Indeed, there are several reasons against the alternate terminologies in naming the same phenomenon. One obvious reason concerns the conceptual homogeneity in research.

There is a sound argument for differentiating addiction from dependence (O'Brien et al., 2006). While the term *dependence* is often, and perhaps carelessly, used as a synonym for addiction, the latter includes the former and also includes *compulsion* (Goodman, 1990). Accordingly, a general formula for addiction may be: *addiction = dependence + compulsion*. Goodman specifies that not all dependencies and compulsions may be classified as an addiction. Therefore, this chapter will use the term *exercise addiction* because it is the most appropriate for describing morbidity since it incorporates both dependence and compulsion.

6.2 Early studies

The idea that exercise could become addictive surfaced over half a decade ago, during a study by Baekeland (1970). The author studied sleep in 14

DOI: 10.4324/9781003173595-6

Table 6.1 The various terms used for denoting 'unhealthy' exercise behavior.

Terms used	In the title of papers in Google Scholar (Number of papers up to October 2021)
Compulsive exercise	195
Dysfunctional exercise	3
Exercise abuse	9
Exercise addiction	481
Exercise dependence	458
Excessive exercise	194
Morbid exercise	4
Obligatory exercise	56
Obsessive exercise	5
Pathological exercise	43

regularly exercising college students on two exercise days and four days of abstinence from exercise over one month. The results showed that the participants' sleep patterns mirrored increased anxiety during the exercise deprivation period. Furthermore, the participants reported impaired sleep patterns, increased need for social contact, and increased sexual tension. However, the author did not mention the term 'addiction' or 'dependence' as its synonym in this early paper; instead, he attributed his finding to an inner drive surfacing as an instinctual discharge. Accordingly, exercise can be perceived as a means of discharge for the aggressive drive. It generates increased self-esteem and feelings of mastery; the pausing of exercise triggers an increase in compensatory drives (i.e., sexual), which, after satisfaction, dampen the inner pressure. This explanation is in accord with a recently proposed catharsis theory of stress, suggesting that exercise could be an 'instinctual' means of coping with stress (Szabo et al., 2021). It also agrees, at least in part, with most psychophysiological models proposed for exercise addiction discussed in Chapter 11.

In 1976, Glasser presented running as a positive addiction. The term 'exercise addiction' penetrated the academic literature in the late 1970s. Burgess and Pargman (1977) proposed that stimulus-seeking and extraversion are principal determinants of exercise addiction. They tested the relationships between these constructs and exercise frequency in 90 age- and education-matched men in three groups, 30 regular, 30 occasional, and 30 non-exercisers. In accord with the authors' hypothesis, the results suggested that regular and occasional exercise are associated with higher scores of 'thrills' and 'adventure seeking' and lower scores of neuroticism compared to no-exercise. The authors interpreted the results as indicating that stimulus-seeking could be an incentive for physical activity and athletic involvement. Still, it cannot distinguish participants exercising with different volumes of exercise, and it is not a determinant of exercise addiction.

Two years later, Sachs and Pargman (1979) defined exercise addiction as a psychological or physiological dependence on habitual physical activity. These authors suggested that a specific characteristic of exercise addiction is the emergence of withdrawal symptoms 24–36 hours after the unsatisfied need (or urge) to exercise. The nature of these withdrawal symptoms could be both psychological and physiological. Sachs and Pargman interviewed dedicated runners about their motives for running, perceived role as a runner, the significance of running, running volume, and exercise addiction. They found that primary motives for running were health, being in shape, controlling body weight, and unwinding. Addicted runners perceived their role to be an essential part of their daily lives, and if prevented from running, they experienced withdrawal symptoms. Finally, the interviewed participants felt motivated to maintain running because of their addiction to exercise and belief that running is the only way to have a healthy cardiovascular system. Sachs and Pargman's conceptualization of exercise addiction was often cited in the later literature. Still, the paralleling of *addiction* with *dependence* was criticized (Szabo, 2010) for reasons discussed earlier in this chapter.

One of the still often-cited papers on exercise addiction, referred to as 'exercise dependence,' was published in 1987 by De Coverley Veale, who proposed the first criteria for diagnosing exercise addiction. While positive addiction criteria for running addiction were earlier presented by Glasser (1976), they did not address the dysfunctional nature of the problematic exercise. In contrast, De Covereley Veale's criteria were based on the characteristic dependence syndromes. An abbreviated (modified) version of these criteria is shown in Table 6.2.

In addition to offering the very first set of diagnostic criteria for exercise addiction, De Coverley Veale (1987) also differentiated between primary and secondary exercise addiction. In Chapter 10, we look at these classifications more closely. Generally, in primary exercise addiction, exercise

Table 6.2 The first criteria for problematic exercise or exercise addiction.

1.	Stereotypical exercise behavior
2.	Salience, exercise has the highest priority
3.	Tolerance, more exercise is needed over time
4.	Withdrawal symptoms when exercise is not possible
5.	Relief or control of withdrawal symptoms with exercise
6.	Awareness of a compulsion to exercise
7.	Relapse after a period of abstinence
Associated Features	
8.	Exercise is continued despite injury, or exercise causes conflict with others
9.	Dieting and weight loss for better exercise performance

Note: Modified on the basis of De Coverley Veale (1987), Table 1, p. 736.

is the means to achieve an exercise-related goal without associated eating disorders. Secondary exercise addiction reflects dependence on exercise that is performed for the sake of controlling or losing weight. Therefore, it is related to various eating disorders. The topic merits special consideration later in this book because, as understood by these authors, in secondary exercise addiction (dependence), the exercise behavior merely serves as a means (vehicle) for achieving a weight-related goal.

6.3 The first published case

Addiction to exercise only occurs when there is established *harm* to the person's physical, social, or psychological life (Juwono & Szabo, 2020). However, despite over 1000 papers published in exercise addiction (Szabo & Kovacsik, 2019), only about a dozen individual case studies are published in the academic literature. The first case of exercise addiction was published in 1995 by Veale. This clinician presented the case of Anna (a pseudonym; Szabo, 2015), who at the time was a 27-year-old university-educated woman, single and unemployed. Anna did not seek help for her problematic exercise behavior, but she responded to a call by Veale, who wished to talk to people who consider themselves addicted to exercise. Anna trained for marathon races and had a great personal best time of 2 hours 40 minutes. Her regular weekly exercise comprised 15 miles of cycling every day and running twice a day except on two days of the week when she ran only once.

Anna also engaged in anaerobic exercise (weight training) twice a week. Although her total amount of running was not excessive, according to Veale (1995), she had no other interests in life. Running or exercise meant life itself. Anna realized that her running is compulsive (quote: 'I've got to do it,' p. 3; Veale, 1995). Her running was motivated by negative reinforcement. She would experience withdrawal symptoms that included depressed mood, insomnia, restlessness, and uncertainty when she was forced to adjust her training due to an injury. Anna even ended up in a casualty department due to her severe withdrawal symptoms, but she did not receive psychiatric help. These withdrawal symptoms point to an addictive pattern in her exercise behavior. Anna's life was running; she described her life goals as (quote: 'to run till I die,' page. 3; Veale, 1995). She had a dream to represent her country in the Olympic games. This attitude, reflecting that everything revolves around the exercise in her life, shows salience (refer to Table 6.2). Another typical symptom of addiction was that Anna continued to exercise despite injury or health difficulties. Indeed, she was running while having severe back pain and other health problems. According to Veale, once, she ran a marathon with a high fever from German measles. She did such things more than once. On another occasion, when she had a fever, she was forced to give up after 16 miles. Conflict is also evident in her case (refer to 'associated features' in Table 6.2). Anna has lost her partner because of her excessive exercise. She also had frequent arguments and conflicts with her family members about her training volume that has damaged her health.

She was unemployed because she did not want work to conflict with her training routine. Anna manifested no psychiatric or eating disorders. However, she was concerned about her weight and appearance because she considered herself overweight for a runner. She was vegetarian and sometimes skipped lunch. Still, she could not be diagnosed with an eating disorder. Her laboratory (blood) tests were normal, and so were her menstrual cycles. There was a family history of depression from her mother's side, and she also had a history of a depressive episode at the age of 18. Veale (1995) suggested that her exercise was a means of preventing a recurrence of her depression (coping). Anna displayed all components of addiction based on the components model introduced in Chapter 5 (Griffiths, 2005). Her case fits well the interactional model of exercise addiction (Egorov & Szabo, 2013), presented later in Chapter 11. Her running pattern showed both mastery (performance) and therapeutic (health) orientation. If Veale was right in his diagnosis, the symptoms could be traced back to Anna's depression or fear of depression. However, it may also be a means of coping with losses (i.e., partner) or compensation for neglecting other necessary and possibly rewarding aspects of life (recall that Anna's life was running itself). The negative consequences were clear in Anna's case.

Only a few more cases have been published since Anna's story came to light. Since the ratio of the known (published) cases of exercise addiction to the number of publications in the area is extremely low, the few published cases warrant separate discussion. In fact, as proposed in a later chapter, well-understood case studies are the infrastructure of the research on exercise addiction. Therefore, to examine their fit into exercise addiction models and identify common symptoms that could be targeted in rehabilitation, we dedicate Chapter 13 in this book to the presentation and evaluation of the published cases of exercise addiction.

6.4 Early psychometric assessment of exercise addiction

A valid means of assessment was necessary to study exercise addiction from the beginning of the growing interest in the field. Initially, scholars relied on exercise frequency (Burgess & Pargman, 1977) and in-depth interviews (Sachs & Pargman, 1979) to examine exercise addiction. While today it is known that the former is unlikely to be related to exercise addiction (Szabo & Kovacsik, 2019), in-depth interviews are still the most robust and recommended method for identifying exercise addiction as a behavioral dysfunction (Szabo et al., 2015). However, in-depth interviews are not economical because they are time-consuming. Furthermore, they only provide useful idiographic information in a particular case (see Szabo, 2018) with limited generalization. Therefore, scholars sought a more efficient assessment of exercise addiction that is adoptable in nomothetic research fulfilling the scientific criteria.

In lack of thorough knowledge about exercise addiction, some research-ers considered it a positive addiction (Glasser, 1976) akin to a high level of exercise commitment. On the basis of this conceptualization, Carmack and Martens (1979) developed the Commitment to Running Scale and used it for assessing commitment to running in 250 male and 65 female runners with different levels of running skills and experience. The authors found that the 12-item scale possessed good psychometric properties. Addition-ally, their results unveiled that perceived addiction, history of running, and state of mind were significant predictors of commitment to running. Car-mack and Martens interpreted the findings as supportive of the concept of *positive* addiction to exercise. However, commitment and addiction to exer-cise are different behavioral concepts and manifestations (Szabo, 2010), as discussed in the next chapter.

Hailey and Bailey (1982) realized the conceptual dilemma caused by the commitment to running viewed as a 'positive addiction.' This view gener-ated confusion between desirable exercise behavior and addiction to exer-cise, which is dysfunctional (Goodman, 1990). Consequently, these scholars developed their 14-item instrument to measure 'negative' addiction in run-ners. Unfortunately, the authors did not conduct a psychometric evaluation of the Negative Addiction Scale. However, examining 60 male participants, they found that runners with less than one year of running history reported less addiction than runners who ran for more than a year.

6.5 Research interest in exercise addiction

Research interest in exercise addiction has grown substantially since the 1980s. A *Google Scholar* advanced search, using the exact terms 'exercise addiction' and 'exercise dependence' *anywhere in the published paper text,* yielded a progressive increase in the number of publications. While only a minority of these papers may focus *specifically* on exercise addiction, a pro-portional relationship between the primary and secondary attention dedi-cated to the subject may be expected. These findings gathered on May 1, 2021 (until the end of 2020), and October 10, 2021 (to the exact date), are illustrated in Figure 6.1. The swift growth in the number of publications divulges extensive interest in the subject.

Earlier, Szabo et al. (2015) performed an analysis of published papers on PubMed and Google Scholar over a 3-year period (from January 2011 to January 2014). They found 128 papers that *specifically* examined exer-cise addiction. The authors calculated that this number reflects about 40 publications per year in that period. The 128 papers were published in 89 different journals, suggesting that exercise addiction is studied in a mul-tidisciplinary field of research. Most studies originated from three English-speaking nations (Figure 6.2). Still, the figure illustrates that research

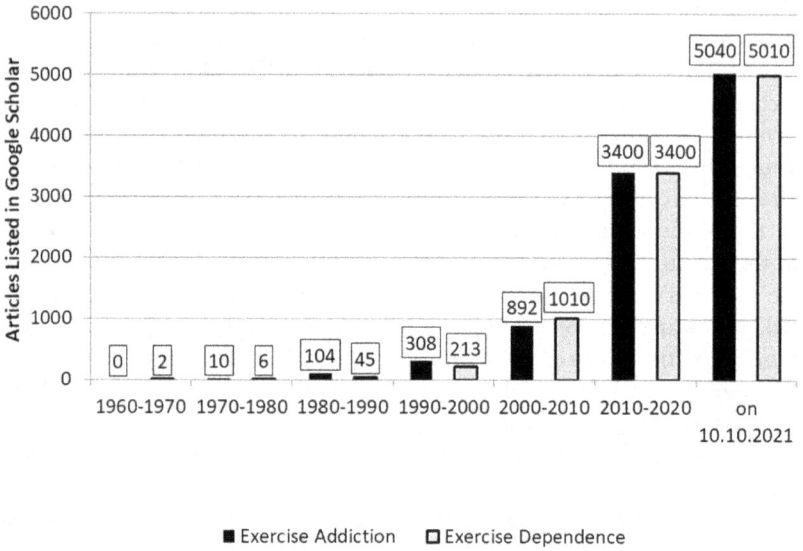

Figure 6.1 Diagram illustrating the growth of publications in exercise addiction from 1960 to October 10, 2021.

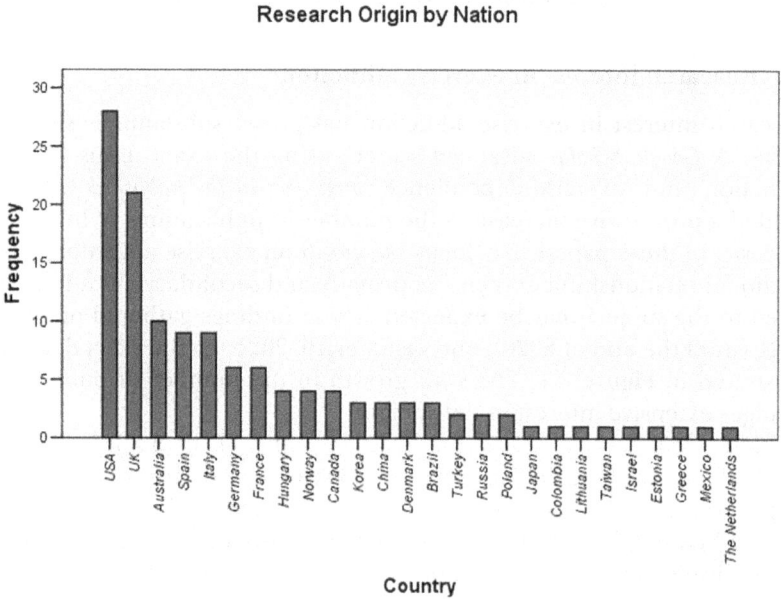

Figure 6.2 Diagram illustrating the origin and number of publications on PubMed and Google Scholar in exercise addiction from January 2011 to January 2014 (Szabo et al., 2015).

interest in the topic, at the time of the study, has spread to nearly 30 nations. This figure is much larger today as international collaboration is facilitated through partnership via various online contact platforms.

6.6 Key points

1. Exercise dependence is not the same as exercise addiction.
2. Exercise addiction research started with the identification of exercise deprivation.
3. Early studies used interviews and questionnaires to gain insight into exercise addiction.
4. Early research often confounded exercise addiction with a high commitment to exercise.
5. The number of research publications on exercise addiction is growing at a fast rate.

6.7 References

Baekeland, F. (1970). Exercise deprivation. *Archives of General Psychiatry, 22*(4), 365. doi:10.1001/archpsyc.1970.01740280077014

Boone, T. (1990). Obsessive exercise; Some reflections. *Journal of Physical Education, Recreation & Dance, 61*(7), 45–49. doi:10.1080/07303084.1990.10604579

Burgess, S. S., & Pargman, D. (1977). *Stimulus-seeking, extraversion, and neuroticism in regular, occasional, and non-exercisers.* Paper presented at the 1977 Annual Meeting of North American Society for the Psychology of Sport and Physical Activity (Abstract from: ERIC: #ED141301).

Carmack, M. A., & Martens, R. (1979). Measuring commitment to running: A survey of runners' attitudes and mental states. *Journal of Sport Psychology, 1*, 25–42. doi:10.1123/jsp.1.1.25

Cockerill, I. M., & Riddington, M. E. (1996). Exercise dependence and associated disorders: A review. *Counselling Psychology Quarterly, 9*(2), 119–129. doi:10.1080/09515079608256358

Davis, C. (2000). Exercise abuse. *International Journal of Sport Psychology, 31*(2), 278–289.

De Coverley Veale, D. M. W. (1987). Exercise dependence. *British Journal of Addiction, 82*(7), 735–740. doi:10.1111/j.1360-0443.1987.tb01539.x

Eberle, S. G. (2004). *Compulsive exercise: Too much of a good thing?* National Eating Disorders Association. Retrieved from: https://uhs.berkeley.edu/sites/default/files/bewell_cmpvexc.pdf

Egorov, A. Y., & Szabo, A. (2013). The exercise paradox: An interactional model for a clearer conceptualization of exercise addiction. *Journal of Behavioral Addictions, 2*(4), 199–208. doi:10.1556/jba.2.2013.4.2

Glasser, W. (1976). *Positive addiction.* New York, NY: Harper & Row.

Goodman, A. (1990). Addiction: Definition and implications. *British Journal of Addiction, 85*(11), 1403–1408. doi:10.1111/j.1360-0443.1990.tb01620.x

Griffiths, M. D. (2005). A 'components' model of addiction within a biopsychosocial framework. *Journal of Substance Use, 10*(4), 191–197. doi:10.1080/14659890500114359

Hailey, B. J., & Bailey, L. A. (1982). Negative addiction in runners: A quantitative approach. *Journal of Sport Behavior, 5*(3), 150–154.

Hausenblas, H. A., & Downs, S. D. (2002). Exercise dependence: A systematic review. *Psychology of Sport and Exercise, 3*(2), 89–123. doi:10.1016/s1469-0292(00)00015-7.

Juwono, I. D., & Szabo, A. (2020). 100 cases of exercise addiction: More evidence for a widely researched but rarely identified dysfunction. *International Journal of Mental Health and Addiction.* (Online first). doi:10.1007/s11469-020-00264-6

O'Brien, C. P., Volkow, N., & Li, T.-K. (2006). What's in a word? Addiction versus dependence in DSM-V. *American Journal of Psychiatry, 163*(5), 764–765. doi:10.1176/ajp.2006.163.5.764

Pasman, L., & Thompson, J. K. (1988). Body image and eating disturbance in obligatory runners, obligatory weightlifters, and sedentary individuals. *International Journal of Eating Disorders, 7*(6), 759–777. doi:10.1002/1098-108X(198811)7:6<759::AID-EAT2260070605>3.0.CO;2-G

Sachs, M. L., & Pargman, D. (1979). Running addictions: A depth Interview approach. *Journal of Sport Behavior, 2,* 143–155.

Szabo, A. (2000). Physical activity as a source of psychological dysfunction. In S. J. H. Biddle, K. R. Fox, & S. H. Boutcher (Eds.), *Physical activity and psychological well-being* (pp. 130–153). London: Routledge.

Szabo, A. (2010). *Addiction to exercise: A symptom or a disorder?* New York, NY: Nova Science Publishers.

Szabo, A. (2015). *The bright and dark sides of exercise behaviour: Untangling the paradox.* Doctoral dissertation of the Hungarian Academy of Sciences. Hungary, Budapest. Retrieved from: http://real-d.mtak.hu/886/7/dc_912_14_doktori_mu.pdf

Szabo, A. (2018). Addiction, passion, or confusion? New theoretical insights on exercise addiction research from the case study of a female body builder. *Europe's Journal of Psychology, 14*(2), 296–316. doi:10.5964/ejop.v14i2.1545

Szabo, A., Demetrovics, Z., & Griffiths, M. D. (2018). Morbid exercise behavior: Addiction or psychological escape? In H. Budde & M. Wegner (Eds.), *The exercise effect on mental health* (pp. 277–311), New York, NY: Routledge. doi:10.4324/9781315113906-11

Szabo, A., Griffiths, M. D., Marcos, R. D. L. V., Mervó, B., & Demetrovics, Z. (2015). Focus: Addiction: Methodological and conceptual limitations in exercise addiction research. *The Yale Journal of Biology and Medicine, 88*(3), 303. Retrieved from: www.ncbi.nlm.nih.gov/pmc/articles/PMC4553651/

Szabo, A., & Kovacsik, R. (2019). When passion appears, exercise addiction disappears. *Swiss Journal of Psychology, 78*(3–4), 137–142. doi:10.1024/1421-0185/a000228

Szabo, A., Tóth, E., Kósa, L., Laki, Á., & Ihász, F. (2021). Increased exercise effort after artificially-induced stress: Laboratory-based evidence for the catharsis theory of stress. *Baltic Journal of Sport and Health Sciences, 4*(119), 24–30. doi:10.33607/bjshs.v4i119.1016

Veale, D. (1995). Does primary exercise dependence really exist? In J. Annett, B. Cripps, & H. Steinberg (Eds.), *Exercise addiction: Motivation for participation in sport and exercise: Proceedings of British Psychology, Sport and Exercise Psychology Section* (pp. 71–75). Leicester, UK: British Psychological Society.

7 Commitment versus addiction in sports and exercise

7.1 Exercise motivation: a behaviorist perspective

Commitment to exercise and sport is very different from addiction to exercise, regardless of training volume. Motivation for exercise behavior is another distinguishing feature between healthy commitment and dysfunctional addiction. People exercise for specific and usually very personal reasons. The reason is generally associated with some psychological reward obtained through an altered physical or social state like being in shape, looking good, being with friends, staying healthy, building muscle, and losing weight. The personal experience of the anticipated reward strengthens the exercise behavior through conditioning.

Scholars of the behaviorist school of thought postulate that behavior, in general, can be explained through reinforcement and punishment. Accordingly, the operant conditioning theory posits three principles of behavior: 1) positive reinforcement, 2) negative reinforcement, and 3) punishment (Bozarth, 1994). Positive reinforcement is a motivational incentive for doing something to *gain a reward* that is something pleasant or desirable (e.g., increased muscle tone). The reward then turns into a motivational incentive, which increases the likelihood of that behavior being repeated. In contrast, negative reinforcement is a motivational incentive for doing something to *avoid* a harmful or unpleasant outcome (e.g., gaining weight). The successful avoidance or reduction of harm is the reward, which increases the probability of the behavior in the future. Consequently, both positive and negative reinforcers act as *rewards* that increase one's incentive for a behavior (Bozarth, 1994). However, their mechanism is different because, in behaviors motivated via positive reinforcement, there is some gain resulting from an action (e.g., feeling great). Consequently, they are driven by positive expectancies. In contrast, negatively reinforced behaviors are driven by negative expectancies and, therefore, to avoid their fulfillment, the behavior must be obligatorily performed (e.g., feeling guilty or fat if a planned exercise session is missed; *must* exercise to avoid such feelings).

Punishment refers to situations in which the delivery of a noxious or an unpleasant agent or event, or alternately the removal of a pleasant or desired

DOI: 10.4324/9781003173595-7

agent or action, reduces the probability of a behavior being repeated. In contrast to reinforcement, punishment suppresses the behavior, and therefore, exercise or physical activity should never be used (by teachers, parents, peers, or coaches) as a form of punishment. Paradoxically, exercise addiction can be perceived as self-punishing behavior. It is a relatively rare form of addiction that requires substantial physical effort, often to the point of exhaustion and pain, in contrast to the instantly rewarding passive addictions like alcohol, tobacco, or drug abuse. Therefore, affected people may have unique personality characteristics (Bircher et al., 2017).

People addicted to exercise may be motivated by negative reinforcement (e.g., to avoid withdrawal symptoms) as well as positive reinforcement (e.g., mere pleasure, the runner's high feeling, which has limited empirical support at this time [Pierce, 1994; Szabo, 2010], or experiencing and expecting successive athletic success even beyond the person's skills and abilities [Egorov & Szabo, 2013]). However, negative reinforcement, or avoidance-motivated behavior, is not a general characteristic of the committed exercisers (Szabo, 2010). Indeed, committed individuals maintain their habitual exercise regimen to benefit from the activity. On the contrary, addicted exercisers must perform it, or otherwise, something unwanted might happen to them. Their exercise becomes an 'obligation' (also reflected by the popular term 'obligatory exercise') that needs to be fulfilled or else an unwanted life event might occur, like the inability to cope with stress, maintain weight, or be cheerful. Every time a person undertakes a behavior to avoid something negative, harmful, or unpleasant, the incentive for that behavior is fueled by negative reinforcement. In these situations, the person involved *must do it* in contrast to wants to do it. Therefore, commitment to exercise may involve a freely chosen *gain-oriented* reason and a pressured *avoidance-oriented* reason.

There are many examples in several sports areas in which a behavior initially driven by positive reinforcement (gain-oriented) could turn into negatively reinforced behavior (avoidance-oriented). For example, an excellent football player who starts playing the game for fun and derives pleasure from participation after being discovered as a talent and offered a service contract with a team becomes a professional player expected to perform upon signing the contract. An unfulfilled external expectancy triggers internal pressure to conform and the associated obligatory feeling (i.e., *I must do better this time*). Consequently, the new motivational source is avoidance-oriented as the player tries to overcome the negative consequences of unsatisfactory performance. Although the player might still enjoy playing (especially when all goes well), the external pressure to perform well (Gaspar & Szabo, 2019) adds a new, negatively reinforcing, incentive to the motivation of the football player. The internal pressure eliciting an avoidance-aimed motivation for the play is different from the same motivational orientation in addictive behaviors. Its main source is primarily external (conforming to what is expected by others). In contrast, in addictions, the source is mainly internal (conforming to the person's internal needs like handling stress or trauma). Table 7.1 presents the critical differences between the underlying motives in exercise behaviors driven by positive (gain-oriented) and negative (avoidance-oriented) reinforcements.

In contrast to commitment, Duncan (1974), in the context of substance abuse, suggested that addiction is nearly identical with, and semantically is just another term for, avoidance or escape behavior when the unpleasant feeling is being negatively reinforced by drug-taking. The addictive substance or behavior acts as a temporary pain reliever by providing relief or momentary comfort. Individuals addicted to exercise, in this view, seek a means – with which they had past relieving experience – that gives them the chance to escape from chronic emotional distress and struggle, which might be caused by mental dysfunction, or by psychosocial stress, or by a discomforting social or physical environment. In Duncan's view, all addictions represent similar negatively reinforced behaviors. However, this argument may not always be valid in exercise addiction, at least based on the interactional model (Egorov & Szabo, 2013) discussed in Chapter 11.

Duncan argued that negative reinforcement is a powerful mechanism in maintaining high-frequency and long-persistent behaviors. Animals that could have escaped a noxious stimulus or event by pressing a bar (negative reinforcement) will often do so to the point of ignoring other, even instinctual activities like eating, sleeping, and sexual activity. Avoidance behaviors are highly resistant to extinction, and even when they appear to have been finally eliminated, they tend to reoccur spontaneously. Consequently, the relapse rate in addictions, regardless of the form of addiction, is very

Table 7.1 Exercise behaviors are motivated via positive and negative reinforcement.

Positive reinforcement	*Negative reinforcement*
Origin: Behaviorist school of thought	**Origin:** Behaviorist school of thought
Definition: Positive reinforcement strengthens a behavior because a tangible or intangible *gain* results from the behavior	**Definition:** Negative reinforcement strengthens a behavior because a harmful condition is stopped or *avoided* as a consequence of the behavior
Examples:	**Examples:**
'I feel revitalized after exercise' (*gains* good feeling)	'I run *to avoid* circulatory problems that my parents had'
'I like to decrease my running time on the same distance' (*gains* skill and confidence)	'I go to the gym *to avoid* getting fat'
'I lift weights to look good' (*gains* physical benefits, good looks)	'I have to run my 10 miles every day, or else I feel guilty and irritated' (*avoids* the feeling of guilt and irritation)

high. In Duncan's view, the intensity, compulsiveness, and predisposition to relapse, common characteristics of addictions, result from the fact that the behavior is maintained by negative reinforcement.

Although positive reinforcement like the runners' high and brain reward systems has been implicated in explaining exercise addiction, the motivational incentive in addiction may be more closely connected to the prevention, escape, or avoidance of something unwanted (Baker et al., 2004). Accordingly, the process of addiction, especially in the later or the actual addiction phase, is more likely motivated by negative reinforcement in which the affected individual must exercise to avoid an unwanted consequence. This *obligatory* (must) aspect of the behavior sets it apart from the healthy commitment to exercise.

7.2 Commitment to exercise

Commitment to exercise is a construct and relative measure of an individual's devotion to an activity, philosophy, or movement. It estimates the strength of adherence to the activities that are a part of people's daily lives. For committed individuals, satisfaction, enjoyment, and achievement derived from their activity are internal motivators that make them stick to their sport or exercise training (Chapman & De Castro, 1990; Locke & Schattke, 2019). Sachs (1981) believed that commitment to exercise results from the cognitive-intellectual analysis of the rewards, including social relationships, health, social status, or money gained from the activity. Committed exercisers, according to Sachs: 1) exercise mainly for extrinsic rewards, 2) view their exercise as an important, but not the central part of their lives, and 3) may not experience painful withdrawal symptoms when they cannot exercise for some reason (Summers & Hinton, 1986). The critical point is that committed exercisers control their activity (Johnson, 1995) rather than being controlled by the activity. In contrast to committed exercisers, addicted exercisers are: 1) more likely to exercise for intrinsic rewards, 2) aware that exercise is the central part of their lives, and 3) experience *severe* withdrawal symptoms when they cannot exercise (Sachs, 1981; Summers & Hinton, 1986).

7.3 Commitment to running

Running is the most popular recreational physical activity in many nations[1] (Fitbit Co., 2021). Therefore, commitment to running is high around the world. The level of commitment to running is a measure of the probability that could predict the maintenance of running behavior in lack of some barriers, such as injuries, illness, or other hindering commitments. This measure reflects the intensity of effort (Brehm & Self, 1989) invested in running based on motivational theories. For the committed runner, feelings like satisfaction, enjoyment, and achievement derived from running are incentives that motivate the continuity of the behavior (Chapman & De Castro, 1990). These incentives are primarily internal and, therefore, contradict Sachs (1981), who thought that committed runners run for external rewards, which nevertheless can also have motivating roles. A high commitment was seen as beneficial for the individual, and its highest level was considered as positive addiction (Glasser, 1976). By penetrating the media, the term has spread among runners who proudly declared that they are addicted to running while referring to their uttermost commitment to their habit.

7.4 Obligatory running

Obligatory runners (Sachs, 1981; Summers & Hinton, 1986) are individuals who, over time, feel *obliged* to run or otherwise feel unwell. At this stage, running is no longer a pleasurable leisure activity for them or even an achievement goal-oriented task; it is a chore that must be fulfilled. Obligatory exercise, in general, has three dimensions: 1) *tolerance*, manifested in increased dose or volume of exercise, 2) *deprivation feelings*, emerging as negative psychological states when missing a workout, and 3) *salience*, manifested in more and more preoccupation with exercise (Ackard et al., 2002). In contrast to committed runners, according to Sachs (1981), obligatory runners: 1) are more likely to run for intrinsic rewards, 2) view running as the most crucial part of their everyday lives, and 3) are prone to experience strong deprivation sensations when they are unable to run. However, as we noted in the previous section, committed runners are also likely to run for intrinsic reasons. Locke and Schattke (2019) suggest that intrinsic motivation means *liking the doing* and that extrinsic motivation refers to *doing something as a means to an end.*

Therefore, the source or form of the person's motivation for running, exercise, or sport, in general, is an essential distinguishing factor between commitment and addiction to exercise. On the one hand, committed exercisers perform their activity because they *like* the feeling associated with their action. Therefore, they are motivated internally and rewarded through positive reinforcement. On the other hand, obligatory exercisers strive to achieve a reward manifested in a *means to an end* via negative reinforcement, exemplified in the avoidance of withdrawal symptoms, or through much-desired rewards, such as experiencing the runners' high feeling (Pierce, 1994; Szabo, 2010).

Therefore, addiction to running, or obligatory running, can be relatively well distinguished from commitment. The former was also termed 'negative addiction' to point at its morbid features (Morgan, 1979) and imply a transition from commitment, which can be erroneously interpreted as a previous phase to addiction. However, addiction surfaces when the agent or behavior starts to control the person. De Coverley Veale (1987) forwarded the criteria for exercise addiction, as discussed in Chapter 6. These are: 1) stereotypic exercise behavior, 2) salience, 3) tolerance, 4) severe withdrawal symptoms, 5) intentional avoidance of withdrawal symptoms, 6) awareness of compulsive exercise, 7) relapse after abstinence, 8) weight loss for the sake of performance, 9) continuation of exercise despite injuries, and 10) conflicts due to the excessive exercise. Therefore, in contrast to committed exercise, addictive exercise is considered dysfunctional, requiring medical intervention (Weinstein & Weinstein, 2014). Indeed, exercise addiction is associated with mental dysfunctions such as depression (Levit et al., 2018) and eating disorders (Trott et al., 2020).

7.5 The relationship between committed and obligatory running or addictive exercise

Addiction to running can only take place if the runner is highly committed. However, this type of commitment is instead obsession and compulsion (Wyatt, 1997). The association between commitment to exercise and obsessive-compulsive personality was reported only in men (Davis et al., 1993). Sachs (1981) warned that not all committed runners become addicted, and regular or daily running cannot be associated with addiction. Sachs and Pargman (1984) proposed a two-dimensional model to describe the relationship between exercise addiction and commitment to exercise/running. The former has a psychobiological base while the latter has a cognitive-rational base for running. The four quadrants emerging from the two-dimensional model are 1) low commitment and low dependence, 2) high commitment and low dependence, 3) high commitment and high dependence, and 4) high dependence and low commitment (see Figure 7.1). In

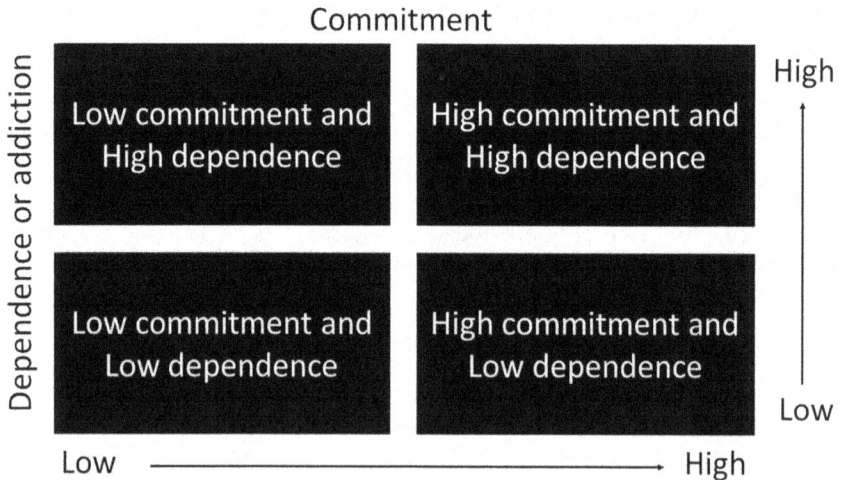

Figure 7.1 Model explaining the relationship between commitment to running and addiction to running. We draw the current figure upon the work of Sachs and Pargman (1984).

this model, commitment and addiction to running are considered separate but closely interrelated concepts.

A decade later, Conboy (1994) tested the model and found that highly committed and highly dependent runners were the least prone to withdrawal symptoms or deprivation feelings. In contrast, runners who reported a high level of dependence and low commitment were the most prone to experience withdrawal symptoms. However, Conboy's study has a problem; the author adopted an instrument to assess the *commitment* to running (i.e., the Commitment to Running Scale; Carmack & Martens, 1979) to measure obligatory running. Therefore, we suppose that addictive running was not measured in this work. In our recent longitudinal study of young university students adopting various new sports with a training frequency of once per week, commitment, as reflected by passion criteria,[2] and withdrawal symptoms did not correlate at the beginning of the study, or four and 12 weeks later, respectively (Kovacsik et al., 2020). However, the mere once-per-week exercise frequency and the beginner status in a newly adopted sport prevent these findings from extrapolating to the regular exercisers or experienced athletes.

Other early studies in the field project equivocal findings. Thaxton (1982) reported that commitment to running was not related to perceived addiction scores. In contrast, Summers et al. (1983) found that runners who perceived themselves as addicted to running also exhibited a high commitment to running. Supporting this finding, Chapman and De Castro (1990) showed a positive correlation between committed and obligatory running. However, the latter correlation was based on relatively small sample size (n = 47), and the scale used for assessing exercise addiction was developed and psychometrically evaluated on the same sample. Therefore, while the theoretical distinction between committed and obligatory or addicted running exists (e.g., Chapman & De Castro, 1990; Sachs, 1981), the relationship between the two needs further clarification.

Recent investigations appear to support the expected association between commitment and addiction to exercise. Kovacsik et al. (2020) examined 149 university students enrolled in a new sport over 12 weeks. Measurements obtained at baseline (before the start of the study), four weeks later, and at the end of the study showed that commitment, as reflected by passion criteria, and the risk of exercise addiction correlated positively in all instances accounting for 29.2%–37.2% of the shared variance between the two. In another recent large international study of 1,079 participants, de la Vega et al. (2020) found a statistically significant positive correlation between passion criteria, assumed to reflect commitment to exercise (Szabo, 2018) and the risk of exercise addiction, accounting for 24% of shared variance between the two variables. This relationship is logical and expectable because greater or deeper involvement in an activity is paralleled by greater commitment. However, seemingly in accord with the model in Figure 7.1, the *strength* of the association can be expected to vary. In other words, in people exhibiting no or low risk of exercise addiction, the correlation between exercise addiction and commitment would be weaker than in individuals at high risk of exercise addiction. In accord with Thaxton's (1982) results, an alternative line of thought is that addiction is fueled by dependence and compulsion rather than commitment. Consequently, among individuals at risk of addiction, the commitment would no longer be related to the risk of addiction. The model in Figure 7.1 can still be correct because it depicts the relationship between a component of addiction (dependence) rather than addiction *per se.*

   To further investigate the relationship between exercise addiction and commitment, we reanalyzed our recent cross-sectional data (Kovacsik et al., 2019) obtained from 360 regular exercisers (who reported a continuous exercise history of at least two years along with a minimum of three exercise workouts each week). First, we categorized the sample into three groups of exercise addiction according to Terry et al. (2004): 1) *asymptomatic* (n = 64), 2) *symptomatic* (n = 281), and 3) *at risk* (n = 15). Subsequently, we performed separate correlations between the risk of exercise addiction and commitment levels, again based on passion criteria. In accord with the alternative thought about the link between addiction and commitment, the results of the correlations were statistically significant in the former two groups, but not in the 'at risk' for exercise addiction group. While these results may lend partial support for commitment to exercise not being a motivational source in exercise addiction, which is in accord with the obligatory nature of the behavior, they are only tentative because they are based on few observations. Indeed, only 15/360 of the sample could be classified as *at risk* of exercise addiction in the study of Kovacsik et al. (2019). Still, these results point in the direction that commitment to exercise and addiction are different constructs.

7.6 Commitment to sport

In contrast to the earlier discussion of commitment pertaining primarily to recreational exercisers, commitment in competitive athletes is different. The Sport Commitment Model (SCM; Scanlan et al., 2016) explains athletes' persistence and dedication in sport. Scanlan et al. (2016) defined sport commitment as a time-enduring and constantly persistent (motivational?) *psychological state.* The duality, like in passion, emerges in the SCM too. The developers define *enthusiastic* commitment as 'the psychological construct representing the desire and resolve to persist in a sport over time' (p. 235). In contrast, the other pillar of dedication and adherence to a sport is the *confined* commitment, which the authors conceptualize as 'the psychological construct representing perceptions of obligation to persist in a sport over time' (p. 235). Therefore athletes, and in our view recreational exercisers too, can persevere in their sport or exercise because they are internally motivated to do so (want to) or because they are under some internal or external pressure (need to or must).

Scanlan et al. point out that people can be both enthusiastic and confined in an overall commitment, and the levels of these forms of commitment may change over time. Enthusiastic and constrained commitment are examples of functional and obligatory types of involvements. Scholars may think of these two forms as healthy and as unhealthy or pressured commitment. We use the word *pressured* because obligatory (confined) commitment is not necessarily unhealthy or dysfunctional. For example, an individual *must* prepare for a major competition, but at the same time, the feeling of 'I want to' usually also prevails. In fact, in such situations, an individual may score high on both forms of commitments, while later in a training situation, a fall in confined commitment could be observed.

In recreational exercise, an example would be when a person commits to a partner to exercise together. In this case, the person presumably *wants to* exercise but is also pressured (*must*) to do so because of the commitment (e.g., 'I can't let my partner down') to the other. Alternately, recreational running participation in street races or various non-processional competitions could temporarily heighten both forms of commitment. However, in the context of the risk of exercise addiction, it can be anticipated that a closer relationship would exist between confided commitment and exercise addiction as opposed to the link between enthusiastic commitment and addiction. This association is analogous to the relationship between obsessive passion and the risk of exercise addiction (Kovacsik et al., 2019).

The SCM has seven constituents (Figure 7.2). The first, *sport enjoyment*, refers to the enjoyable, satisfactory, and positive affective experiences stemming from the performance of the sports activity. The second, *valuable opportunities*, incorporates those special privileges and gains that can be accessed only via continuous sport participation. The third constituent, *other priorities*, refers to those obligations and appealing alternatives which could interfere with continued sport participation. The fourth component, *personal investments*, is further categorized into two subcategories: 1) loss of personal resources invested in the sport that are irrecoverable upon the termination of the athletic career and 2) quantity of the available personal resources invested in the sport. The fifth constituent, *social constraints*, involves social norms, expectations, and related pressures that create a feeling of obligation to perform (short term) or to remain (long term) in a sport. The sixth component, *social support*, is classified into three subcategories: 1) social support-mirroring the emotional support manifested in attention, encouragement, and empathy provided by significant others; 2) social support-informational (instructional) refers to the provision of helpful information, such as mentoring, guidance, or advice provided by significant others; and 3) social support-instrumental that involves the provision of material resources or instrumental assistance by significant others. Finally, the seventh and last constituent, the *desire to excel*, has two subcategories: 1) mastery achievement, implying the wish or striving to grow and achieve mastery; and 2) sport-competition (social) achievement reflecting in the inner need and striving to win and demonstrate superiority over opponents in sport. On the basis of these components, the authors developed the 58-item Sport Commitment Questionnaire-2 (Scanlan et al., 2016). A strength of this tool is that 11 items gauge specifically enthusiastic (6) and confined (5) commitment, making it helpful in studying their association with internal-external motivation, harmonious-obsessive passion, and high-low risk of exercise addiction.

We believe that personal factors, including unique constraints, task-ego orientation, personality traits (i.e., perfectionism, narcissism, and extraversion), and psychological needs (i.e., self, esteem/concept, anxiety/stress-coping) could also affect one's commitment. So, we added *personal factors* as a hypothetical additional component to SCM in Figure 7.2. We also propose interactions between the various components that eventually affect the form and level of commitment. For example, *personal factors* directly affect commitment, sport enjoyment, and personal investment while mutually affecting each other with a desire to excel, social support, and valuable opportunities. The *desire to excel* influences commitment and the consideration of other priorities, and it is in a mutually influencing relationship with personal factors. *Social support* directly affects commitment and the desire

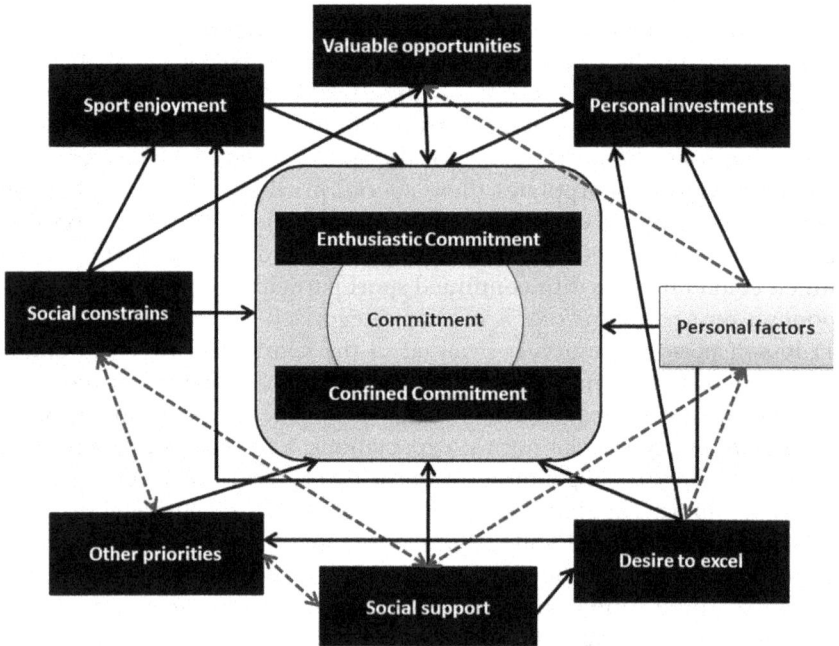

Figure 7.2 The Sport Commitment Model (Scanlan et al., 2016), as perceived by the current authors. The illustrated model here is different from that presented by the developers by having an additional component (personal factors) and showing the possible interactions between the components in the model.

to excel, and it is in a mutually influencing association with other priorities, social constraints, and personal factors. *Other priorities* affect commitment, and it is in a mutually impacting relationship with social support and social constraints. Social constraints directly impact commitment, sport enjoyment, and valuable opportunities while being in a mutually influencing relationship with other priorities and social support. *Sport enjoyment* has a direct effect on personal investment and commitment. *Valuable opportunities* directly affect commitment and are in a mutual association with personal factors. Last, *personal investment* is a determinant of commitment.

Research on the commitment to exercise and exercise addiction yields a relatively clear picture of the relationship. The two concepts are very different. One is healthy, the other is dysfunctional (Szabo, 2010). Furthermore, based on the closer examination of the manifestation of committed exercise/sport behavior (Scanlan et al., 2016), it is likely that the reported relationship between commitment and the risk of exercise addiction is attributable not to an overall (general) level of commitment but a specific commitment, like confined commitment. Future research should establish the relationship between the forms of commitment, interactions between its determinants, relationships to forms of passion, and the risk of exercise addiction. Motivational incentives should also be scrutinized in this type of research (Kovacsik et al., 2020).

7.7 Key points

1. Commitment to sport/exercise is different from addiction.
2. Motivational incentives also differentiate addiction from commitment.
3. The relationship between addiction and commitment is two-dimensional.
4. Commitment to sport is not the primary driving force in exercise addiction.
5. The SCM also needs to consider personality factors.

Notes

1. Cycling may be more popular around the world, but for many people cycling represents a means of commuting rather than exercise.
2. Passion criteria implies the rating of four criteria items on the Passion Scale assumedly (Szabo, 2018) also reflecting a high level of commitment [1] I spend a lot of time doing my activity; 2) I love my activity; 3) my activity is important for me; and 4) my activity is a passion for me; Carbonneau et al., 2008].

7.8 References

Ackard, D. M., Brehm, B. J., & Steffen, J. J. (2002). Exercise and eating disorders in college-aged women: Profiling excessive exercisers. *Eating Disorders: The Journal of Treatment & Prevention, 10*(1), 31–47. doi:10.1080/106402602753573540

Baker, T. B., Piper, M. E., McCarthy, D. E., Majeskie, M. R., & Fiore, M. C. (2004). Addiction motivation reformulated: An affective processing model of negative rein-forcement. *Psychological Review, 111*(1), 33–51. doi:10.1037/0033-295X.111.1.33

Bircher, J., Griffiths, M. D., Kasos, K., Demetrovics, Z., & Szabo, A. (2017). Exer-cise addiction and personality: A two-decade systematic review of the empirical literature (1995–2015). *Baltic Journal of Sport and Health Sciences, 3*(106), 19–33. doi:10.33607/bjshs.v3i106.30

Bozarth, M. A. (1994). Physical dependence produced by central morphine infu-sions: An anatomical mapping study. *Neuroscience & Biobehavioral Reviews, 18*(3), 373–383. doi:10.1016/0149-7634(94)90050-7

Brehm, J. W., & Self, E. A. (1989). The intensity of motivation. *Annual Review of Psy-chology, 40*(1), 109–131. doi:10.1146/annurev.ps.40.020189.000545

Carbonneau, N., Vallerand, R. J., Fernet, C., & Guay, F. (2008). The role of passion for teaching in intrapersonal and interpersonal outcomes. *Journal of Educational Psychology, 100*(4), 977–987. doi:10.1037/a0012545

Carmack, M. A., & Martens, R. (1979). Measuring commitment to running: A sur-vey of runners' attitudes and mental states. *Journal of Sport Psychology, 1*, 25–42. doi:10.1123/jsp.1.1.25

Chapman, C. L., & De Castro, J. M. (1990). Running addiction: Measurement and associated psychological characteristics. *The Journal of Sports Medicine and Physical Fitness, 30*(3), 283–290

Conboy, J. K. (1994). The effects of exercise withdrawal on mood states of runners. *Journal of Sport Behaviour, 17*(3), 188–203.

Davis, C., Brewer, H., & Ratusny, D. (1993). Behavioral frequency and psychological commitment: Necessary concepts in the study of excessive exercising. *Journal of Behavioral Medicine, 16*, 611–628. doi:10.1007/BF00844722

De Coverley Veale, D. M. W. (1987). Exercise dependence. *British Journal of Addic-tion, 82*(7), 735–740. doi:10.1111/j.1360-0443.1987.tb01539.x

de la Vega, R., Almendros, L. J., Barquín, R. R., Boros, S., Demetrovics, Z., & Szabo, A. (2020). Exercise addiction during the COVID-19 pandemic: An inter-national study confirming the need for considering passion and perfectionism. *International Journal of Mental Health and Addiction.* (Online first). doi:10.1007/s11469-020-00433-7

Duncan, D. F. (1974). Drug abuse as a coping mechanism. *American Journal of Psy-chiatry, 131*(6), 724–724. doi:10.1176/ajp.131.6.724

Egorov, A. Y., & Szabo, A. (2013). The exercise paradox: An interactional model for a clearer conceptualization of exercise addiction. *Journal of Behavioral Addictions, 2*(4), 199–208. doi:10.1556/jba.2.2013.4.2

Fitbit Co. (2021). *Fitbit health & activity index™*. Retrieved from: www.fitbit.com/global/us/activity-index

Gaspar, Z., & Szabo, A. (2019). Burnout in football coaching. In E. Konter, J. Beck-mann, & T. M. Loughead (Eds.), *Football psychology: From theory to practice* (pp. 150–162). New York, NY: Routledge. doi:10.4324/9781315268248-13

Glasser, W. (1976). *Positive addiction.* New York, NY: Harper & Row.

Johnson, R. (1995). Exercise dependence: When runners don't know when to quit. *Sports Medicine and Arthroscopy Review, 3*(4), 267–273.

Kovacsik, R., Griffiths, M. D., Pontes, H. M., Soós, I., de la Vega, R., Ruíz-Barquín, R., . . . Szabo, A. (2019). The role of passion in exercise addiction, exercise volume, and exercise intensity in long-term exercisers. *International Journal of Mental Health and Addiction, 17*(6), 1389–1400. doi:10.1007/s11469-018-9880-1

Kovacsik, R., Tóth-Király, I., Egorov, A., & Szabo, A. (2020). A longitudinal study of exercise addiction and passion in new sport activities: The impact of motivational factors. *International Journal of Mental Health and Addiction.* (Online first). doi:10.1007/s11469-020-00241-z

Levit, M., Weinstein, A., Weinstein, Y., Tzur-Bitan, D., & Weinstein, A. (2018). A study on the relationship between exercise addiction, abnormal eating attitudes, anxiety and depression among athletes in Israel. *Journal of Behavioral Addictions, 7*(3), 800–805. doi:10.1556/2006.7.2018.83

Locke, E. A., & Schattke, K. (2019). Intrinsic and extrinsic motivation: Time for expansion and clarification. *Motivation Science, 5*(4), 277–290. doi:10.1037/mot0000116

Morgan, W. P. (1979). Anxiety reduction following acute physical activity. *Psychiatric Annals, 9*, 141–147. doi:10.3928/0048-5713-19790301-06

Pierce, E. F. (1994). Exercise dependence syndrome in runners. *Sports Medicine, 18*(3), 149–155. doi:10.2165/00007256-199418030-00001

Sachs, M. L. (1981). Running addiction. In M. Sacks & M. Sachs (Eds.), *Psychology of running* (pp. 116–126). Champaign, IL: Human Kinetics.

Sachs, M. L., & Pargman, D. (1984). Running addiction. In M. L. Sachs & G. W. Buffone (Eds.), *Running as therapy: An integrated approach* (pp. 231–252). Lincoln, NE: University of Nebraska Press.

Scanlan, T. K., Chow, G. M., Sousa, C., Scanlan, L. A., & Knifsend, C. A. (2016). The development of the Sport Commitment Questionnaire-2 (English version). *Psychology of Sport and Exercise, 22*, 233–246. doi:10.1016/j.psychsport.2015.08.002

Summers, J. J., & Hinton, E. R. (1986). Development of scales to measure participation in running. In L. E. Unestahl (Ed.), *Contemporary Sport Psychology* (pp. 73–84). Orebro, Sweden: Veje Publishing.

Summers, J. J., Machin, V. J., & Sargent, G. I. (1983). Psychosocial factors related to marathon running. *Journal of Sport Psychology, 5*(3), 314–331. doi:10.1123/jsp.5.3.314

Szabo, A. (2010). *Addiction to exercise: A symptom or a disorder?* New York, NY: Nova Science Publishers.

Szabo, A. (2018). Addiction, passion, or confusion? New theoretical insights on exercise addiction research from the case study of a female body builder. *Europe's Journal of Psychology, 14*(2), 296–316. doi:10.5964/ejop.v14i2.1545

Terry, A., Szabo, A., & Griffiths, M. (2004). The Exercise Addiction Inventory: A new brief screening tool. *Addiction Research & Theory, 12*(5), 489–499. doi:10.1080/16066350310001637363

Thaxton, L. (1982). Physiological and psychological effects of short term exercise addiction on habitual runners. *Journal of Sport Psychology, 4*(1), 73–80. doi:10.1123/jsp.4.1.73

Trott, M., Jackson, S. E., Firth, J., Jacob, L., Grabovac, I., Mistry, A., . . . Smith, L. (2020). A comparative meta-analysis of the prevalence of exercise addiction in adults with and without indicated eating disorders. *Eating and Weight Disorders – Studies on Anorexia, Bulimia and Obesity, 26*(1), 37–46. doi:10.1007/s40519-019-00842-1

Weinstein, A., & Weinstein, Y. (2014). Exercise addiction- diagnosis, bio-psychological mechanisms and treatment issues. *Current Pharmaceutical Design, 20*(25), 4062–4069. doi:10.2174/13816128113199990614

Wyatt, L. M. (1997). *Obsessive-compulsiveness and disordered eating in obligatory and non-obligatory exercisers (Unpublished doctoral dissertation).* California School of Professional Psychology, Los Angeles, California. Retrieved from: https://www.proquest.com/docview/304376256?pq-origsite=gscholar&fromopenview=true

8 Psychological manifestations of exercise deprivation

8.1 Difference between deprivation feelings and withdrawal symptoms

It is essential to distinguish between instances of missing something or painfully craving for something. For example, some athletes who had to retire because of aging, injury, or other reasons might miss their sport and occasionally experience feelings of deprivation. Likewise, if one plans to exercise one afternoon but that plan is crossed over by a relative's visit or a work commitment, the person may experience deprivation feelings. Those who could not go to the gym, swimming pool, play tennis, football, or any other adopted exercise during the COVID-19 pandemic most likely have experienced uncomfortable feelings of *deprivation*. These feelings are perhaps best described as a set of emotions encompassing longing for something that is part of the person's life, sorry for the self, possibly guilt, helplessness, disappointment, and a sort of emptiness or void in life. Simply stated, 'something is missing.'

Withdrawal symptoms are more intense than deprivation sensations, despite being often used as synonyms to those. The difference is that when one is experiencing withdrawal symptoms, the uncomfortable feelings emerge at both psychological and physiological levels and can be painful. In contrast, deprivation feelings are primarily experienced psychologically, but they are still disappointing, uncomfortable, and uncontrollable experiences. Early studies pinpoint that the withdrawal symptoms, although very marking, are merely one of the several symptoms of exercise addiction (Brown, 1993; Griffiths, 1997). Still, preliminary investigations of exercise addiction relied on the presence or experience rather than the type, frequency, and intensity of withdrawal symptoms (Szabo, 1995; Szabo et al., 1997).

Most regular exercisers report some negative psychological symptoms when they cannot exercise for any reason (Szabo et al., 1996; Szabo et al., 1997). Indeed, 25 years ago, Szabo and his colleagues (1996) conducted a study online and found that even people involved in physically less demanding types of exercise, like bowling, reported deprivation symptoms when

DOI: 10.4324/9781003173595-8

their habitual activity could not be performed for some reason. Yet, the intensity or severity of the symptoms reported by bowlers was less than that of aerobic dancers, weight trainers, cross-trainers, and fencers (Szabo et al., 1996). However, even the latter may have only experienced deprivation rather than withdrawal symptoms despite the higher rating manifested by these participants. Although Szabo (2010) raised this important point, some scholars, even these days (e.g., Quraishi & Chahal, 2021; Weinstein et al., 2017), do not elaborate on the difference between feeling deprived of something (exercise) and experiencing withdrawal symptoms, which, in our opinion, are relatively different in terms of the intensity or severity of the experience, despite related psychosomatic manifestations as illustrated in Figure 8.1. In brief, deprivation feelings are acute (momentary) negative psychological states that may manifest in minor or moderate psychophysiological changes and dissipate relatively quickly. On the contrary, withdrawal symptoms are very severe and hard-hitting manifestations of an unfulfilled need or urge, resulting in recurring or lasting debilitative physical symptoms and psychological hardship. It should be noted that some withdrawal symptoms can be short-lived and intense. Therefore, the two represent the opposite ends of a spectrum ranging from minor discomfort to severe morbidity.

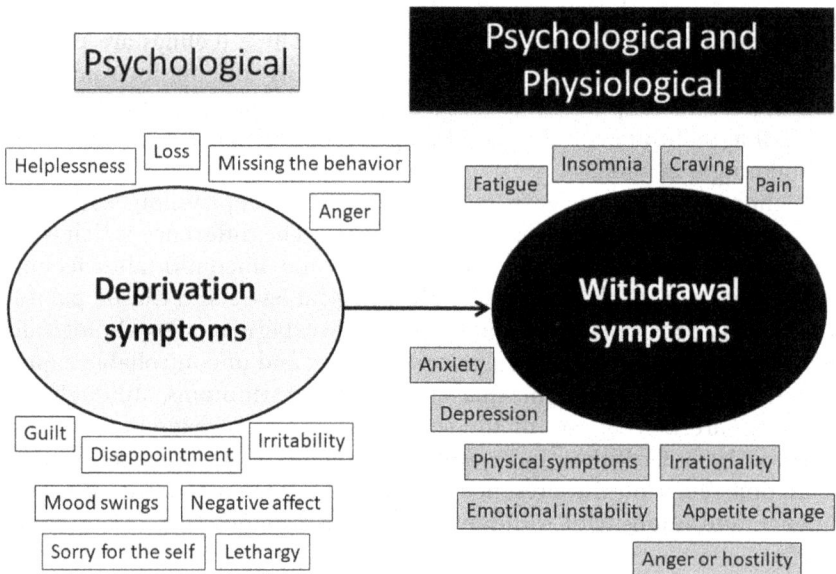

Figure 8.1 The differences between feelings of deprivation and withdrawal symptoms are illustrated on a continuum ranging from relatively light to severe. Please note that there may be conceptual and semantic overlap between listed factors, but still their 'intensity' is greater in withdrawal symptoms than in deprivation feelings.

This clarification is necessary to appreciate that the mere perception of deprivation cannot be linked to exercise addiction. However, the *intensity* of these symptoms is a distinguishing factor in separating healthy committed from morbidity-evidencing addicted exercisers. In their early conceptualization of exercise addiction, Cockerill and Riddington (1996) did not mention deprivation feelings or withdrawal symptoms on the list of symptoms associated with the disorder. In fact, in many forms of sports and physical activity, deprivation feelings may simply suggest that exercise exerts a positive effect on its practitioner. This repeatedly experienced positive effect is missed to various extents when an interruption in the regular activity is necessary for an unplanned or unwanted reason.

8.2 Psychophysiological responses to exercise deprivation

For a while, it has been known that the interruption of habitual physical activity results in negative feelings reflected by changes in mood and affect (Chan & Grossman, 1988; Gauvin & Szabo, 1992; Wingate, 1993). The term 'affect' refers to the subjective psychological feeling state resulting from the *impact of a situation*. Russell (2003) views affect as: 'A neurophysiological state that is consciously accessible as a simple, nonreflective feeling that is an integral blend of hedonic (pleasure – displeasure) and arousal (sleepy – activated) values' (p. 147). It is like a stream of dynamic change in one's neuropsychophysiological state in response to the ongoing events (Duncan & Barrett, 2007). For example, when uncontrollable factors prevent the fulfillment of one or more planned training or exercise sessions, the emerging affective states reflect the feelings of deprivation (Robbins & Joseph, 1985).

In examining deprivation from physical activity, it is essential to understand whether the *physiological* or *psychological outcome* (associated with self-gratification, social interaction, or other forms of reward) is the source of the deprivation feelings (Szabo, 1995). Placebo and nocebo effects, via conditioned behaviors, could also lead to a sense of void or deprivation (Szabo, 2013). For example, runners report deprivation sensations when they cannot run. But practitioners of a physically less demanding sport like bowling also experience negative feelings when they cannot attend their regular bowling session (Szabo et al., 1996).

The physiological adaptations to bowling cannot be compared to running. Hence, the perceived deprivation feelings in the former may be of psychological rather than physiological origin, most likely generated by nocebo effects. These effects are directionally opposite to placebo effects (Horváth et al., 2021) and result from negative beliefs and expectations connected to the missing of the conditioned (i.e., habitual) behavior. For example, an individual whose daily exercise is part of a weight management plan may lose control over something perceived as very important in life when deprived of exercise. Then, thoughts and expectations associated with the loss trigger a nocebo effect manifested in negative mood and affect. In Table 8.1, presenting a summary of the intervention studies examining exercise deprivation, it is evident that apart from one work (Szabo & Gauvin, 1992), which only studied heart rate and psychosocial stress reactivity as related to exercise deprivation, all other studies have disclosed a negative psychological effect attributable to exercise deprivation.

The physiological changes linked to exercise deprivation are less commonly reported, as shown in Table 8.1, because focused research on such measures is still rare (Krivoschekov, & Lushnikov, 2017). The few relevant results are controversial. After one week of exercise deprivation, Szabo and Gauvin (1992) could not disclose debilitative effects on heart rate and psychosocial stress reactivity. In contrast, Aidman and Woollard (2003) reported increased mood disturbance and resting heart rate after 24 hours of deprivation in club-level runners. Such differences could stem from the type of participants examined in the two studies. While Szabo and Gauvin (1992) examined university students committed to various exercises, Aidman and Woollard (2003) studied club-level runners. Testing adults from multiple exercise activities, Kop et al. (2008) found increased negative psychological states in response to a 2-week exercise deprivation period but no significant changes in various inflammatory markers.

Apart from increased mood disturbance, Poole et al. (2011) also found decreased interleukin 6 (IL-6) after two weeks of exercise deprivation in regular exercisers. However, the IL-6 levels were significantly related to mood changes, and, consequently, the authors concluded that the decreased IL-6 was due to the increased negative mood. (This finding may be puzzling because, in general, decreased IL-6 is associated with psychological improvement.) In a more recent study, aimed at assessing the physiological changes associated with one week of exercise deprivation in 50 football players, differences were observed in those who exhibited a high risk of exercise addiction (Krivoschekov, & Lushnikov, 2017). Twelve participants in this group had lower brain electric activity (i.e., lower α-rhythm amplitude and power) and exhibited higher muscular tension, sympathetic activity, anxiety, and depression in contrast to the other players. These authors' findings suggest, in accord with our conjecture (Figure 8.1), that the group affected by exercise addiction might have experienced *withdrawal symptoms* beyond and above the deprivation sensations (feeling states) reported by the control group. Therefore, the impact of exercise deprivation on the proposed continuum, ranging from mild psychological deprivation feelings to psychophysiological withdrawal symptoms, appears to be determined by the level of involvement in the activity.

8.3 Exercise deprivation in the highly committed exercisers

Indeed, training deprivation may be more irritating in individuals who are highly committed to their adopted physical activity. In an early investigation,

Chapman and De Castro (1990) reported a positive relationship between the *intensity* of the deprivation feelings and the level of commitment in male runners. In other words, a higher commitment was related to more frequent and stronger deprivation sensations. This early study is important because it is pioneering research demonstrating a *positive relationship* between the *magnitude* of the negative feelings experienced during exercise deprivation and the level of involvement in exercise behavior. Although this association infers no causal relationship, it supports the notion that the *intensity of the symptoms* on the deprivation-withdrawal spectrum is likely determined by the level of commitment to the sport or exercise activity.

8.4 Reason for exercise

Limited information concerning the role of exercise motives in the occurrence and severity of exercise deprivation feelings stems from early cross-sectional work with runners (Robbins & Joseph, 1985). In this study, participants who ran for health reasons (therapeutic runners, as referred to by the authors) reported more intense deprivation sensations for the periods when they were unable to run than runners who ran for a mastery reason, characterized by development and performance goals. Robbins and Joseph (1985) introduced the notions of *therapeutic running* and *mastery running* to describe two principal incentive categories behind one's personal goals in the running. The former is linked to health-related reasons, while the latter includes mainly other reasons, such as a challenge or self-fulfillment.

It is unknown whether health, as a reason for physical activity, is related to the intensity or severity of deprivation sensations. However, a recent study (de la Vega et al., 2020) showed that the proportion of people (79.3%) at the high risk of exercise addiction were exercising for health or therapeutic reasons. Accordingly, it can be expected that deprivation feelings, possibly culminating in withdrawal symptoms, would be more significant in this population because when they lose exercise, they also lose control over the management of their health concern. Indeed Fernandez et al. (2020) in a review of the effects of abstinence across various behavioral addictions found that across all behaviors, exercise was related to the clearest pattern of withdrawal-related symptoms, mainly mood disturbances.

8.5 Control over adherence to exercise deprivation

Until the last decade before the new millennium, there was little or no control over exercise deprivation intervention. Morris et al. (1990) and later Gauvin and Szabo (1992) tried to overcome this problem by contacting the participants regularly and stressing the need for adherence to the treatment. While in these studies, the participants were asked to stop exercising, they were told that it was *voluntary*. So, if they feel that they must exercise,

Table 8.1 Summary of the close to half-a-decade intervention research on exercise deprivation in chronological order.

Intervention studies on the effects of exercise deprivation

Year/Author(s)	Aim	Participants	Length of exercise deprivation	Effects of exercise deprivation
1970 – Baekeland	To study the effect of exercise deprivation on sleep	14 healthy college students who trained at least 3 days/week	One month	Increased mood disturbance, less appetite, worse sleep, sexual tension, and an increased need to be with others
1982 – Thaxton	To examine mood responses to a brief exercise deprivation	33 male and female regular runners	One day (24-hours)	Increased mood disturbance
1982 – Tooman	To study the effects of exercise deprivation on muscle tension, mood, and anxiety	40 male and female regular runners	Two days	Increased mood disturbance, confusion, state anxiety, and tension
1986 – Bahrke et al.	To study the effects of exercise deprivation on mood	13 males who exercised regularly at least 3 times per week	Six weeks	Increase in mood disturbance and anxiety
1988 – Chan & Grossman	To examine the psychological effect of exercise withdrawal on runners	60 male and female regular runners	Four weeks	Increase in mood disturbance, lower self-esteem, and increase in depressive symptoms
1990 – Morris et al.	To study emotional effects of exercise deprivation	40 male regular runners	Two weeks	Decrease in general well-being, increase in depressive symptoms and anxiety

Intervention studies on the effects of exercise deprivation

Year/Author(s)	Aim	Participants	Length of exercise deprivation	Effects of exercise deprivation
1992 – Gauvin and Szabo	To study *in situ* the effects of exercise deprivation on well-being	21 male and female college students who exercised regularly	One week	Increased reporting of physical symptoms
1992 – Szabo and Gauvin	To study the effects of exercise deprivation on heart rate and psychosocial stress response	24 physically active males and females	One week	No effects on heart rate or stress reactivity
1994 – Conboy	To study the effects of exercise deprivation on mood on non-running days	61 male and female runners	Non-running days	Increased mood disturbance on no-running days
1996 – Mondin et al.	To study emotional effects of exercise deprivation	10 male and female habitual exercisers	Three days	Increased mood disturbance, anxiety, and depressive symptoms
1997 – Matthews	To assess responses to exercise deprivation in exercise addicts and nonaddicts	27 exercise addicts and 32 nonaddicts, both genders	Three days	Increased mood disturbance
1998 – Szabo et al.	To study the effects of running deprivation on mood and anxiety on non-running days	40 male and female regular runners	Non-running days	Increased state anxiety and exhaustion accompanied by decreased tranquility, positive engagement, and revitalization on non-running days

(*Continued*)

Table 8.1 (Continued)

Year/Author(s)	Aim	Participants	Length of exercise deprivation	Effects of exercise deprivation
Intervention studies on the effects of exercise deprivation				
2001 – Szabo and Parkin	To investigate the effects of training deprivation among brown and black belt karate practitioners	20 competing male and female martial artists	One week	Increased mood disturbance, negative affect, depression, anger, and tension, and slight decrease in vigor and positive affect
2003 – Aidman and Woollard	To test the effects of training deprivation on mood	60 male and female regular runners	One day	Increased mood disturbance and elevated heart rate
2004 – Glass et al.	To study the effects of exercise deprivation on somatic symptoms	18 male and female regular exercisers	One week	Increased fatigue, depressive symptoms, and anxiety
2006 – Berlin et al.	To test the effects of exercise deprivation on mood, fatigue, and depression	40 male and female regular exercisers	Two weeks	Increased mood disturbance, depressive symptoms, and fatigue
2008 – Hausenblas et al.	To investigate the effects of exercise deprivation on affect	40 male and female regular exercisers	Three days	Increased mood disturbance while deprivation and rest days produced similar symptoms
2008 – Kop et al.	To study the effects of exercise deprivation on inflammatory markers mood, and fatigue	40 male and female regular exercisers	Two weeks	Increased negative mood while various inflammatory markers did not increase

Intervention studies on the effects of exercise deprivation

Year/Author(s)	Aim	Participants	Length of exercise deprivation	Effects of exercise deprivation
2008 – Niven et al.	To test the effects of exercise abstinence on affect and body dissatisfaction	58 women regular exercisers	Three days	Increased tension and body dissatisfaction accompanied by decreased energetic arousal and hedonic tone
2011 – Poole et al.	To test the effects of exercise deprivation on mood and well-being	26 male and female regular exercisers	Two weeks	Increased negative mood and mood disturbance accompanied by decreased general well-being; IL-6 decreased
2009 – Zeller et al.	To investigate the impact of exercise deprivation on life quality	26 male and female athletes	One week	Decreased vitality, emotional, and physical functioning
2013 – Ablin et al.	To test the effects of sleep and exercise deprivation on pain, fatigue mood, somatic symptoms, and cognition	87 male and female regular runners	Ten days	Increased fatigue in response to the exercise deprivation
2016 – Antunes et al.	To study the effects of exercise deprivation in the context of exercise addiction	18 male regular runners	Two weeks	Increased depression, fatigue, confusion, anger, and less vigor among the group of runners exhibiting exercise addiction symptoms

(*Continued*)

Table 8.1 (Continued)

Intervention studies on the effects of exercise deprivation

Year/Author(s)	Aim	Participants	Length of exercise deprivation	Effects of exercise deprivation
2017 – Krivoschekov and Lushnikov	To identify various psychophysio-logical during exercise deprivation in the context of exercise addiction	50 male football players	One week	Decreased brain electric activity, increased muscular tension, sympathetic activity, anxiety, and depression in participants exhibiting exercise addiction symptoms

Note: IL-6, interleukin 6.

they may do so without negative consequences, but no significant dropout was reported. Additionally, Gauvin and Szabo (1992) also implemented an indirect 'psychological control' by estimating participants' aerobic fitness (VO$_2$ max) before and immediately after exercise deprivation. This test was performed to lead participants to believe that noncompliance would surface via some changes in their level of physical fitness.

Nowadays, more accurate control can be exerted over the activity levels during an experimental deprivation period by using, for example, easily accessible and relatively inexpensive accelerometers (Antunes et al., 2016; Berlin et al., 2006; Poole et al., 2011) or similar activity monitors (Ablin et al., 2013). These tools are helpful in experimental work. They might have contributed to an increase in controlled studies in the area. Indeed, since 2000, numerous experimental investigations have been performed in this field (Table 8.1).

8.6 The participants in exercise deprivation research

Participants in exercise deprivation research are aware of the beneficial effects of exercise. Consequently, they may associate periods of exercise deprivation with negative subjective states. These beliefs, not independent of expectations, can be conveyed through their responses to the collected data. In experimental studies, it is almost impossible to blind participants from the research hypothesis. However, the extent to which the knowledge of the hypothesis may influence the results in this field is unclear. Possible answers could be gathering qualitative data, through in-depth interviews, after the conclusion of the study. Another possible method of dealing with this issue is to present the deprivation period positively, such as rest, revitalization, or energy conservation for an upcoming major event or competition and, consequently, trying to create positive expectations.

This approach can induce a *placebo* rather than nocebo effect, which might buffer the negative effects of exercise deprivation. One study employed this method (Szabo & Parkin, 2001) and found a significant increase in mood disturbance after one week of training deprivation in martial artists. Therefore, the extreme to which the 'positive perspective' delivery of an exercise deprivation intervention is helpful in this type of investigation is still unclear. Even though the participants in Szabo and Parkin's study were presented with a rest period in the positive sense, how they perceived the actual intervention was not determined in the course of the work. An *imposed* rest period before competition may not be perceived as positive even though its delivery is presented in a positive way.

8.7 Methodological issues in exercise deprivation research

Single or isolated time-delimited assessment of feeling states and other measures in exercise deprivation research may be largely affected by the situation (Szabo & Ábel, 2021). This method was used in most intervention studies in this field. However, at least two studies (Gauvin & Szabo, 1992; Hausenblas et al., 2008) used the ecological momentary assessment (EMA; Hausenblas et al., 2008), also known as the experience sampling method (ESM; Gauvin & Szabo, 1992), which collects data at random times on several occasions during the days of the study. These protocols have the advantage of providing a 'moving picture' instead of a single snapshot about participants feeling states and may reduce the situational impact on assessment.

Not comparable to EMA/ESM, but still better than single-point measurements, Szabo and Parkin (2001) adopted daily assessments of mood during every evening prior to bedtime throughout the experiment. However, results obtained by their method may also reflect only momentary (i.e., experienced in the evening) subjective states as opposed to general, or typical, states experienced across the days of the deprivation and baseline periods. Indeed, an overall 'good day' may be spoiled by a negative event before bedtime – preceding the time of completion of the questionnaires – and bias the participants' responses. The EMA/ESM may overcome this concern.

The wider application of multiple *in situ* sampling in this area of research could yield more reliable data. Three forms of data collection methods, 1) pre- to post-deprivation, 2) single daily appraisals of psychological states in the evening, and 3) experience sampling several times a day, may yield answers to three different questions: 1) How one felt at the moment before and after deprivation? 2) How participants appraise their days in the deprivation and exercise periods?, and 3) What sort of psychological states are projected by the aggregate measures that were taken at random times in the daily life of the individual? It may be apparent that comparability of findings from studies using different data collection methods is difficult, if not impossible. Figure 8.2 illustrates these protocols. The two-point assessment misses all events during the exercise deprivation period. The daily assessment could compare the *overall* appraisal of control and intervention days. The EMA/ESM yields several measures during both control and intervention days and provides to most reliable data on the effects of the intervention.

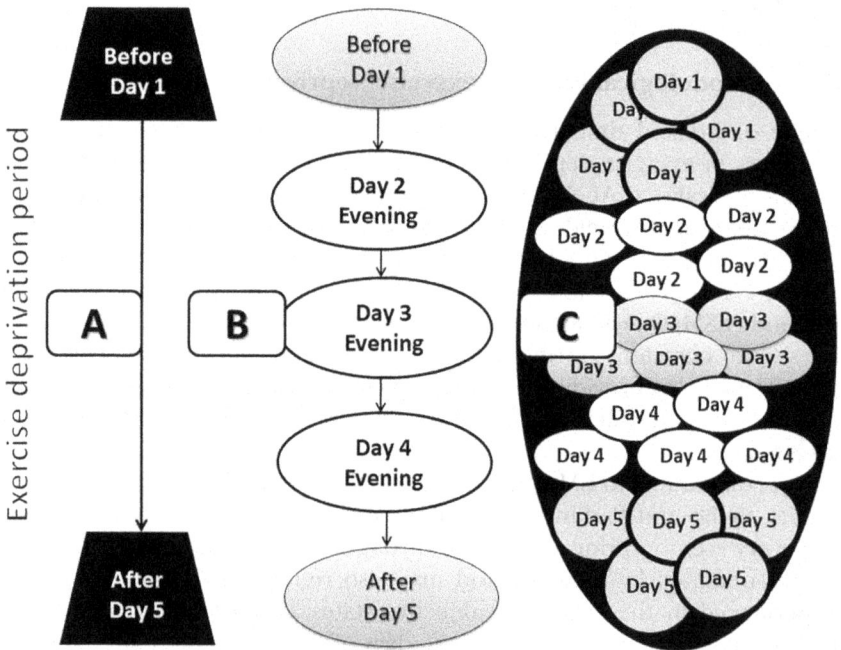

Figure 8.2 Illustration of 5-day intervention studies on exercise deprivation with two pre- (baseline) and postintervention measures (A), with five daily assessments before bedtime (B), and with ecological momentary assessment (EMA), or experience sampling method (C) using five random assessments over a 5-day experimental period.

8.8 Deprivation in committed versus addicted exercisers

Commitment is a healthy attitude toward an activity or ideology, while addiction is a dysfunctional behavior. The underlying causes or triggers of the discomforts experienced by committed and addicted exercisers, as a consequence of exercise deprivation, are different among these individuals. The former may experience various discomforts for reasons of 1) *social deprivation*, if their exercise is in a social context, 2) *inability to give time to the self*, in case of exercisers who engage in an exercise activity for the sake of self-care, contemplation, or reflection, 3) *inability to cope with stress*, in case of exercisers who adopt an activity for coping with the daily hassles and challenges, 4) *inability to control health issues*, in case of exercisers who participate in activities for a health-related reason, and 5) *unwanted change* in the usual lifestyle routine.

While it may be argued that exercise addicts may experience withdrawal symptoms for comparable reasons to committed exercisers, there is a fine line between the two that should be observed. The former will continue exercising even when contraindicated, while the latter will not do so. People addicted to exercise will jeopardize family and work relationships to meet the need of exercising, but healthy exercisers will not do so (Morgan, 1979). Because they cannot live without exercise, like smokers or workaholics, *exercise addicts will not participate in exercise deprivation research* simply because they cannot stop exercising (Baekeland, 1970). In contrast, committed exercisers may be interested in these types of studies either for intellectual curiosity or to better understand the meaning of their exercise to them.

8.9 Key points

1. Deprivation and withdrawal symptoms differ in their impact severity.
2. A sense of deprivation in response to missed training is experienced by all committed athletes and exercisers.
3. Individuals addicted to exercise experience severe withdrawal symptoms.
4. Experimentally induced exercise deprivation is difficult to implement.
5. EMA is the best method for studying the impact of exercise deprivation.

8.10 References

Ablin, J. N., Clauw, D. J., Lyden, A. K., Ambrose, K., Williams, D. A., Gracely, R. H., & Glass, J. M. (2013). Effects of sleep restriction and exercise deprivation on somatic symptoms and mood in healthy adults. *Clinical and Experimental Rheumatology, 31*(6 Suppl 79), S53–S59.

Aidman, E. V., & Woollard, S. (2003). The influence of self-reported exercise addiction on acute emotional and physiological responses to brief exercise deprivation. *Psychology of Sport and Exercise, 4*(3), 225–236. Doi:10.1016/s1469-0292(02)00003-1

Antunes, H. K. M., Leite, G. S. F., Lee, K. S., Barreto, A. T., Santos, R. V. T. dos, Souza, H. de S., . . . de Mello, M. T. (2016). Exercise deprivation increases negative mood in exercise-addicted subjects and modifies their biochemical markers. *Physiology & Behavior, 156*, 182–190. Doi:10.1016/j.physbeh.2016.01.028

Baekeland, F. (1970). Exercise deprivation. *Archives of General Psychiatry, 22*(4), 365. Doi:10.1001/archpsyc.1970.01740280077014

Bahrke, M. S., Thompson, C., & Thomas, T. (1986). Mood alterations following aerobic exercise withdrawal. *Indiana Alliance for Health, Physical Education, Recreation and Dance Journal, 15*(2), 8–10.

Berlin, A. A., Kop, W. J., & Deuster, P. A. (2006). Depressive mood symptoms and fatigue after exercise withdrawal: The potential role of decreased fitness. *Psychosomatic Medicine, 68*(2), 224–230. Doi:10.1097/01.psy.0000204628.73273.23

Brown, R. I. F. (1993). Some contributions of the study of gambling to the study of other addictions. In W. R. Eadington & J. A. Cornelius (Eds.), *Gambling behavior and problem gambling* (pp. 241–272). Reno: University of Nevada Press.

Chan, C. S., & Grossman, H. Y. (1988). Psychological effects of running loss on consistent runners. *Perceptual and Motor Skills, 66*(3), 875–883. Doi:10.2466/pms.1988.66.3.875

Chapman, C. L., & De Castro, J. M. (1990). Running addiction: Measurement and associated psychological characteristics. *The Journal of Sports Medicine and Physical Fitness, 30*(3), 283–290.

Cockerill, I. M., & Riddington, M. E. (1996). Exercise dependence and associated disorders: A review. Counselling Psychology Quarterly, 9(2), 119–129. doi:10.1080/09515079608256358

Conboy, J. K. (1994). The effects of exercise withdrawal on mood states in runners. *Journal of Sport Behavior, 17*(3), 188–204.

De la Vega, R., Almendros, L. J., Barquín, R. R., Boros, S., Demetrovics, Z., & Szabo, A. (2020). Exercise addiction during the COVID-19 pandemic: An international study confirming the need for considering passion and perfectionism. *International Journal of Mental Health and Addiction.* (Online first). Doi:10.1007/s11469-020-00433-7

Duncan, S., & Barrett, L. F. (2007). Affect is a form of cognition: A neurobiological analysis. *Cognition & Emotion, 21*(6), 1184–1211. Doi:10.1080/02699930701437931

Fernandez, D. P., Kuss, D. J., & Griffiths, M. D. (2020). Short-term abstinence effects across potential behavioral addictions: A systematic review. *Clinical Psychology Review, 76.* (Online first). 101828. Doi:10.1016/j.cpr.2020.101828

Gauvin, L., & Szabo, A. (1992). Application of the experience sampling method to the study of the effects of exercise withdrawal on well-being. *Journal of Sport Exercise Psychology, 14*(4), 361–374. Doi:10.1123/jsep.14.4.361

Glass, J. M., Lyden, A. K., Petzke, F., Stein, P., Whalen, G., Ambrose, K., . . . Clauw, D. J. (2004). The effect of brief exercise cessation on pain, fatigue, and mood symptom development in healthy, fit individuals. *Journal of Psychosomatic Research, 57*(4), 391–398. Doi:10.1016/s0022-3999(04)00080-7

Griffiths, M. D. (1997). Exercise addiction: A case study. *Addiction Research, 5*(2), 161–168. Doi:10.3109/16066359709005257

Hausenblas, H. A., Gauvin, L., Downs, D. S., & Duley, A. R. (2008). Effects of abstinence from habitual involvement in regular exercise on feeling states: An ecological momentary assessment study. *British Journal of Health Psychology, 13*(2), 237–255. Doi:10.1348/135910707x180378

Horváth, Á., Köteles, F., & Szabo, A. (2021). Nocebo effects on motor performance: A systematic literature review. *Scandinavian Journal of Psychology*. (Online first). Doi:10.1111/sjop.12753

Kop, W. J., Weinstein, A. A., Deuster, P. A., Whittaker, K. S., & Tracy, R. P. (2008). Inflammatory markers and negative mood symptoms following exercise withdrawal. *Brain, Behavior, and Immunity, 22*(8), 1190–1196. Doi:10.1016/j. bbi.2008.05.011

Krivoschekov, S. G., & Lushnikov, O. N. (2017). The functional state of athletes addicted to exercises during exercise deprivation. *Human Physiology, 43*(6), 678–685. Doi:10.1134/s0362119717040077

Matthews, J. K. (1997). *The impact of planned and unplanned lay-offs from training on withdrawal symptoms of exercise-addicted individuals.* Doctoral dissertation. The University of Tennessee, Knoxville, TN.

Mondin, G. W., Morgan, W. P., Piering, P. N., Stegner, A. J., Stotesbery, C. L., Trine, M. R., & Wu, M. Y. (1996). Psychological consequences of exercise deprivation in habitual exercisers. *Medicine & Science in Sports & Exercise. 28*(9), 1199–1203. Doi:10.1097/00005768-199609000-00018

Morgan, W. P. (1979). Anxiety reduction following acute physical activity. *Psychiatric Annals, 9*, 141–147.

Morris, M., Steinberg, H., Sykes, E. A., & Salmon, P. (1990). Effects of temporary withdrawal from regular running. *Journal of Psychosomatic Research, 34*(5), 493–500. Doi:10.1016/0022-3999(90)90023-w

Niven, A., Rendell, E., & Chisholm, L. (2008). Effects of 72-h of exercise abstinence on affect and body dissatisfaction in healthy female regular exercisers. *Journal of Sports Sciences, 26*(11), 1235–1242. Doi:10.1080/02640410802027378

Poole, L., Hamer, M., Wawrzyniak, A. J., & Steptoe, A. (2011). The effects of exercise withdrawal on mood and inflammatory cytokine responses in humans. *Stress, 14*(4), 439–447. Doi:10.3109/10253890.2011.557109

Quraishi, S., & Chahal, A. (2021). The role of sports physiotherapist in confronting exercise addiction. *Journal of Lifestyle Medicine, 11*(2), 47–51. Doi:10.15280/jlm.2021.11.2.47

Robbins, J. M., & Joseph, P. (1985). Experiencing exercise withdrawal: Possible consequences of therapeutic and mastery running. *Journal of Sport Psychology, 7*(1), 23–39. Doi:10.1123/jsp.7.1.2

Russell, J. A. (2003). Core affect and the psychological construction of emotion. *Psychological Review, 110*(1), 145–172. Doi:10.1037/0033-295X.110.1.145

Szabo, A. (1995). The impact of exercise deprivation on well-being of habitual exercisers. *The Australian Journal of Science and Medicine in Sport, 27*, 68–75.

Szabo, A. (2010). *Addiction to exercise: A symptom or a disorder?* New York, NY: Nova Science Publishers.

Szabo, A. (2013). Acute psychological benefits of exercise: Reconsideration of the placebo effect. *Journal of Mental Health, 22*(5), 449–455. Doi:10.3109/09638237.2012.734657

Szabo, A., & Ábel, K. (2021). General psychosocial measures are affected by the situation preceding assessment: The "arbitrary distinction" between state and trait measures is still unresolved. *Psychologija, 63*, 86–100. Doi:10.15388/psichol.2021.29

Szabo, A., Frenkl, R., & Caputo, A. (1996). Deprivation feelings, anxiety, and commitment in various forms of physical activity: A cross-sectional study on the Internet. *Psychologia: An International Journal of Psychology in the Orient, 39*(4), 223–230.

Szabo, A., Frenkl, R., & Caputo, A. (1997). Relationships between addiction to running, commitment to running and deprivation from running: A study on the internet. *European Yearbook of Sport Psychology, 1*, 130–147.

Szabo, A., Frenkl, R., Janek, G., Kálmán, L., & Lászay, D. (1998). Runners' anxiety and mood on running and non-running days: An in situ daily monitoring study. *Psychology, Health & Medicine, 3*(2), 193–199. Doi:10.1080/13548509808402235

Szabo, A., & Gauvin, L. (1992). Reactivity to written mental arithmetic: Effects of exercise lay-off and habituation. *Physiology & Behavior, 51*(3), 501–506. Doi:10.1016/0031-9384(92)90171-w

Szabo, A., & Parkin, A. M. (2001). The psychological impact of training deprivation in martial artists. *Psychology of Sport and Exercise, 2*(3), 187–199. Doi:10.1016/s1469-0292(01)00004-8

Thaxton, L. (1982). Physiological and psychological effects of short-term exercise addiction on habitual runners. *Journal of Sport Psychology, 4*(1), 73–80. Doi:10.1123/jsp.4.1.73

Tooman, M. E. (1982). *The effect of running and its deprivation on muscle tension, mood, and anxiety*. Doctoral dissertation. Pennsylvania State University, University Park, PA.

Weinstein, A. A., Koehmstedt, C., & Kop, W. J. (2017). Mental health consequences of exercise withdrawal: A systematic review. *General Hospital Psychiatry, 49*, 11–18. Doi:10.1016/j.genhosppsych.2017.06.001

Wingate, C. F. (1993). Exploring the Karate way of life: Coping, commitment, and psychological well-being among traditional karate participants. Doctoral dissertation. Temple University, Philadelphia.

Zeller, L., Weitzman, D., Buskila, D., & Abu-Shakra, M. (2009). The effect of exercise cessation in well-trained athletes on non-articular tenderness masseurs. *Medicine & Science in Sports & Exercise, 41*(5), 302. Doi:10.1249/01.mss.0000355470.17769.18

9 Exercise addiction

Definition and conceptualization

We have presented the general concept of exercise addiction in Chapter 6 after its contextual classification within behavioral addictions in Chapter 5. This chapter elaborates on exercise addiction by looking at it more closely and hopefully placing it into proper research and clinical frameworks. We already know that exercise addiction is a form of obligatory exercise characterized by exaggerated training volume associated with losing control over an initially healthy behavior. Why and how does this loss of self-control occur? Several models attempt to answer these questions, but a closer examination of the drastic transition from constructive to destructive behavior is warranted.

9.1 Stress and exercise

As suggested by the cognitive appraisal hypothesis (Szabo, 1995; see Chapter 11), exercise is often used as a means of coping with stress. However, people use many different ways to handle the various challenges in their lives. Escape into alcohol or drugs is also a form of escape from reality, which is stressful for the affected person. Stress is subjective and largely depends on the appraisal of the situation causing the stress while the form of coping varies depending on the available resources to the person, and attitudes or experiences with those resources, along with the attributed importance, impact, or stakes (Folkman et al., 1986). Then the never-ending dilemma is the prediction of the coping mechanism in a given situation. For example, why would one person choose to unwind with music after a stressful event while another may drink whiskey after the same situation? Still, another individual might do both, relax to music and have whiskey to augment perceived coping efficacy.

Three general coping categories are identified: *constrictive, destructive,* and *social* (Jonason et al., 2020). Exercise, depending on its context, can be classified within any of the three categories. These categories represent higher-order means of coping with stress and are reflected by a similar but distinctive battery of lower-order or *generally used* coping strategies, such as avoidance, projection, exercise, travel, reading, listening to music, chatting

DOI: 10.4324/9781003173595-9

with friends, praying, superstitious and esoterically oriented practices, and acceptance through rationalization and many others. Therefore, exercise classified as a lower-order coping strategy can be part of any of the three higher-order strategies. It is constructive when done in moderation with full control over it; it is destructive when it becomes addictive to the point of salience, loss of control, and negative health consequences (i.e., injuries and social losses); and it is social when the stress-relieving effect is primarily achieved through being part of a group or team in which the problem can be shared or support can be secured. However, even in lack of discussion of the stressful situation, mere social involvement could have a stress-relieving role. Higher-order coping strategies are associated with individual traits. For example, in a recent study, social coping was linked to extraversion, narcissism, and interpersonal trust (Jonason et al., 2020). In the same work, constructive coping was negatively associated with 'dark traits' such as Machiavellianism, psychopathy, sadism, and spitefulness. Conversely, destructive coping was connected to a high incidence of dark personality traits. It is, therefore, relatively evident that personality factors are strong determinants in the choice and manifestation of coping with stress.

On the basis of the transactional model of stress and coping (Lazarus & Folkman, 1984), scholars can isolate *problem-oriented coping*, which begs for action to change or control the stressful situation, from *emotion-oriented coping*, which calls for cognitive reinterpretation to achieve emotional control (Beer & Moneta, 2012). It should be stressed that both orientations can be inherent parts of all three higher-order coping strategies. Problem-focused coping is only possible when the individual thinks, believes, or is convinced that the stress-causing situation is manageable through an action. For example, the plantar fasciitis caused by the running shoe can be alleviated by changing the shoe. Problem-oriented coping is a response to an active stress situation, which the individual perceives to be manageable through action.

However, even passive forms of stress comprised by situations over which the person has little or no *direct* control, such as the COVID-19 pandemic, can be perceived by some to be manageable through an action. For example, Vogel et al. (2021) found that physical activity was associated with less subjectively experienced stress during isolation. In this case, the action (deliberate exercise) is directed toward an unaffectable passive event through the belief and expectancy that helps in dealing with the unfavorable situation. The immediate effects may mirror placebo effects (Szabo, 2013). The expected reward (relief) is obtained through the performance of exercise. On the long term, these effects can make the situation *mentally* more bearable even though exercise does not change the pandemic's unfolding. Consequently, the *attributed* active nature of the stress and selected coping method are based on a *subjective appraisal* of the situation determined by past experiences and personality traits (Figure 9.1).

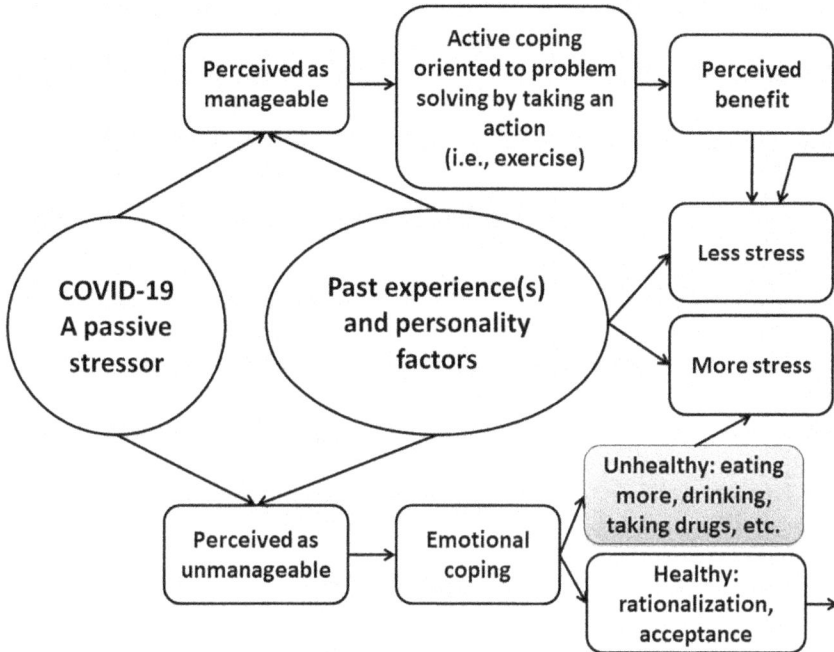

Figure 9.1 The diagram illustrates how a passive stressor can elicit either a problem-oriented or emotionally focused coping strategy with the emerging consequences.

Accordingly, a COVID-19 or any lockdown can represent active stress for some and passive for others, even though the situation itself is relatively passive because there is only little or no control over its unfolding and consequences. As perceived, passive stress requires emotion-focused coping because the affected individual sees no way to manage the situation through action. Therefore, according to Lazarus and Folkman (1984), coping is dictated by varied cognitive appraisals of the situation even though the situation is specific. In contrast to the example of the plantar fasciitis caused by the wrong running shoe that can be simply replaced to solve the stress, COVID-19 causes stress that cannot be *directly* managed via an activity, but action taken due to the belief that it will help can *indirectly* generate a benefit as illustrated in Figure 9.1. This path through beliefs and expectations can surface as placebo effects resulting from an action. In contrast, emotion-oriented coping can be both positive and negative. In the former case, the person accepts the situation and hopes for the best outcome in the stressful situation. Uses rationalization to comfort the self-thought responsible for emotional feeling states. A negative emotion-oriented coping may be characterized by hopelessness and helplessness and compensatory behaviors aimed at emotion regulation, like eating, drinking, smoking, or distraction such as TV watching, Internet overuse, and the like. Passive coping is not void of action because eating and watching TV are also actions, but they are oriented to easing pain stemming from the stress rather than combating stress itself. Indeed, Vogel et al. (2021) found that managing COVID-19 situation using outdoor and indoor exercise was related to lower reported stress while managing stress with TV/movie watching, sleeping, or eating was associated with more stress.

Even though exercise is not the only means to cope with significant stress, it is a powerful defense weapon against it because it increases self-efficacy (Neace et al., 2020), resilience (Arida & Teixeira-Machado, 2021), and stress resistance itself (Greenwood et al., 2012). Most exercisers know this fact, and, therefore, many of them use exercise for therapeutic purposes. A study based on a convenience sample recruited on social media has shown that over two-thirds of the exercisers gave a *health-related* reason for their exercise motive (Szabo et al., 2019). This finding is in line with the 'Exercise is Medicine' movement, described in Chapter 1, initiated and supported by the American College of Sports Medicine (ACSM; Jonas & Phillips, 2012).

9.2 Therapeutic exercise

The well-known health benefits of exercise are critical incentives for participation above and beyond social, esthetic, skill development, growth, and leisure or competitive reasons. The main reasons for exercise can be classified into two general categories. The first is connected *directly* (i.e., improved cardiorespiratory fitness) or *indirectly* (i.e., feeling more self-confident after exercise-induced changes in body form and composition) to a health-related incentive. The other is a more general category that includes anything else than health, with mastery and enjoyment (self-challenge, skill learning, development, control over life experiences, joy, fun, social relatedness, etc.) possibly being the best terms for it. A while ago, Robbins and Joseph (1985) introduced the concepts of 'therapeutic' and 'mastery' running that were expanded to other forms of exercises (Szabo et al., 2019).

Therapeutic exercise can be driven by reward-seeking via both positive and negative reinforcement (Szabo, 2010). Engaging in exercise for prevention when the individual is still healthy is more likely driven by positive reinforcement (the reward) emerging as a form of *gain* in health. It is like a growing bank account, making the individual believe (with a valid reason) that health gets better and better while it also equips the self with greater resilience and overall resistance to various health risks. However, when health is already at risk, based on the 'health belief model' (Rosenstock, 1974), exercise becomes a means of avoiding or dealing with the health hazard. These motives could be extrinsic (originating externally) or intrinsic (stemming from the self). For example, there is a general consensus that exercise alleviates both state anxiety (Ensari et al., 2015) and depression (Daley, 2008). This knowledge, coupled with expectancy and experience, could motivate one to exercise via both negative reinforcement to *avoid* the worsening of the condition or if cured to prevent a relapse, but also through positive reinforcement in which the reward is the gain of feeling better and appraising health as being improved.

Health-related behavioral rewards are sought intrinsically, but considering others (family, partner), work demand, status growth, or maintenance (survival needs) could also be the primary reasons for engaging in exercise, in which case the behavior is externally motivated. According to the study of Robbins and Joseph (1985), runners who experienced the therapeutic effects of running have learned to rely on it when the need arises (a typical conditioned effect). Therefore, a situation-driven switch between two forms of motives and reward expectancies may occur. In case of extreme stress or trauma, the social image-conscious exerciser, who knows about and has experienced the therapeutic effects of exercise, is likely to adopt the tested behavior as a means of coping or escape (Egorov & Szabo, 2013) because the behavior is perceived to be a socially accepted form of 'positive addiction' (Glasser, 1976) in contrast to using drugs or alcohol, which are behaviors linked to a negative social stigma.

9.3 Mastery exercise

Mastery exercise is driven by a reward that is unrelated to health. It is a source of self-fulfillment, self-challenge, a sense of accomplishment, and novelty (Robbins & Joseph, 1985). Popular magazines and books cite personal accounts of athletes achieving incredible, almost superhuman, goals resulting in self-fulfillment. It also includes social pleasure if the exercise is performed in team or group settings, but the 'here and now' experience is the ultimate reward generated via positive reinforcement (Allen-Collinson & Leledaki, 2014). This very positive feeling (similar or possibly even identical to the runners' high experience discussed in Chapter 4) often generates *flow*, which, as stated earlier, is thought to be the optimal or the peak human experience (Csikszentmihalyi, 2017). While health-conscious therapeutic exercisers can also experience flow, *the health-related expectation* associated with exercise persists as the principal driving force behind their exercise behavior, or else they no longer would be therapeutic exercisers.

As common sense suggests, academic research underpins that outcome expectations significantly affect exercise behavior (Mothes et al., 2016; Resnick et al., 2000; Resnick & Spellbring, 2000). Early work has shown that outcome expectations were strong predictors of exercise behavior, even stronger than perceived self-efficacy (Jette et al., 1998). Obviously, the reason for one's exercise cannot be isolated from outcome expectancies. However, the perception of the fulfillment of the outcome expectancy (i.e., obtaining the sought reward) mediates the components of one's exercise behavior ranging from the form of exercise (i.e., swimming versus yoga [Berger & Owen, 1992]) to the amount of exercise performed. *Tolerance* plays an important role in the latter, especially when the expected and previously experienced reward is no longer derived from a particular exercise volume (Griffiths, 2005). Increased tolerance paired with craving for exercise is an early sign of exercise addiction.

9.4 Terminology: exercise addiction, dependence, compulsion, and obligatory exercise

It is important to stress that as we shall see in Chapter 11, based on the interactional model of exercise addiction (Egorov & Szabo, 2013), both therapeutic and mastery exercise can lead to exercise addiction. The transition in both cases takes place when one loses control over the exercise behavior. In therapeutic exercise, the individual is *dependent* on exercise to manage personal health issues. In mastery exercise, there is a strong and perhaps unrealistic drive to achieve athletic or exercise goals above one's personal limits while the extent of dependence on the sport or exercise is not totally obvious. One may argue that mastery exercisers *depend* on certain performance and achievement goals, or athletic results, to feel valued and appreciated or to achieve self-actualization based on Maslow's hierarchical model of needs (Maslow, 1962). However, in that case, the outcome goals (i.e., reward) are no longer mastery-oriented. Instead, mastery goals are only a means to achieve a therapeutic (in this case, psychological) need. Therefore, the exercise behavior is connected to an aspect of one's *psychological health* and well-being. Accordingly, we see dependence primarily as an aspect of therapeutic exercise on the path of addiction. In contrast, we conjecture that the lack of acceptance of personal limits and unrealistic expectations, along with the false appraisal of personal resources, are the stages of addiction in mastery exercise in which mastery goals are unrelated to health issues.

As mentioned in Chapter 6, while the term *exercise dependence* is often used as a synonym for addiction, the latter includes the former in addition to compulsion (Goodman, 1990). Accordingly, addiction may be described as a two-dimensional concept encompassing dependence and compulsion. Consequently, when exercise addiction is referred to as exercise 'dependence,' one misses an integral component of exercise addiction: the urge or compulsion, being the main propelling force behind the disorder. In accord with Goodman, not all dependencies and compulsions may be classified as addiction (see Figure 9.2). Both high dependence and high compulsion are necessary for identifying exercise addiction.

What about *obligatory exercise*? This term was adopted a while ago by Pasman and Thompson (1988). The term *obligatory* matches well the addictive aspects of exercise. It suggests a loss of control over exercise manifesting in

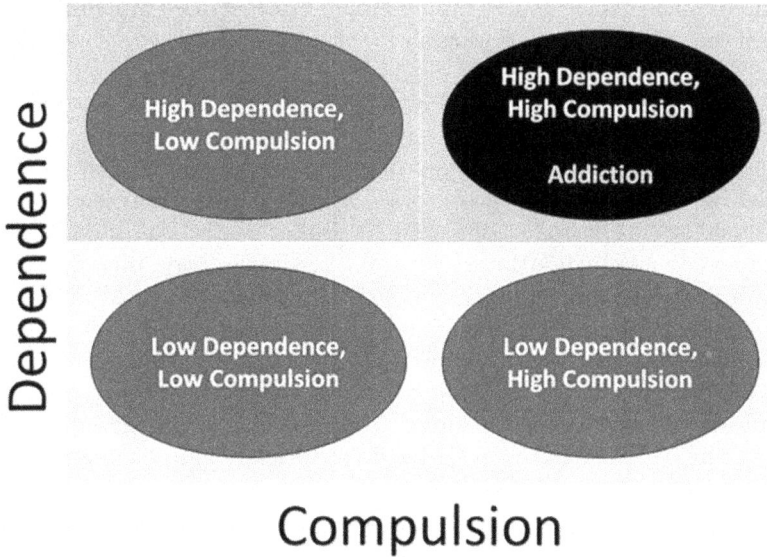

Figure 9.2 A two-dimensional model of exercise addiction.

exercise tolerance, salience, and withdrawal symptoms (Ackard et al., 2002). The person is *obliged* to exercise, or something very unpleasant, harmful, or painful consequences may occur. This interpretation implicitly implies that it includes compulsion (must do) for some reason (i.e., to manage stress), with this specific reason mirroring the dependence. Therefore, the term obligatory also reflects that the behavior controls the individual rather than vice versa. Consequently, it matches well the concept of addiction. Still, for consistency, easier resource identification, research homogeneity, and a more uniform and universal definition, the term 'exercise addiction' may be the most preferred.

9.5 The components model of exercise addiction

The six symptoms comprised in the components model of addictions were briefly presented in Chapter 5 in the *general context* of behavioral addictions. Table 5.2 in that chapter lists these symptoms compared to two other frameworks in the conceptualization of behavioral addictions. Here we describe the components model in *specific relevance* to exercise behavior. The six components comprise one of the most popular assessment tools, the Exercise Addiction Inventory (EAI), used to measure the risk of exercise addiction as discussed in Chapter 12 of this book. Given that most research in the field relies on the components model and the EAI, it is essential to look at its components separately and examine whether they are sufficient to screen the risk of exercise addiction.

9.5.1 Tolerance

Tolerance is one of the six components in the often-cited components model of addictions (Griffiths, 2005). It is a symptom that is evident in substance and behavioral addictions. It should not be confused with the 'training effect,' which surfaces as more skilled and energy-efficient exercise behavior. The training effect does not cause an increased need to do more exercise but provides an opportunity for enjoying more the exercise because of increased progress in skill acquisition and the progressively lower energy cost of the activity. However, tolerance results from *no longer experiencing* the previously experienced reward at a constant volume of exercise (Szabo, 2010). The person feels compelled to do more exercise to reexperience the desired effects. Similar to the impact of substance tolerance, the increase in the amount of exercise jeopardizes the individual's health. Tolerance is one of the three dimensions of obligatory exercise discussed in Chapter 7, the other two being withdrawal symptoms and salience (Ackard et al., 2002).

9.5.2 Withdrawal symptoms

Another of the six typical symptoms of addictions in the components model is withdrawal symptoms (Griffiths, 2005). These psychological symptoms were discussed in detail in the context of exercise deprivation in Chapter 8. Reiterating briefly, they are very unpleasant psychological and physical feeling states, which occur when exercise (especially therapeutic and obligatory exercise) is discontinued or its volume is significantly reduced. The most commonly reported withdrawal symptoms are illustrated in the previous chapter in Figure 8.1. The intensity of the feeling states is severe in obligatory exercisers to the extent that they really feel miserable when the need for exercise cannot be fulfilled. The manifestation of these symptoms in obligatory exercisers is largely different from the symptoms experienced by the committed exercisers who simply feel a void or that something is missing when exercising is not possible for a reason. Obligatory exercisers have to exercise to overcome withdrawal symptoms even at the expense of other possibly more important life obligations. Yet, the presence of salience, which is another aspect of obligatory exercise (Ackard et al., 2002), suggests that exercise has the principal role in obligatory exercisers' lives. Therefore, all other life obligations assume a secondary place.

9.5.3 Salience

This symptom is present when the physical activity or exercise becomes the most important activity for the person. The preoccupation with it during the daily activities dominates the individual's thinking, feelings (i.e., urges and cravings), and behavior (i.e., worsening of the social relations). For instance, even when people are not engaged in exercise, they might think of the next time they will be. The mind of the addicted individual wanders off to exercise during other daily activities like driving, having meals, attending meetings, and even between conversations with friends. The closer is the planned time for exercise, the greater is the urge and even anxiety or fear from not starting on time. The addicted exerciser is literally obsessed with exercise, and regardless of the time of the day, place, or activity performed, their mind is directed toward exercise during most waking hours.

9.5.4 Mood modification

This symptom reflects subjective experiences resulting from engaging in a particular activity. It could be perceived as a coping strategy (i.e., they experience an arousing buzz or a high, or paradoxically tranquilizing feelings, escape, or numbing). Most exercisers report positive feeling states and pleasant exhaustion after a session of exercise. However, the person addicted to exercise would seek mood modification not necessarily for the gain or the positive mental effect of exercise but rather for modifying or avoiding the negative psychological feeling states they would experience if their exercise sessions were missed. Fear of not feeling well or going down (psychologically) is a strong incentive for exercise perceived as the vehicle that could prevent unwanted negative mood experiences. Mood modification plays a role in the conditioning effects stemming from exercise. The feeling good and uplifting experience after a workout is the reward, which is sought (and received) again and again. The expectancies become stronger over time, and the response becomes conditioned, which could account for the placebo effects of acute exercise (Szabo, 2013). Therefore, some individuals can achieve a certain level of mood modification by merely undertaking their habitual activity regardless of its volume. Research shows that even only three minutes (!) of light exercises could trigger positive psychological changes (Szabo et al., 2013). However, the dose–response relationship in addictive exercise behavior requires more effort, perceived as sufficient by the affected individual, to yield a subjective effect. This need for greater effort stems from the belief that exerting more work triggers a more significant effect. Specifically, total physical exhaustion may be necessary for the addicted mind that it had enough (for the sought reward). Similar to alcohol use, one may become friendly and funny, or alternately aggressive and unbearable, just by sipping alcohol while another may need to drink till reaching the state of tipsiness to exhibit the same behavior.

9.5.5 Conflict

This symptom represents the conflicts between the exercise addicts and others around them (interpersonal conflict), conflicts with other daily activities (job, social life, hobbies, and interests), or from within the individual them-selves (intrapersonal or intrapsychic conflict) which are concerned with the particular activity. Interpersonal conflict usually results from neglect of the relationship with friends or family because of the exaggerated time and preoccupation devoted to exercise. Conflict in daily activities arises because of the abnormally high priority given to exercise in contrast to important survival activities like cleaning, taking care of bills, working, or studying for exams. Intrapsychic conflict occurs when the addicted person has realized that fulfilling the need to exercise takes a toll on other life obligations, but they are unable to cut down or control the exercise behavior. Whether intra- or interpersonal, the conflict triggers feelings of stress, which are most frequently handled by the addicted individual through even more exercise. Therefore, the exercise behavior continues to be increased in a vicious circle, generating more stress, which is relieved with more exercise.

9.5.6 Relapse

This symptom reflects the tendency for repeated reversions to earlier exer-cise patterns after a break, whether voluntary or involuntary. The phenom-enon is similar to symptoms seen in alcoholics who stop drinking for some time and then start over again and drink as much – if not more – than before their break from drinking. Relapse could be observed after injury (which is involuntary) or after a planned reduction in exercise volume due to a personal decision to halt the unhealthy pattern of exercise behavior or as a consequence of professional advice. Upon resumption of the activity, addicted individuals could soon exercise as much or even more as before reducing their exercise volume. Therefore, relapse prevention is one of the most significant challenges in addiction medicine.

9.6 Other signs and symptoms of exercise addiction

The components model is based on six *typical* components or symptoms. Still, for a more accurate evaluation of the risk of exercise addiction, some other behavioral manifestations observed in maladaptive exercise should also be considered. Some of these components (see below) are included in the addiction components as subcomponents (e.g., loss of control and negative life consequences are subsumed within the conflict component; Griffiths, 2013).

9.6.1 Loss of control over life activities

The internal drive or urge for exercise becomes psychologically so intense that it preoccupies attention in most waking hours by dominating the person's thoughts. Consequently, the affected individual is unable to pay attention or concentrate on other daily activities properly. Until that urge is satisfied, other life activities are poorly performed or neglected. Upon fulfillment of the need to exercise, the affected person may function well and take care of some other mundane obligations. Still, normal functioning is limited to the period encompassing the acute effects of the previous exercise session or until the urge for another bout of exercise starts to rise again. Therefore, these regular functioning periods are relatively short due to a lack of control over the cravings to exercise.

9.6.2 Loss of control over exercise behavior

This is a phenomenon where vows cannot be kept. The exerciser cannot resist the vital need to exercise. While they may try to set limits in their exercise patterns, they cannot respect those self-set limits. In short, lack of control denotes the inability to exercise with moderation. This phenomenon is also observable in alcoholics (and in most addictions in general) who vow not to get drunk again after several incidences of heavy drinking and some severe consequences of such drinking patterns. However, on the same day later, after making such a vow, they get drunk again. The inability to keep exercise in control, despite an inner desire to do that, results in feelings of powerlessness, loss of willpower, and guilt. Such feelings yield the thought of failure to do it (control it) anyway, so why bother trying to control the habit. This thought process, characterized by guilt, and associated learned helplessness (or possibly a feeling of sorry for the self for which the addictive behavior provides some sort of relief or compensation), then grants green light to the addicted behavior.

9.6.3 Negative, non-injury-related life consequences

Negative life events may occur because of overexercising. For example, suppose life activities are ignored or superficially performed due to excessive exercise and too much preoccupation with exercise in the long term. In that case, negative life consequences may emerge involving even loss of employment, poor academic performance, breakup in relationships and friendships, and other repercussions generally considered undesirable on the person's life. Untreated, exercise addiction can have serious consequences.

9.6.4 Risk of self-injury

At times of mild injuries, the addicted exerciser cannot abstain from exercise and, therefore, assumes the risk of self-injury by maintaining their physical activity. In more severe cases, the affected individual needs to see a medical professional who may advise the person to refrain from exercising until full recovery occurs. Despite the medical advice, the person addicted to exercise will likely resume her or his exercise immediately upon experiencing minor alleviation in the discomfort associated with the injury – or in the early stages of recovery – therefore, exposing her or himself to further and possibly more severe injuries triggering often irreversible health damages.

9.6.5 Social selection and withdrawal

This symptom reflects the behavioral tendency by which the addicted person identifies with others who approve their exercise behavior and avoids the company of those who criticize their physical activity pattern. Such social gravitation is generally observed in individuals suffering from other forms of behavioral (e.g., gambling) or substance (e.g., alcohol) addictions.

9.6.6 Lack of compromise

This symptom is closely related to the loss of control. Although there may be several warning signs associated with the neglect of family or work responsibilities due to excessive exercise, these signs are often insufficient to trigger a decision to compromise. Consequently, other life commitments remain ignored, even though the affected person is aware that the result may be worse than undesirable.

9.6.7 Denial

This symptom represents a psychological defense mechanism known as rationalization. People addicted to their exercise explain or justify the problem via a conscious search for why exercise training is beneficial even in a massive volume. The mass media and scientific reports provide ample reasons for rationalization. The ACSM guidelines for exercise and the positive correlation between the dose of exercise and general health (Haskell et al., 2007) are excellent anchors for justifying the excessive amounts of physical activity.

9.6.8 Awareness of the problem

The exercise addict may know well that there are problems with exercise behavior through feedback from other people or some adverse life events directly resulting from overexercising. However, they feel powerless to act against the problem. This feeling may trigger giving up and giving in (to the addiction) reactions, eventually resulting in the deterioration of self-image that feelings of worthlessness may accompany.

9.6.9 Other classifications

As discussed in Chapter 5 in the general context of behavioral addictions, Grüsser and Thalemann (2006) presented another classification for behavioral addictions (Table 5.2) based on 15 relatively common charac-teristics of several forms of addictions. These scholars conjectured that these symptoms might serve diagnostic purposes for behavioral addictions, including exercise addiction. Nevertheless, the authors have emphasized that all cases need to be examined *individually* to determine whether the heavy involvement with the given behavior is indeed addictive or just an excessive one (nonpathological or related to another dysfunction). Indeed, symptoms alone may not be sufficient for the correct diagnosis, but a col-lection of typical and severe symptoms, in conjunction with the history of negative consequences, due to the excessive indulgence in a given behavior may pinpoint the presence of addiction.

9.7 Clinical diagnosis

Due to insufficient empirical evidence for mental dysfunction, exercise addiction is not listed in the fifth edition of the *Diagnostic and Statisti-cal Manual of Mental Disorders* (*DSM-5*; American Psychiatric Association, 2013). Therefore, based on *DSM-5*, no clinical diagnosis is possible for the dysfunction at this time. Still, authors have borrowed the *DSM-5* criteria for another behavioral addiction, namely gambling disorder, to identify the problem (Cook et al., 2014; Downs et al., 2004; Szabo, 2018). Szabo (2018), in line with a previous theoretical note (Szabo et al., 2015), stressed that these categories could embed relatively different interpretations from the part of elite athletes in contrast to recreational exercisers in who the ten-dency of addiction was noted initially (Table 9.1). In a recent systematic review of the literature, Juwono et al. (2021) have found that elite athletes consistently score higher on psychometric measures of exercise addiction but argue that this general finding is an artifact. Their argument reflects the general knowledge that addictions are governed by strong urges beg-ging for immediate gratification, which does not fit into the disciplined and highly organized athletic training.

9.8 Exercise addiction in recreational exercisers and elite athletes

Only relatively few studies have examined the risk of exercise addiction in athletes. These studies report prevalence rates ranging from 2.7% (Zeulner et al., 2016) to as high as >40% in another study (Smith et al., 2010). The lowest rate matches the results of a population-wide study (Mónok et al., 2012). Still, the estimated *average* risk of exercise addiction in athletes is too high (Szabo et al., 2015). According to Juwono et al. (2021), risk rates over 30% make no sense because such rates imply that one in three ath-letes might be addicted to exercise. Instead, as suggested by Szabo et al. (2015) and Szabo (2018), athletes are likely to interpret the items assessing exercise addiction differently from nonathletes (refer to Table 9.1) because

Table 9.1 Adaptation of the *DSM-5* criteria for gambling disorder to exercise addiction and the possible interpretation of each criterion by the elite athlete (last column in bold letters).

DSM-5 Gambling Disorder criteria	*DSM-5 criteria adopted to Exercise Addiction in recreational athletes*	*What the symptom-criteria might mirror in the case of elite athletes*
Need to gamble with an increasing amount of money to achieve the desired excitement	The person needs to exercise more to achieve the same satisfaction as before	**The athlete needs to train more and more to reach higher goals**
Restless or irritable when trying to cut down or stop gambling	Restless or irritable when must cut down or stop exercising	**Feels bad when losing training for an unwanted or unexpected reason**
Repeated unsuccessful efforts to control, cut back on, or stop gambling	Repeated unsuccessful efforts to control and cut back on exercise	**Does not usually want to cut down on training (unless injured)**
Frequently thinks about gambling (such as reliving past gambling experiences, planning the next gambling venture, and thinking of ways to get money to gamble)	Frequently thinks about exercise (such as reliving past experiences, planning the next exercise session, and thinking of ways to get more exercise)	**Must plan and evaluate workouts and schedule the days around the training**
Often resorts to gambling when feeling distressed	Often exercises when feeling distressed	**May rely on exercise or training to deal with stress**
After losing money when gambling, the person often returns to get even (referred to as 'chasing' one's losses)	After insufficient or missed exercise (felt loss), pushes hard to make up for it	**Self-imposed conformity and pressure manifested in obsessive passion. It is part of elite athletes' training**
The person is lying to conceal gambling activity	The person is lying to conceal problematic exercise behavior	**It is not applicable in most cases of elite athletes**
The person jeopardizes or loses a significant relationship, job, or educational/career opportunity because of gambling	The person jeopardizes or loses a significant relationship, job, or educational/career opportunity because of exercise	**Being an elite athlete takes sacrifices**
The person is relying on others to help with money problems caused by gambling	The person relies on others to help with issues caused by excessive exercise	**Due to the demand for training, time constraints, and travel to competitions, they may rely on others' help**

Note: Items 6 and 9 are unique to gambling disorder criteria and our substitutes are not fully comparable.

these tools were mainly developed for the assessment of the problematic behavior in noncompetitive recreational exercisers.

While nonathletes can engage in escape behaviors, including exercise, whenever the urge arises, athletes train by following a rigidly and often externally controlled schedule that requires their personal life to be scheduled around their training regimen. As Juwono et al. (2021) argue, urges of addiction cannot be fulfilled on a prescribed schedule. Indeed, smokers would have a hard time if they were to follow a daily schedule in smoking. Therefore, these higher scores of the risk of exercise addiction in athletes reported in the literature should reflect something other than pathological tendencies. Instead, according to Juwono et al., these high scores might reflect keen passion, commitment, and dedication to the sport in which the athlete wants to excel and around which the athlete's life revolves.

We share these views, and in addition, we stress that even high scores on various assessment tools might not reflect exercise addiction because these scores are significantly affected by several other factors. In recognition of dysfunctional or addictive exercise behavior, there should be clear evidence of loss of control over exercise training and its negative consequences (self-harm). Because of the substantial influence of passion, commitment, or even perfectionism (Çakın et al., 2021), the estimated risk of exercise addiction does not reflect any pathology, and this is an important reason why the dysfunction cannot be included in the *DSM* or other diagnostic references.

9.9 Key points

1. Sports and exercise are some of the many behavioral means of coping with stress.
2. Exercise addiction is more closely connected with therapeutic than mastery exercise.
3. Exercise addiction involves both high compulsion and high dependence.
4. Obligatory exercise is a term used for denoting that the behavior controls the person.
5. In theory, exercise addiction in *externally controlled* organized sports is nonexistent.

9.10 References

Ackard, D. M., Brehm, B. J., & Steffen, J. J. (2002). Exercise and eating disorders in college-aged women: Profiling excessive exercisers. *Eating Disorders: The Journal of Treatment & Prevention, 10*(1), 31–47. Doi:10.1080/106402602753573540

Allen-Collinson, J., & Leledaki, A. (2014). Sensing the outdoors: A visual and haptic phenomenology of outdoor exercise embodiment. *Leisure Studies, 34*(4), 457–470. Doi:10.1080/02614367.2014.923499

American Psychiatric Association (2013). *Diagnostic and statistical manual of mental disorders* (5th ed.). Arlington, VA: Author.

Arida, R. M., & Teixeira-Machado, L. (2021). The contribution of physical exercise to brain resilience. *Frontiers in Behavioral Neuroscience, 14.* (Online first). Doi:10.3389/fnbeh.2020.626769

Beer, N., & Moneta, G. B. (2012). Coping and perceived stress as a function of positive metacognitions and positive meta-emotions. *Individual Differences Research, 10*(2), 105–116. Doi:10.1037/t10305-000

Berger, B. G., & Owen, D. R. (1992). Mood alteration with yoga and swimming; aerobic exercise may not be necessary. *Perceptual and Motor Skills, 75,* 1331–1343. Doi:10.2466/pms.1992.75.3f.1331

Çakın, G., Juwono, I. D., Potenza, M. N., & Szabo, A. (2021). Exercise addiction and perfectionism: A systematic review of the literature. *Current Addiction Reports, 8*(1), 144–155. Doi:10.1007/s40429-021-00358-8

Cook, B., Hausenblas, H., & Freimuth, M. (2014). Exercise addiction and compulsive exercising: Relationship to eating disorders, substance use disorders, and addictive disorders. *Eating Disorders, Addictions and Substance Use Disorders,* 127–144. Doi:10.1007/978-3-642-45378-6_7

Csikszentmihalyi, M. (2017). *Finding flow. The psychology of engagement with everyday life.* Gildan: Audio Book.

Daley, A. (2008). Exercise and depression: A review of reviews. *Journal of Clinical Psychology in Medical Settings, 15*(2), 140–147. Doi:10.1007/s10880-008-9105-z

Downs, D. S., Hausenblas, H. A., & Nigg, C. R. (2004). Factorial validity and psychometric examination of the exercise dependence scale-revised. *Measurement in Physical Education and Exercise Science, 8*(4), 183–201. Doi:10.1207/s15327841mpee0804_1

Egorov, A. Y., & Szabo, A. (2013). The exercise paradox: An interactional model for a clearer conceptualization of exercise addiction. *Journal of Behavioral Addictions, 2*(4), 199–208. Doi:10.1556/jba.2.2013.4.2

Ensari, I., Greenlee, T. A., Motl, R. W., & Petruzzello, S. J. (2015). Meta-analysis of acute exercise effects on state anxiety: An update of randomized controlled trials over the past 25 years. *Depression and Anxiety, 32*(8), 624–634. Doi:10.1002/da.22370

Folkman, S., Lazarus, R. S., Dunkel-Schetter, C., DeLongis, A., & Gruen, R. J. (1986). Dynamics of a stressful encounter: Cognitive appraisal, coping, and encounter outcomes. *Journal of Personality and Social Psychology, 50*(5), 992–1003. Doi:10.1037/0022-3514.50.5.992

Glasser, W. (1976). *Positive addiction.* Oxford, England: Harper & Row.

Goodman, A. (1990). Addiction: Definition and implications. *British Journal of Addiction, 85*(11), 1403–1408. Doi:10.1111/j.1360-0443.1990.tb01620.x

Greenwood, B. N., Spence, K. G., Crevling, D. M., Clark, P. J., Craig, W. C., & Fleshner, M. (2012). Exercise-induced stress resistance is independent of exercise controllability and the medial prefrontal cortex. *European Journal of Neuroscience, 37*(3), 469–478. Doi:10.1111/ejn.12044

Griffiths, M. D. (2013). Is "loss of control" always a consequence of addiction? *Frontiers in Psychiatry, 4.* Doi:10.3389/fpsyt.2013.00036

Griffiths, M. D. (2005). A 'components' model of addiction within a biopsychosocial framework. *Journal of Substance Use, 10*(4), 191–197. Doi:10.1080/14659890500114359

Grüsser, S. M., & Thalemann, C. N. (2006). *Verhaltenssucht Diagnostik, Therapie, Forschung*. Bern: Huber

Haskell, W. L., Lee, I. M., Pate, R. R., Powell, K. E., Blair, S. N., Franklin, B. A., . . . Bauman, A. (2007). Physical activity and public health: Updated recommendation for adults from the American College of Sports Medicine and the American Heart Association. *Circulation, 116*(9), 1081. Doi: 10.1249/mss.0b013e3180616b27

Jette, A., Lachman, M., Giorgetti, M., Assmann, S., Harris, B., . . . Krebs, D. (1998). Effectiveness of home-based, resistance training with disabled older persons. *The Gerontologist, 38*, 412–422.

Jonas, S., & Phillips, E. M. (2012). *ACSM's Exercise is Medicine™: A clinician's guide to exercise prescription*. Philadelphia, PA: Wolters Kluwer, Lippincott Williams & Wilkins.

Jonason, P. K., Talbot, D., Cunningham, M. L., & Chonody, J. (2020). Higher-order coping strategies: Who uses them and what outcomes are linked to them. *Personality and Individual Differences, 155*, 109755. Doi:10.1016/j.paid.2019.109755

Juwono, I. D., Tolnai, N., & Szabo, A. (2021). Exercise addiction in athletes: A systematic review of the literature. *International Journal of Mental Health and Addiction*. (Online first). Doi:10.1007/s11469-021-00568-1

Lazarus, R. S., & Folkman, S. (1984). *Stress, appraisal, and coping*. New York, NY: Springer Publishing.

Maslow, A. H. (1962). *Toward a psychology of being*. Princeton: D. Van Nostrand Company.

Mónok, K., Berczik, K., Urbán, R., Szabo, A., Griffiths, M. D., Farkas, J., . . . Demetrovics, Z. (2012). Psychometric properties and concurrent validity of two exercise addiction measures: A population-wide study. *Psychology of Sport and Exercise, 13*(6), 739–746. doi:10.1016/j.psychsport.2012.06.003

Mothes, H., Leukel, C., Jo, H.-G., Seelig, H., Schmidt, S., & Fuchs, R. (2016). Expectations affect psychological and neurophysiological benefits even after a single bout of exercise. *Journal of Behavioral Medicine, 40*(2), 293–306. Doi:10.1007/s10865-016-9781-3

Neace, S. M., Hicks, A. M., DeCaro, M. S., & Salmon, P. G. (2020). Trait mindfulness and intrinsic exercise motivation uniquely contribute to exercise self-efficacy. *Journal of American College Health*, 1–5. (Online first). Doi:10.1080/07448481.20 20.1748041

Pasman, L., & Thompson, J. K. (1988). Body image and eating disturbance in obligatory runners, obligatory weightlifters, and sedentary individuals. *International Journal of Eating Disorders, 7*(6), 759–777. Doi:10.1002/1098-108X (198811)7:6<759::AID-EAT2260070605>3.0.CO;2-G

Resnick, B., Palmer, M. H., Jenkins, L. S., & Spellbring, A. M. (2000). Path analysis of efficacy expectations and exercise behaviour in older adults. *Journal of Advanced Nursing, 31*(6), 1309–1315. Doi:10.1046/j.1365-2648.2000.01463.x

Resnick, B., & Spellbring, A. M. (2000). Understanding what motivates older adults to exercise. *Journal of Gerontological Nursing, 26*(3), 34–42. Doi:10.3928/0098-9134-20000301-08

Robbins, J. M., & Joseph, P. (1985). Experiencing exercise withdrawal: Possible consequences of therapeutic and mastery running. *Journal of Sport Psychology, 7*(1), 23–39. Doi: 10.1123/jsp.7.1.2

Rosenstock, I. M. (1974). The health belief model and preventive health behavior. *Health Education Monographs, 2*(4), 354–386. Doi:10.1177/109019817400200405

Smith, D., Wright, C., & Winrow, D. (2010). Exercise dependence and social physique anxiety in competitive and non-competitive runners. *International Journal of Sport and Exercise Psychology, 8*(1), 61–69. doi:10.1080/1612197X.2010.9671934

Szabo, A. (1995). The impact of exercise deprivation on wellbeing of habitual exercisers. The *Australian Journal of Science and Medicine in Sport, 27*, 68–75.

Szabo, A. (2010). *Addiction to exercise: A symptom or a disorder?* New York, NY: Nova Science Publishers.

Szabo, A. (2013). Acute psychological benefits of exercise: Reconsideration of the placebo effect. *Journal of Mental Health, 22*(5), 449–455. Doi:10.3109/09638237.2012.734657

Szabo, A. (2018). Addiction, passion, or confusion? New theoretical insights on exercise addiction research from the case study of a female body builder. *Europe's Journal of Psychology, 14*(2), 296–316. Doi:10.5964/ejop.v14i2.1545

Szabo, A., Boros, S., & Bősze, J. P. (2019). Are there differences in life-satisfaction, optimism, pessimism and perceived stress between therapeutic and mastery exercisers? A preliminary investigation. *Baltic Journal of Sport and Health Sciences, 3*(114). Doi:10.33607/bjshs.v3i114.807

Szabo, A., Gaspar, Z., & Abraham, J. (2013). Acute effects of light exercise on subjectively experienced wellbeing: Benefits in only three minutes. *Baltic Journal of Health and Physical Activity, 5*(4). Doi:10.2478/bjha-2013-0024

Szabo, A., Griffiths, M. D., Marcos, R. D. L. V., Mervó, B., & Demetrovics, Z. (2015). Focus: Addiction: Methodological and conceptual limitations in exercise addiction research. *The Yale Journal of Biology and Medicine, 88*(3), 303–308.

Vogel, E. A., Zhang, J. S., Peng, K., Heaney, C. A., Lu, Y., Lounsbury, D., . . . Prochaska, J. J. (2021). Physical activity and stress management during COVID-19: A longitudinal survey study. *Psychology & Health*, 1–11. (Online first). Doi:10.1080/08870446.2020.1869740

Zeulner, B., Ziemainz, H., Beyer, C., Hammon, M., & Janka, R. (2016). Disordered eating and exercise dependence in endurance athletes. *Advances in Physical Education, 6*(02), 76–87. doi:10.4236/ape.2016.62009

10 Primary and secondary forms of exercise dependence

10.1 Primary exercise dependence refers to exercise addiction

There would be no problem if the terms *addiction* and *dependence* were not used as synonyms in the literature. However, some scholars implicitly categorize exercise addiction into *primary* and *secondary* forms (e.g., Cook et al., 2013; Trott et al., 2021), despite a justified call against such classification (Szabo et al., 2018). However, most investigations in this field focus primarily on the dysfunction in which individuals lose control over their exercise behavior, which takes control over their lives. This rare (Mónok et al., 2012), and currently clinically not diagnosable (see Chapter 9), psychological disorder is considered to be a behavioral addiction (Egorov & Szabo, 2013) that includes the two pillars of addictions in general, which are *compulsion* and *dependence* (Goodman, 1990; Szabo, 2010). Due to its latter component, exercise addiction is also often defined (incompletely) as *primary exercise* dependence (Bamber et al., 2000; Cook et al., 2013; Trott et al., 2021).

Primary exercise dependence is merely a symptom of exercise addiction that can trigger negative life consequences, including those listed in the components model of addiction (Griffiths, 2005) and excessive exercise behavior resulting *directly* in immediate psychological gratification (Bamber et al., 2000). In this case, the exercise consequences are the *direct* rewards manifested in pleasure or psychological relief derived from the behavior. However, high dependence on exercise could also be observed as a comorbidity in eating disorders, including anorexia, bulimia nervosa, and others in which weight loss or body shaping are the primary objectives of exercise behavior (Bamber et al., 2000). In these instances, excessive exercise behavior is termed *secondary exercise dependence*, but many scholars often confound this *symptom* with (secondary) exercise addiction, a *dysfunction*.

10.2 Secondary exercise dependence refers to instrumental exercise

Secondary exercise addiction does not exist. As discussed in Chapter 9, exercise addiction, or its part, primary exercise dependence, is not an

DOI: 10.4324/9781003173595-10

independent category of mental dysfunction in the *Diagnostic and Statistical Manual of Mental Disorders* (*DSM-5*; American Psychiatric Association, 2013). However, the *DSM-5* recognizes *excessive exercise* (conceptualized as behavior that interferes with important life activities, occurs at an inappropriate time or place, or is performed despite injury, or against medical advice) as a diagnostic *symptom* for restricting subtype of anorexia nervosa and bulimia nervosa. Consequently, the relationship between excessive exercise and eating disorders has been clinically established, but this relationship does not denote an *addiction to exercise behavior*. Therefore, extreme exercise behavior may only be considered a symptom of eating disorders from a clinical perspective. This view agrees with the conclusion of an earlier monograph by Szabo (2010), suggesting that excessive physical activity is unlikely to be a *cause* of a specific psychological dysfunction but rather a symptom of the latter. This conjecture, however, today may not be accurate based on the published cases (which are still few to be considered supportive of inclusion in *DSM-5*) and recently unveiled 100 testimonials on the Internet (Juwono & Szabo, 2020).

Secondary exercise dependence as a clinical *symptom* in eating disorders is not an addiction to the exercise behavior but an *instrumental action* in weight or body shape control. Muscle dysmorphia, too, is a dysfunction in which exercise is *instrumental* in building muscles (Foster et al., 2015). Instrumental exercise, nevertheless, can be excessive. The instrumental use of exercise in weight loss stems from scientific results, penetrating the widespread popular knowledge, affirming that exercise is energy-demanding and, consequently, calorie-burning physical work. Physical activity promotes weight loss, primarily through aerobic activities, such as running, cycling, swimming, and other exercises. Usually, a light or moderate exercise load is necessary for an extended period. Heart rate (Burke, 1998) can be used in determining the workload. High-intensity exercise burns more fat (Burke, 1998), but fatigue onsets much faster. So, for example, it is better to burn 600 calories in one hour, which supposedly is the starting point of exhaustion, than 450 in half an hour at a higher exercise intensity inducing earlier fatigue and exhaustion. Still, individuals affected by eating disorders tend to exercise harder than those without a dysfunction (Höglund & Normén, 2002). In eating disorders, individuals use exercise as an additional *means* (an instrument) to dieting to increase the amount or to speed up the process of weight loss by increasing their caloric expenditure in addition to caloric restraint. Alternately, they may exercise to compensate for caloric intake through food, which in some cases may result in a vicious circle. Indeed, both incentives may provide more psychological relief than actual physiological results in several instances, as demonstrated in a recent randomized control trial summarized below.

Martin et al. (2019) examined energy expenditure compensation response in regular physical exercise. The authors randomly assigned 198 men and women to three interventions over 24 weeks. The interventions consisted of a control group that did not exercise and a low and a high caloric expenditure group. At baseline and after 24 weeks, the dependent measures included the total energy expenditure, total energy intake, and body composition. As expected, energy expenditure has increased in both exercise groups, but no compensatory metabolic or physical activity changes were noted. Still, the weight loss was merely 36% and 41% of the predicted values in the low- and high-calorie expenditure groups, respectively. This finding suggests that compensation for exercise-burned calories occurred at both exercise levels. However, the results also showed that 42% of the low-exercise expenditure group participants and 24% of those in the high exercise expenditure group did not lose any weight. Some of them have even gained weight. These findings suggest that the participants compensated for exercise-induced energy expenditure by increasing their energy intake in this form of instrumental exercise.

The study by Martin et al. (2019) demonstrated that when exercise is *instrumental* in weight loss, its efficacy may be less than that believed or expected by the person, and occasionally the performance of the exercise activity may provide psychological relief mediated by a placebo effect (Szabo, 2013). Similarly, more challenging exercise associated with eating disorders (Höglund & Normén, 2002) may be more beneficial *mentally* than physically in the context of its objective. These observations question the efficacy of excessive exercise in eating disorders unless a very stringent *control* over the exercise behavior is maintained, which carefully considers both the calorie intake and expenditure balance and the exercise-induced time-to-exhaustion at various workloads. Then, due to careful planning, the *loss of control* over the exercise behavior, which is a characteristic of exercise addiction, is unlikely to occur in instrumental exercise.

10.3 Exercise addiction versus instrumental exercise

Based on our current knowledge about its clinical significance, secondary exercise dependence (not addiction) is a *symptom*. In contrast, primary exercise addiction has no clinical classification, but it is researched as a *dysfunction*. More than two decades ago, the state of knowledge was similar when Bamber et al. (2000) suggested that primary exercise dependence may not even exist to merit scholarly attention. Despite this assertion, Veale (1995) affirmed that (primary) exercise addiction exists, but it is rare. This assertion of rarity was corroborated by a population-wide study revealing that *the risk* of exercise addiction was approximately 0.3%–0.5% in the Hungarian population (Mónok et al., 2012). However, these numbers are still significant considering that about 1/400 to 1/200 people may be affected. Some studies even reported a prevalence of exercise addiction greater than 40% (Lejoyeux et al., 2008), which would be enormous if it would reflect actual clinical cases (Szabo et al., 2015). However, these numbers are not alarming because all prevalence studies are based on questionnaires assessing only the level of *risk of exercise addiction*, which eventually may never turn into medical attention-requiring dysfunction.

Dysfunctional exercise cannot be established with questionnaires alone but only in conjunction with in-depth interviews (Müller et al., 2014). In most eating disorders, various psychological problems resulting in distorted and unacceptable body image and low self-concept are also involved. At the same time, excessive exercise is only a *symptom* reflecting an instrumental role. Interviews should reveal the relatively significant difference between exercise as escape behavior and pain-avoidance (exercise addiction) or gratification seeking, yielding *immediate effects* in contrast to the exercise for weight control or distorted body image (eating disorders) resulting in *delayed effects*. Therefore, exercise addiction that is clinically not recognized yet but still generates substantial research publications (Szabo & Kovacsik, 2019) should be untangled from *instrumental exercise*, a symptom of eating disorders, muscle dysmorphia, or body dissatisfaction. Still, considering their manifestation, both behaviors meet conceptual classifications that render them excessive or even morbid. When one does not distinguish between exercise addiction *per se* and instrumental exercise as a *symptom*, the term *morbid exercise behavior* (Alcaraz-Ibáñez et al., 2020; Szabo et al., 2018) may be appropriate.

10.4 Prevalence of exercise addiction versus instrumental exercise

While the prevalence of exercise addiction, in general, has been studied in the literature (Di Lodovico et al., 2019; Marques et al., 2018), the specific prevalence of exercises addiction and instrumental exercise has received research attention only lately. In a meta-analysis including nine studies, Trott et al. (2020) have shown that the incidence of instrumental exercise was almost four times higher than that of exercise addiction. As a caution, these figures only reflect *high risk* rather than clinical diagnosis. The difference in prevalence varied depending on the risk assessment tool used for gauging exercise addiction. Participants with scores above critical values for eating disorders were more than three times likely to be in the *at-risk* category for exercise addiction than those scoring under the critical or cutoff values. These findings show that morbid exercise behavior is manifested about four times more frequently as a symptom of an eating disorder than addiction to the behavior (exercise) itself.

Consequently, Trott et al. (2020) showed that instrumental exercise is more prevalent than exercise addiction. This finding suggests that the prevalence of exercise addiction cases *per se* could be much lower than that reported in the literature. However, the distinctive nature of these cases (Juwono & Szabo, 2020) makes it difficult to generalize from the few published accounts and match the etiology of the individual cases with a theoretical framework. These difficulties hinder the collection of sufficient scientific evidence allowing the dysfunction to be identified as a distinct class of addictive disorder and to be included in a future edition of the *DSM*. However, the most complex issue is that, as stated before, those in the 'high risk' categories are still *not diagnosed* with any disorder, so their medical follow-up is not possible. It is also unlikely that a person identified as an *exercise addict* in a clinical setting (i.e., Kotbagi et al., 2014) would also be screened earlier as being at high risk for exercise addiction in a research setting. Therefore, matching high-risk cases (in research) to dysfunctional patient cases (in practice) and bridging research to clinical practice seems to be a challenging objective. Chapter 12 provides an approach for collaboration between researchers and clinicians to solve this dilemma.

10.5 Commonalities between exercise addiction and instrumental exercise

Exercise addiction has two distinctive features that, in addition to high-risk scores on various screening tools, should affirm the morbid nature of the behavior (Szabo et al., 2018). The first is *loss of control* over the exercise behavior, and the second is a *negative consequence* in the person's physical, psychological, or social health (Juwono & Szabo, 2020). A belief, or expectation, that exercise may yield some unique benefits (*gain*, positive reinforcement) or be the solution for life stress (*avoidance*, negative reinforcement) is another general feature of exercise addiction. These features are different in eating and body concern-related disorders where too much exercise is instrumental in weight loss or body shaping. Indeed, a loss of control may not be present because the dieting person, in general, *must* control the amount of exercise, which is a tool in reaching the desired outcome. For example, one needs to precisely calculate the minimum of calories to be burned to realize a specific short-term goal. Still, doing *as much exercise as possible* to lose as much weight as possible could also be a scenario in eating disorders. However, the loss of control remains obscured because the person 'wants' to exercise as much as the body allows. Griffiths (2013) has argued that a few addicts do not lose control but, in contrast, *over-control* of their behavior, especially among work addicts and in some eating disorders. Similar cases may exist among exercise addicts as well, but it is questionable whether these individuals are addicts or simply too passionate about their exercise?

The loss of control manifests in the 'must do' behavior, or something very unpleasant, distressing, or painful consequence would emerge. What complicates the issue is that the 'must do' is present in eating disorders, too, because if the affected person is not doing the exercise, the risk of not losing or even gaining weight increases. Therefore, the loss of control could occur in both addiction and instrumental exercise. Then this is a common feature that reflects a morbid pattern of exercise (Szabo et al., 2018). Negative consequences to physical, psychological, and social health are also apparent in addiction and instrumental exercise. Fetching far, escape from stress, could be another common symptom of exercise addiction in eating disorders and exercise addiction. In eating disorders, missing exercise can cause stress, similar to exercise addiction in which missing the exercise could generate *additional* stress to that for which exercise is used as a means of coping (Egorov & Szabo, 2013).

Overestimating one's physical abilities and setting unrealistically high goals could be confounded with exercise addiction. Nevertheless, such an unrealistic thought could be the source of stress, and then exercise becomes both an objective and a means of coping. This false belief, leading to 1) compulsive urges and tolerance, 2) frequent and intense exercise sessions at times when the urge becomes unbearable, and 3) exercise tolerance with short-duration relief after the completion of the exercise, represents a morbid pattern of the behavior. In contrast to eating disorders, exercise addiction involves losing control, the uncontrolled urge to exercise, and a compulsion fueled by false expectation(s). These are the morbid aspects of exercise behavior that are not usually observed in eating disorders, which is relatively common morbidity in contrast to exercise addiction.

This connotation is correct if one considers the bridge between instrumental exercise and exercise addiction. As Figure 10.1 depicts, a well-controlled

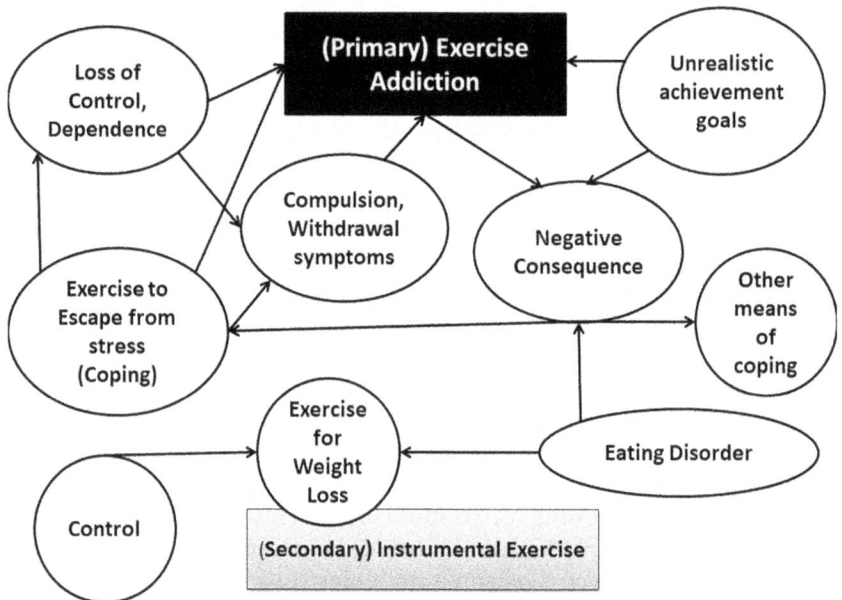

Figure 10.1 The diagram illustrates how instrumental exercise (known as secondary exercise dependence) might turn into (primary) exercise addiction, a form of addictive behavior.

exercise regimen serves for losing and *controlling* weight through burning calories. The number of calories to be burned needs to be calculated in caloric intake and expenditure as the sum of basal metabolism and physical activity. At a certain point, eating disorders are likely to culminate in adverse health, social, and psychological problems for which the already performed exercise *can* provide temporary (pain) relief. At this stage, exercise becomes a means of coping, and the person becomes dependent, exhibiting all the classic symptoms of primary exercise addiction.

Therefore, in contrast to Bamber et al. (2000), we suggest that *instrumental* exercise may turn into addiction (Figure 10.1) when the typical symptoms such as loss of control, dependence, and exercise deprivation-caused withdrawal symptoms are present. As stated, the instrumental exercise in other dysfunctions is not necessarily addictive. Consequently, the term *secondary addiction* is incorrect. Still, instrumental exercise might turn into an addiction, at which point it is no longer instrumental. This distinction, and the commonality between what is called in the literature as primary and secondary exercise dependence, might justify the need for using different terms for the two forms of morbid exercise patterns (Szabo et al., 2018), especially when compared to similar high loads of workouts regimens in athletic training.

10.6 Instrumental exercise in athletes

Given that athletes train on schedule and have little control over their exercise regimen, including exercise characteristics such as frequency, intensity, and duration, the presence of exercise addiction in the athletic population is probably sporadic. This argument can be justified by theoretical rationale; addictive behaviors, in general, are characterized by cravings and urges, which need immediate satisfaction for gratification. These urges cannot be satisfied on a prescribed schedule, like athletic training. Therefore, those who are disciplined enough to control their urges probably cannot be characterized as addicts. Once control is present and successfully applied to a behavior, it is inaccurate to talk about the presence of addiction. Therefore, unless athletes jump out of bed to exercise in the middle of the night or turn their back to life/survival activities to meet the urge of exercise, in addition to their training regimen, it may be illogical to suspect the presence of exercise addiction. Still, research suggests that athletes score higher than nonathletes on exercise addiction inventories. What could be the reason for their higher risk scores compared to recreational exercisers?

One conjecture is that athletes interpret exercise addiction assessment tools differently from nonathletes (Szabo et al., 2015; Szabo, 2018). Another explanation might be that athletes, especially those bound to weight control, are affected by eating disorders to a more considerable extent than leisure exercisers. Therefore, in addition to performance objectives, athletes set weight-control goals as parallel objectives to their training. Indeed, athletes may work harder or longer not merely for the sake of performance but the weight control essential in their sporting performance. Evidence suggests that the prevalence of eating disorders is *two to three times higher* in competitive and elite athletes than in the general population (Money-Taylor et al., 2021; Sundgot-Borgen & Torstveit, 2004). This figure, however, varies with the type and level of sports (Mancine et al., 2020).

Indeed, several studies found an inverse relationship between athletic status and eating disorders in college athletes (Hausenblas & McNally, 2004; Reinking, & Alexander, 2005). Still, the prevalence of disordered eating symptoms appears to be much greater among athletes who score in the *at-risk* category for exercise addiction than those who are not at risk. For example, in a recent study examining a Danish sample of elite athletes, the risk of eating disorders was more than 2.5 times higher in those at risk of exercise addiction than in athletes who were not in the at-risk category (Lichtenstein et al., 2021). Therefore, the higher prevalence of eating disorders and exercise addiction symptoms are coupled in athletes. The untangling of the personal and situational factors that predispose athletes to these 'twin symptoms' is necessary, but the task may prove difficult. Indeed, above and beyond certain personality factors, such as perfectionism (Çakın et al., 2021), athletic (situational) factors such as weight-bound sports, aerobic versus anaerobic training (Pálfi et al., 2021), or team versus individual sports (Haase, 2009; Kovacsik et al., 2018), numerous interactions, and mediating factors are present and influential.

Overall, disordered eating could be accompanied by instrumental exercise in *athletes*, translating into greater exercise addiction risk scores than in nonathletes. Research suggests that the prevalence of *instrumental exercise* is about four times greater than that of exercise addiction (Trott et al., 2020). Can instrumental exercise possibly be conceptualized as a precursor of exercise addiction in this population?

10.7 More reasons for *not* using the primary and secondary classification

Based on the aforementioned discussion, it is evident that (primary) exercise addiction refers to a morbid behavior in which gratification is the *direct* consequence of the exercise behavior. In contrast, secondary exercise dependence, what we call instrumental exercise, is linked to other disorders. A Swedish study with 330 sports and exercise participants investigated the hypothesis that high levels of anxiety, obsessive passion, and physical appearance orientation are associated with the risk for exercise addiction (Back et al., 2019). The researchers found that anxiety and obsessive passion predicted exercise addiction, with anxiety being a more robust predictor. On the basis of these findings, they concluded that a possible interpretation of their results is that the risk of developing exercise addiction could increase either from obsessive passion or as a strategy to cope with anxiety.

This dual path to the dysfunction might be classified as 1) 'primary' when an obsessive passion for exercise drives the disorder or as 2) 'secondary' when exercising functions as a strategy to cope with anxiety. This study's conclusion is an example of the possible different interpretations of the primary and secondary exercise addiction terms, creating possible confusion among the researchers, which is another reason why they should be abandoned.

10.8 Key points

1. Dependence is not the same as addiction, but it is a part of the latter.
2. Exercise addiction (primary) triggers immediate gratification, while instrumental exercise (secondary) is expected to yield delayed effects on body composition.
3. Dependence is a symptom while addiction is a mental dysfunction.
4. Secondary exercise dependence is a form of instrumental exercise.
5. Instrumental exercise can turn into exercise addiction over time.

10.9 References

Alcaraz-Ibáñez, M., Paterna, A., Sicilia, Á., & Griffiths, M. D. (2020). Morbid exercise behaviour and eating disorders: A meta-analysis. *Journal of Behavioral Addictions, 9*(2), 206–224. Doi:10.1556/2006.2020.00027

American Psychiatric Association. (2013). *Diagnostic and statistical manual of mental disorders* (5th ed.). Arlington, VA: Author.

Back, J., Josefsson, T., Ivarsson, A., & Gustafsson, H. (2019). Psychological risk factors for exercise dependence. *International Journal of Sport and Exercise Psychology*, 1–12. (Online first). Doi:10.1080/1612197X.2019.1674902

Bamber, D., Cockerill, I. M., & Carroll, D. (2000). The pathological status of exercise dependence. *British Journal of Sports Medicine, 34*(2), 125–132. Doi:10.1136/bjsm.34.2.125

Burke, E. (1998). *Precision heart rate training*. Champaign, IL: Human Kinetics.

Çakın, G., Juwono, I. D., Potenza, M. N., & Szabo, A. (2021). Exercise Addiction and Perfectionism: A Systematic Review of the Literature. *Current Addiction Reports, 8*(1), 144–155. Doi:10.1007/s40429-021-00358-8

Cook, B., Karr, T. M., Zunker, C., Mitchell, J. E., Thompson, R., Sherman, R., . . . Wonderlich, S. A. (2013). Primary and secondary exercise dependence in a community-based sample of road race runners. *Journal of Sport and Exercise Psychology, 35*(5), 464–469. Doi:10.1123/jsep.35.5.464

Di Lodovico, L., Poulnais, S., & Gorwood, P. (2019). Which sports are more at risk of physical exercise addiction: A systematic review. *Addictive Behaviors, 93*, 257–262. Doi:10.1016/j.addbeh.2018.12.030

Egorov, A. Y., & Szabo, A. (2013). The exercise paradox: An interactional model for a clearer conceptualization of exercise addiction. *Journal of Behavioral Addictions, 2*(4), 199–208. Doi:10.1556/jba.2.2013.4.2

Foster, A., Shorter, G., & Griffiths, M. (2015). Muscle dysmorphia: Could it be classified as an addiction to body image? *Journal of Behavioral Addictions, 4*(1), 1–5. Doi:10.1556/jba.3.2014.001

Goodman, A. (1990). Addiction: Definition and implications. *British Journal of Addiction*, *85*(11), 1403–1408. Doi:10.1111/j.1360-0443.1990.tb01620.x

Griffiths, M. D. (2005). A 'components' model of addiction within a biopsychosocial framework. *Journal of Substance Use*, *10*(4), 191–197. Doi:10.1080/14659890500 114359

Griffiths, M. D. (2013). Is "loss of control" always a consequence of addiction? *Frontiers in Psychiatry*, *4*. Doi:10.3389/fpsyt.2013.00036

Haase, A. M. (2009). Physique anxiety and disordered eating correlates in female athletes: Differences in team and individual sports. *Journal of Clinical Sport Psychology*, *3*(3), 218–231. Doi:10.1123/jcsp.3.3.218

Hausenblas, H. A., & McNally, K. D. (2004). Eating disorder prevalence and symptoms for track and field athletes and non-athletes. *Journal of Applied Sport Psychology*, *16*(3), 274–286. Doi:10.1080/10413200490485630

Höglund, K., & Normén, L. (2002). A high exercise load is linked to pathological weight control behavior and eating disorders in female fitness instructors. *Scandinavian Journal of Medicine & Science in Sports*, *12*(5), 261–275. Doi: 10.1034/j.1600-0838.2002.10323.x

Juwono, I. D., & Szabo, A. (2020). 100 cases of exercise addiction: More evidence for a widely researched but rarely identified dysfunction. *International Journal of Mental Health and Addiction*. Doi:10.1007/s11469-020-00264-6

Kotbagi, G., Muller, I., Romo, L., & Kern, L. (2014). Pratique problématique d'exercice physique: un cas clinique. *Annales Médico-Psychologiques, Revue Psychiatrique*, *172*(10), 883–887. doi:10.1016/j.amp.2014.10.011.

Kovacsik, R., Soós, I., de la Vega, R., Ruíz-Barquín, R., & Szabo, A. (2018). Passion and exercise addiction: Healthier profiles in team than in individual sports. *International Journal of Sport and Exercise Psychology*, *18*(2), 176–186. Doi:10.1080/1612 197x.2018.1486873

Lejoyeux, M., Avril, M., Richoux, C., Embouazza, H., & Nivoli, F. (2008). Prevalence of exercise dependence and other behavioral addictions among clients of a Parisian fitness room. *Comprehensive Psychiatry*, *49*(4), 353–358. Doi:10.1016/j.comppsych.2007.12.005

Lichtenstein, M. B., Melin, A. K., Szabo, A., & Holm, L. (2021). The prevalence of exercise addiction symptoms in a sample of national level elite athletes. *Frontiers in Sports and Active Living*, *3*. Doi:10.3389/fspor.2021.635418

Mancine, R. P., Gusfa, D. W., Moshrefi, A., & Kennedy, S. F. (2020). Prevalence of disordered eating in athletes categorized by emphasis on leanness and activity type – a systematic review. *Journal of Eating Disorders*, *8*(1). (Online first). Doi:10.1186/s40337-020-00323-2

Marques, A., Peralta, M., Sarmento, H., Loureiro, V., Gouveia, É. R., & Gaspar de Matos, M. (2018). Prevalence of risk for exercise dependence: A systematic review. *Sports Medicine*, *49*(2), 319–330. Doi:10.1007/s40279-018-1011-4

Martin, C. K., Johnson, W. D., Myers, C. A., Apolzan, J. W., Earnest, C. P., Thomas, D. M., . . . Church, T. S. (2019). Effect of different doses of supervised exercise on food intake, metabolism, and non-exercise physical activity: The E-MECHANIC randomized controlled trial. *The American Journal of Clinical Nutrition*, *110*(3), 583–592. Doi:10.1093/ajcn/nqz054

Money-Taylor, E., Dobbin, N., Gregg, R., Matthews, J. J., & Esen, O. (2021). Differences in attitudes, behaviours and beliefs towards eating between female bodybuilding athletes and non-athletes, and the implications for eating disorders and disordered eating. *Sport Sciences for Health.* (Online first). Doi:10.1007/s11332-021-00775-2

Mónok, K., Berczik, K., Urbán, R., Szabo, A., Griffiths, M. D., Farkas, J., . . . Demetrovics, Z. (2012). Psychometric properties and concurrent validity of two exercise addiction measures: A population-wide study. *Psychology of Sport and Exercise,* *13*(6), 739–746. doi:10.1016/j.psychsport.2012.06.003

Müller, A., Cook, B., Zander, H., Herberg, A., Müller, V., & de Zwaan, M. (2014). Does the German version of the Exercise Dependence Scale measure exercise dependence? *Psychology of Sport and Exercise,* *15*(3), 288–292. Doi:10.1016/j.psychsport.2013.12.003

Pálfi, V., Kovacsik, R., & Szabo, A. (2021). Symptoms of exercise addiction in aerobic and anaerobic exercises: Beyond the components model of addiction. *Addictive Behaviors Reports, 14,* 100369. Doi:10.1016/j.abrep.2021.100369

Reinking, M. F., & Alexander, L. E. (2005). Prevalence of disordered-eating behaviors in undergraduate female collegiate athletes and non-athletes. *Journal of Athletic Training, 40*(1), 47–51. PMID: 15902324

Sundgot-Borgen, J., & Torstveit, M. K. (2004). Prevalence of eating disorders in elite athletes is higher than in the general population. *Clinical Journal of Sport Medicine,* *14*(1), 25–32. Doi:10.1097/00042752-200401000-00005

Szabo, A. (2010). *Addiction to exercise: A symptom or a disorder?* New York, NY: Nova Science Publishers.

Szabo, A. (2013). Acute psychological benefits of exercise: Reconsideration of the placebo effect. *Journal of Mental Health, 22*(5), 449–455. Doi:10.3109/09638237.2012.734657

Szabo, A. (2018). Addiction, passion, or confusion? New theoretical insights on exercise addiction research from the case study of a female body builder. *Europe's Journal of Psychology, 14*(2), 296–316. Doi:10.5964/ejop.v14i2.1545

Szabo, A., Demetrovics, Z., & Griffiths, M. D. (2018). Morbid exercise behavior: Addiction or psychological escape? In H. Budde & M. Wegner (Eds.), *The exercise effect on mental health,* Chapter 11 (pp. 277–311). New York, NY: Routledge. Doi:10.4324/9781315113906-11

Szabo, A., Griffiths, M. D., Marcos, R. D. L. V., Mervó, B., & Demetrovics, Z. (2015). Methodological and conceptual limitations in exercise addiction research. *The Yale Journal of Biology and Medicine, 88*(3), 303–308.

Szabo, A., & Kovacsik, R. (2019). When passion appears, exercise addiction disappears. *Swiss Journal of Psychology, 78*(3–4), 137–142. Doi:10.1024/1421-0185/a000228

Trott, M., Jackson, S. E., Firth, J., Jacob, L., Grabovac, I., Mistry, A., . . . Smith, L. (2020). A comparative meta-analysis of the prevalence of exercise addiction in adults with and without indicated eating disorders. *Eating and Weight Disorders – Studies on Anorexia, Bulimia and Obesity, 26*(1), 37–46. Doi:10.1007/s40519-019-00842-1

Trott, M., Johnstone, J., McDermott, D. T., Mistry, A., & Smith, L. (2021). The development and validation of the secondary exercise addiction scale. *Eating and Weight Disorders – Studies on Anorexia, Bulimia and Obesity.* (Online first). Doi:10.1007/s40519-021-01284-4

Veale, D. (1995). Does primary exercise dependence really exist? In J. Annett, B. Cripps, & H. Steinberg (Eds.), *Exercise addiction: Motivation for participation in sport and exercise: Proceedings of British Psychology, Sport and Exercise Psychology Section* (pp. 71–75). Leicester, UK: British Psychological Society.

11 Psychophysiological models for exercise addiction

Currently, several models are trying to explain the phenomena of exercise addiction. They all complement each other, and some even share conceptual elements within their dimensions. However, the commonalities are not redundant. Instead, being presented from different perspectives expands the view and, consequently, the comprehension of exercise addiction by broadening our understanding through the emphasis of the most common overlapping elements. Therefore, one model may not be perceived as better than another but simply different. These models can be classified into two general categories: psychological and biological, which implicitly reflect the complementary nature of the extant theories.

11.1 Psychological models

11.1.1 The cognitive appraisal hypothesis

Szabo proposed an early psychological model (1995), which purports that exercise addiction surfaces when exercise becomes a means of coping with mental stress for an individual who has already experienced the stress-relieving benefits of exercise. According to this model, the repeated and often intensive and long-enduring exercise training sessions represent an escape from chronic or persisting stress. However, once the adopted exercise becomes the means of coping with stress, the person involved depends on it to function normally in everyday life. Therefore, when training is not possible for some reason, such as other urgent chores, injury, or illness, withdrawal symptoms occur, which yields additional stress. These withdrawal feelings, characterized by feeling unwell, nervousness, irritability, depression, anxiety, bad mood, lethargy, and other similar affective states, are experienced because the loss of exercise triggers the loss of control over the stressful situation. Therefore, the regular exerciser experiences greater vulnerability to stress through increased negative feelings associated with the inability to exercise. In addition, the augmenting emotional difficulty induces a desire or even craving for exercise to soothe the pain via the resumption of the previous exercise pattern, often at the expense

DOI: 10.4324/9781003173595-11

Exercise is the means of coping with unbearable stress

↓

Lack or exercise means loss of the coping mechanism

↓

Loss of control over the stressful situation

↓

Increased actual or perceived vulnerability to stress

↓

Psychological hardship (withdrawal symptoms)

↓

Strong urge for exercise

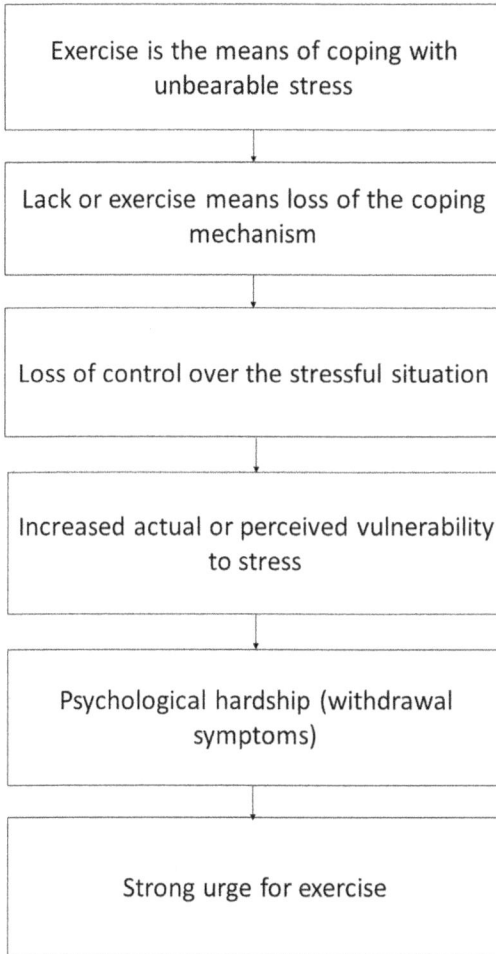

Figure 11.1 The cognitive arousal hypothesis (Szabo, 1995).

of other chores or obligations. Although this model perceives exercise addiction as a means of coping with or escape from stress, it only accounts for the persistence of addiction, but not for its onset. For example, it does not explain why the regular exerciser adopts exercise for coping instead of other means, such as drinking or taking drugs or medication. Accordingly, it does not consider personal factors such as perfectionism (Çakın et al., 2021), motivational factors (Kovácsik et al., 2020), and situational factors that hinder or facilitate the use of exercise for coping with stress. Still, the cognitive arousal hypothesis (Figure 11.1) is a robust model for the persistence of exercise addiction.

11.1.2 The four-phase model

The four-phase model for exercise addiction (Freimuth et al., 2011) is progressive. It is similar to the cognitive appraisal hypothesis, and it accounts for exercise addiction only if regular exercise is adopted for coping with stress. It depicts the progressive change from healthy exercise behavior into maladaptive or addictive exercise. The pleasurable activity characterizes the first phase while the behavior is under control. There are no negative consequences in this phase in general, but rarely muscles soreness or minor strains may occur. In phase two, the psychological benefits of exercise are used especially for mood modification or emotion regulation. Addiction is likely to occur when exercise becomes the primary or the sole means of coping with stress. This part of the model attempts to identify the onset of exercise addiction or the transition from healthy into dysfunctional exercise. Still, it does not specify two critical issues: 1) some distress must exist, whether progressively mounting or suddenly appearing, and b) under what conditions or influences will exercise specifically be adopted for emotion regulation? The third phase involves the onset of a morbid pattern of exercise. It is characterized by the rigid organization of daily activities around exercise, which assumes a primary role in the affected person's life. In this phase, negative consequences may already occur due to excessive exercise. Further, other exercises could be performed either to replace or to complement the usual mode of exercise. Finally, exercise is performed individually, rather than with friends, in a team, or during scheduled fitness classes. Furthermore, the fourth and last stage embeds the typical symptoms of addiction like salience, tolerance, conflict, need for mood modification, withdrawal symptoms, and relapse (Griffiths, 2005).

The four phases (Figure 11.2) were developed to aid clinicians in deciding whether the exercise behavior is healthy, or it is becoming addictive, and when the addictive exercise becomes healthy again. Each phase has three components: motivation (the person's incentive for exercise in that stage), consequences, and frequency/control. Still, the model does not account for the onset and motive beyond emotion regulation. Moreover, it does not explain who and why will become addicted to exercise, which is a shortcoming similar to the cognitive appraisal hypothesis.

11.1.3 The interactional model for exercise addiction

A person-specific model forwarded for the etiology of exercise addiction is the interactional model (Egorov & Szabo, 2013). The model suggests that an interaction between personal values, social image, past exercise experience, and life situation jointly determine whether one will use exercise for coping or resort to other means of dealing with stress. The possible number of interactions between personal and situational factors is vast, and consequently, each case reflects an idiographic mental schema resembling

```
┌─────────────────────────────────────────────┐
│                                               │
│        Phase One: Recreational Exercise       │
│          Rewarding, enjoyable exercise        │
│                                               │
│                                               │
└─────────────────────────────────────────────┘
                       │
                       ▼
┌─────────────────────────────────────────────┐
│                                               │
│           Phase Two: At-Risk Exercise         │
│  Stress-relieving effects of exercise consciously │
│          adopted when the need arises         │
│                                               │
└─────────────────────────────────────────────┘
                       │
                       ▼
┌─────────────────────────────────────────────┐
│                                               │
│        Phase Three: Problematic Exercise      │
│   Life-activities are organized around exercise and │
│        certain negative consequences occur    │
│                                               │
└─────────────────────────────────────────────┘
                       │
                       ▼
┌─────────────────────────────────────────────┐
│                                               │
│          Phase Four: Exercise Addiction       │
│    Loss of control, withdrawal symptoms occur, │
│     and the whole life revolves around exercise │
│                                               │
└─────────────────────────────────────────────┘
```

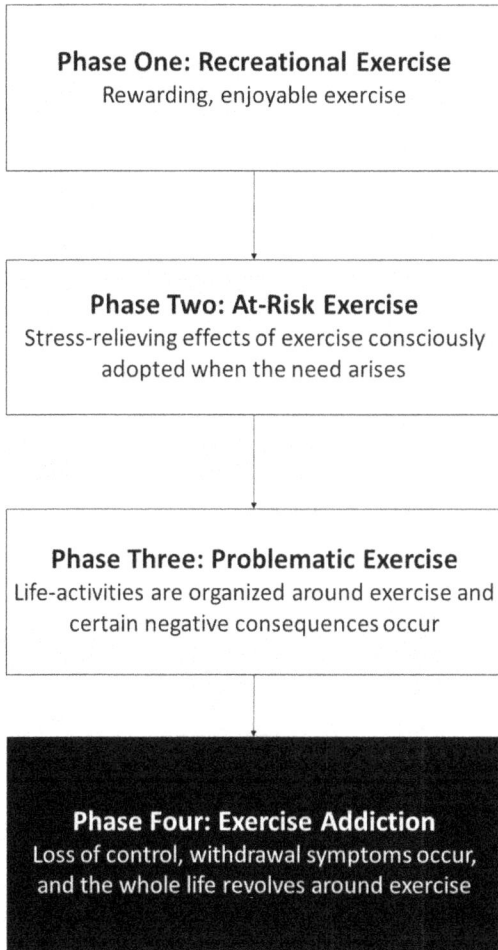

Figure 11.2 The four-phase model for exercise addiction (Freimuth et al., 2011).

a unique *black box* (Figure 11.3). This box is profoundly subjective and can be opened only following a clinical evaluation performed by a mental health professional. Indeed, unlike other chemical or behavioral addictions (except work addiction if the work is physical), exercise addiction has a unique characteristic not present in other addictions, which is the *physical effort* or energy cost.

In the interactional model, a set of personal factors interacts with several situational factors to determine the primary motive for exercise behavior (Figure 11.3). These motives diverge in two directions (Robbins & Joseph, 1985). A health (mental or physical)-motivated individual, for example,

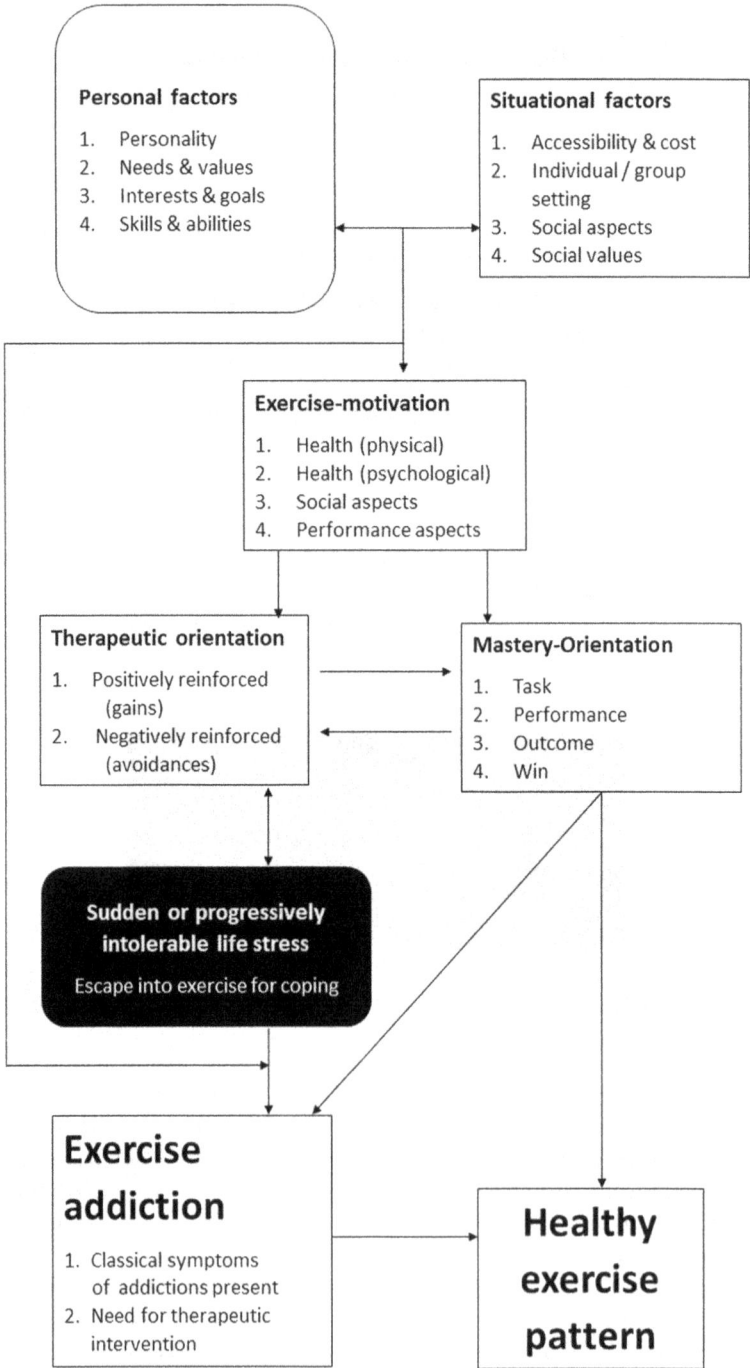

Figure 11.3 The interactional model of exercise addiction (Egorov & Szabo, 2013).

may run for better or improved health (gain health) or to prevent ill health consequences like gaining weight and being lethargic. Both incentives are therapeutic. However, health motives could also have a mastery orientation, like becoming stronger and lifting more weight (performance orientations), concentrating better, and being more productive at work. If better concentration were the aim, a therapeutic orientation would apply, but mastery orientation is the driving force if the expected consequence of the better concentration is performance-related. A vital element is a suddenly emerging reaction, determined by a set of idiographic (i.e., personal and situational) interactions in the black box. This reaction is a response to an ongoing or suddenly appearing life stressor, which causes psychological pain. This component suggests that exercise addiction is not evolutionary or slowly progressing but rather *revolutionary* or suddenly surfacing (Szabo, 2010).

Based on earlier laboratory evidence, exercise could be a cathartic buffer for stress (Szabo & Tsang, 2003). Recently, using a within-participants counterbalanced design, Szabo and his colleagues (2021) found that young research participants walked or jogged faster after artificially induced mental stress than after a control session. The authors proposed a *flight or fight* response to psychosocial stress, which surfaces in a cathartic reaction after the stress exposure. The interactional model purports the conscious use of exercise for coping with stress. Still, it does not rule out the initial subconscious effects that become conscious over time through the repeated experience of *relief from tension*. The switch point may reflect the revolutionary onset of the addiction. Habitual exercisers, when experiencing stress – knowing the mood-improving effects of exercise from experience (Freimuth et al., 2011) – might then resort to exercise to cope with the hardship.

However, not all habitual exercisers will resort to excessive training to reduce stress but instead might adopt passive forms of coping/escape behaviors or chemical addiction(s). Therefore, the interactional model adds particular weight to the personal circumstances that interact with social environmental factors and, therefore, provides a comprehensive view of the genesis of exercise addiction in the affected individuals. Indeed, a positive link was noted between exercise addiction risk scores and personal factors such as trait anxiety (Bircher et al., 2017; Coen & Ogles, 1993), perfectionism (Bircher et al., 2017; Cook, 1996; Lichtenstein et al., 2017), and obsessive compulsiveness (Lichtenstein et al., 2017; Spano, 2001). Furthermore, it appears that neuroticism and extroversion could predict symptoms of exercise addiction (Cook et al., 2020; Hausenblas & Giacobbi Jr., 2004). Finally, gender (Cook et al., 2013) and sex-role orientation (Rejeski et al., 1987) might also have mediating roles. Therefore, many possible combinations of psychological factors interacting with situational variables may render it difficult – if not impossible – to scrutinize exercise addiction using a *nomothetic* approach. Therefore, the interactional model (Figure 11.3) purports that every case of exercise addiction is unique. Consequently, it is best understood via *idiographic* analysis.

11.1.4 The revised interactional model

The interactional model has been recently revised and expended (Dinardi et al., 2021). Like the original model, the revised model includes 'personal factors' and 'situational factors.' Within these domains, the factors represent personal needs and environmental influences. Although not explicitly stated, this conceptualization follows the basic concept of the self-determination theory (Deci & Ryan, 1980; Vallerand, 2000); the individual's motivational orientation results from the interaction of personal and environmental factors. The self-determination theory is a valuable framework for studying exercise motivation.

In the revised model, the domain of 'personal factors' was expanded to include self-concept. This factor is the cognitive reflection of one's self-appraisal that contains ideas, attitudes, and judgments people use to make sense of the world, focus on their goals, understand their self-worth, and decide which aspects of themselves are valuable (Leary & Tangney, 2012). Self-concept could also include elements of identity (e.g., being an athlete) in addition to the appraisals of the self (e.g., being fat). This self-construction is relevant in positively or negatively shaping exercise behavior (de la Vega et al., 2016; Reifsteck et al., 2016; Woolf & Lawrence, 2017). In addition, the domain of 'situational factors' was also expanded with the item '*attractive alternatives.*' This factor considers why an individual chooses to engage in exercise (e.g., for stress management) instead of other alternative activities. Therefore, the situational factors listed in the revised model now resemble more to those described in the Sport Commitment Model (Scanlan et al., 2003). Indeed, the newly added factor, 'attractive alternatives,' is a component of this model.

The domain 'incentives for exercise' was presented in the original model as exercise motivation (Figure 11.3). Its name was changed for semantic accuracy. Four factors were added to the list, the first of which is enjoyment. Enjoyment is often the foremost reason that people exercise (Rodrigues et al., 2020). Second, seeking challenge is another common incentive for exercise, particularly among people who participate in challenging sports and activities, such as ultradistance running, triathlon, cycling, adventure racing, and other endurance sports (Simpson et al., 2017). Those who seek challenges may feel bored in other areas of their lives, disenchanted by mundane routines, or curious about finding their limits. Third, some individuals may also pursue risky activities to experience certain sensations such as feelings of connection with nature, a natural 'high' transcendence, and even suffering (Nogueira et al., 2018). Flow states are often referred to as the ultimate human experience, which can be achieved in various sports and exercise activities (Csikszentmihalyi &

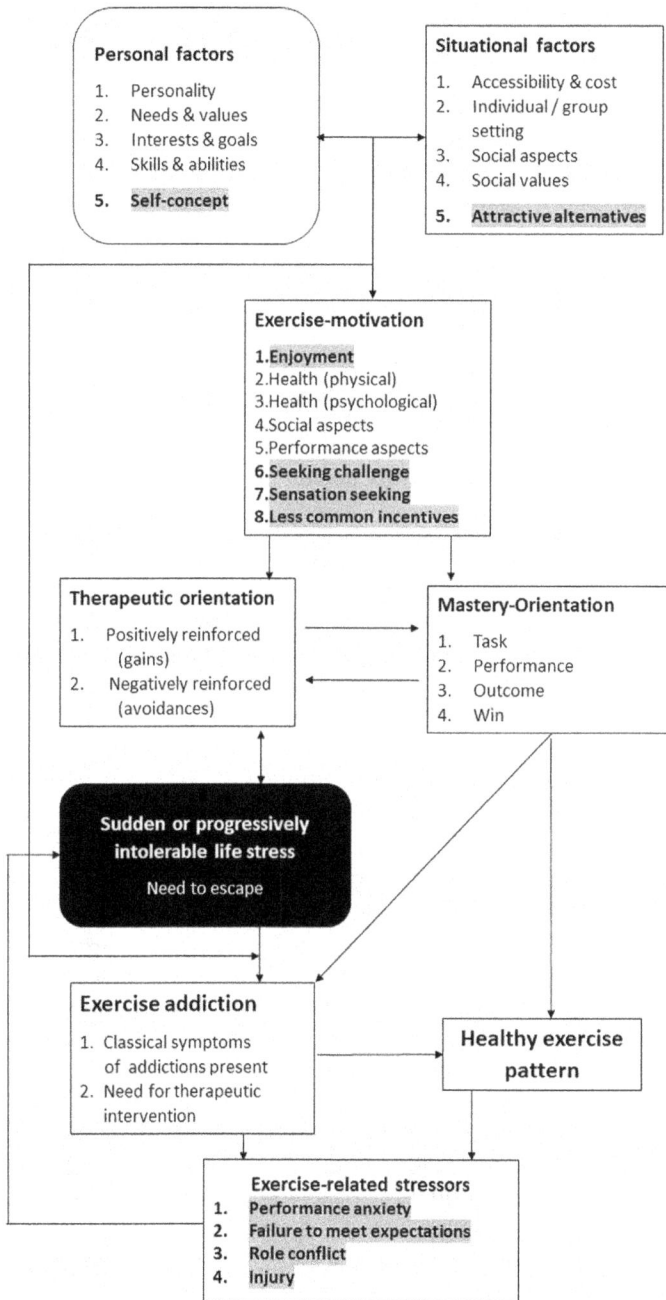

Figure 11.4 The expanded interactional model of exercise addiction (Dinardi et al., 2021). The new elements in the model are highlighted.

Csikzentmihaly, 1990). Last, the factor 'less common reasons' was also added to the revised model to account for the highly idiographic reasons. With the addition of these items, the revised model covers a broader range of incentives for exercise.

'Exercise-related stressors' is a new domain in the revised interactional model. This domain interacts with 'sudden or progressively intolerable stress.' By including this concept, the model accounts for stress resulting from involvement in sports or exercise. Not only is this antithetical to the idea of exercising to relieve stress, but it also necessitates additional stress-coping responses. Individuals who use exercise to escape from stress may result in spiraling further into a pattern of avoidance and escape, creating a dangerous vicious circle. Factors included in this domain are performance anxiety, failure to meet expectations, role conflict, and injury. The last one is a commonly reported factor in exercise addiction.

11.1.5 The Pragmatics, Attraction, Communication, Expectation model

The interactional model for exercise addiction (Dinardi et al., 2021; Egorov & Szabo, 2013) largely agrees with an earlier proposed model, known as the 'Pragmatics, Attraction, Communication, Expectation' (PACE) model, which was forwarded as *a general model* for all addictions (Sussman et al., 2011). When the situation gets out of control, a person might 'gravitate' toward a means of *available coping* reflecting the 'Pragmatics' phase of the PACE model (Sussman et al., 2011; see Figure 11.5). The choice is determined by conscious and subconscious decisions between individuals' characteristics, situational factors, life event antecedents, and current exercise behavior, fitting into the 'Attraction' component of the PACE model. Accordingly, even mastery-oriented exercisers may, at one moment, shift focus to the therapeutic aspects of exercise and get more involved in it to get rid of distress. This change in the attentional focus aligns well with the 'Communication' part of the PACE model, in which experience, interpersonal influences, intrapersonal thoughts, beliefs, and personal convictions all influence the escape path or the means of coping person. For example, lack of experience with alcohol, tobacco, or leisure drugs in conjunction with long exercise history and positive beliefs about exercise (from media, friends, and health values) all interact with unique personal factors during the effort of coping. Therefore, an already 'therapeutic' exerciser in the model is more likely to choose exercise behavior as a means of coping. Then, also in agreement with the PACE model, the greater is the expectation linked to exercise, the more unlikely the exerciser will turn to other forms of addiction. Perceived as a 'positive addiction' (Glasser, 1976), it is much easier to hide behind exercise while maintaining one's reputation in the social environment, unlike other forms of addictions bearing a negative social stigma. The PACE model is illustrated in Figure 11.5.

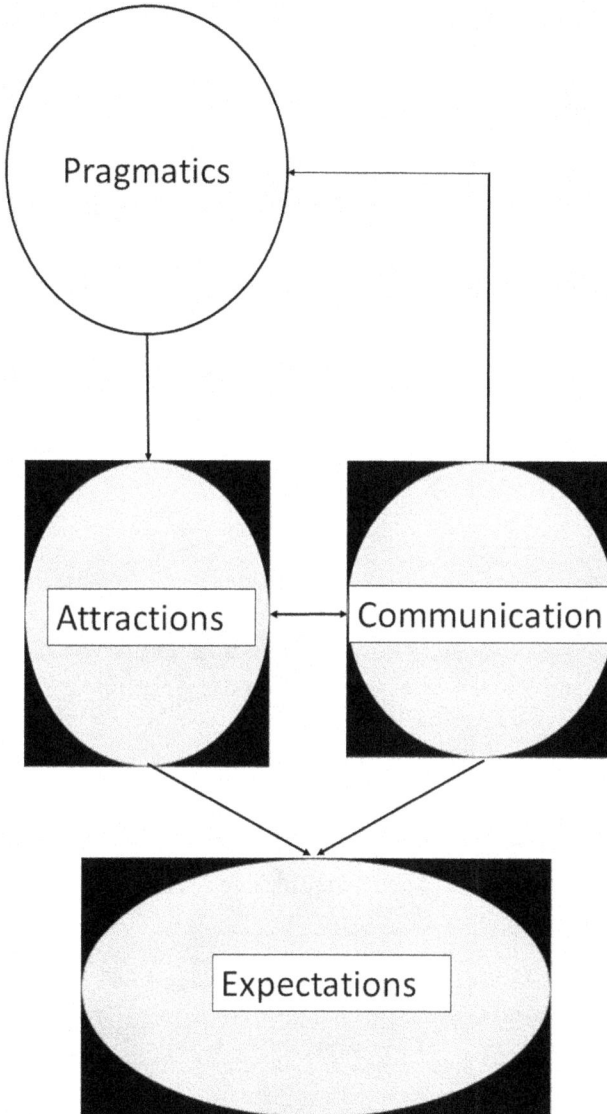

Figure 11.5 Pragmatics, Attraction, Communication, Expectation (PACE) model (Sussman et al., 2011).

11.1.6 The passion model

The most recent psychological model for exercise addiction is the passion model (Lichtenstein et al., 2020b). Recent research has shown a significant overlap between the risk of exercise addiction and passion (Kovacsik et al., 2018a, 2018b; Kovácsik et al., 2020; Lichtenstein et al., 2020a; Lichtenstein et al., 2020b; Parastatidou et al., 2014; Sicilia et al., 2017; Szabo, 2018). In fact, Szabo (2018) proposed that a high risk of exercise addiction often only reflects a high level of commitment and passion for sport and exercise. Lichtenstein et al. (2020b) produced evidence for the three dimensions of passion. They suggested that there is a progressive transition from commitment into the three stages of passion that, in some cases, may culminate in addiction. Based on this conjecture, the model appears to be adequate for explaining the passion–addiction relationship. However, it is still tentative because it is based on a single cross-sectional study of 1225 Danish fitness participants. The passion model is illustrated in Figure 11.6.

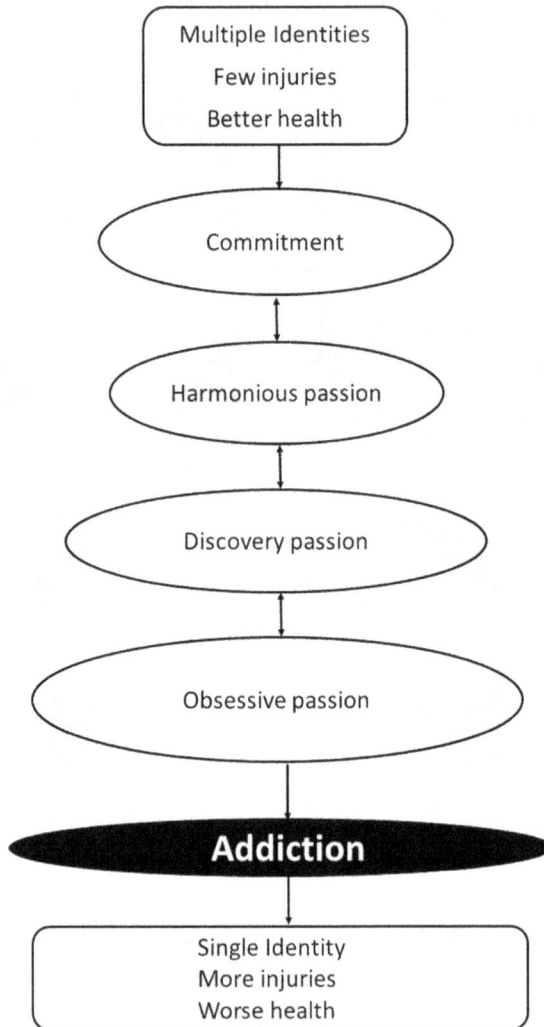

Figure 11.6 The passion model of exercise addiction (Lichtenstein et al., 2020b).

It is a hierarchical model starting from healthy to unhealthy exercise. Commitment and harmonious passion reflect the dedication and enjoyment of the activity in harmony with the person's life. Discovery passion refers to the novelty aspects of the training that yield a subjective reward ranging from avoiding boredom to coping with stress. Finally, obsessive passion surfaces when the individual becomes obsessed with the activity, in this case, exercise. This stage can turn into full-blown addiction, but the factors inducing such a shift are unclear. If addiction occurs, all the typical symptoms and consequences of addictive behaviors also occur. The passion model is a hypothetical psychological model that accounts for the transition in the person's affinity for exercise that could progressively lead to dysfunctional behavior. Its shortcoming is that it does not identify the factors that induce such changes, and therefore the model requires expansion and empirical scrutiny. In the last chapter, we present a modified, less hierarchical version, of the model.

11.2 Biological models

11.2.1 The sympathetic arousal hypothesis

The sympathetic arousal hypothesis is an early physiological model based on bodily adaptation to exercise. Accordingly, the sympathetic adaptation to regular exercise lowers the overall level of arousal (Thompson & Blanton, 1987). Lower levels of arousal may be associated with lethargic, sluggish, or low-energy states. This uncomfortable feeling prompts the person to increase the level of arousal. For the regular exercisers, their exercise activity is the most tangible way to increase arousal. However, since the arousal mediating effects of exercise are relatively short-lasting, increased volumes of exercise are necessary within relatively short periods to generate an optimal state of arousal, leading to tolerance and the onset of an addictive pattern of exercising. An issue with this model is that the sympathetic adaptation to exercise occurs in every regular exerciser while not all exercisers become addicted. The model is illustrated in Figure 11.7.

11.2.2 The biopsychosocial model

The biopsychosocial model differs from several conceptualizations of exercise addiction. This model suggests that certain biological factors, especially Body Mass Index (BMI), mediate the development and maintenance of exercise addiction (McNamara & McCabe, 2012). In this model, the biological factors are closely interconnected with social and psychological factors, which contribute to the etiology of exercise addiction. Social factors in the model may include the coach–athlete relationship, teammate pressure, inequality, cohesion, sociocultural pressure, and social support. Self-esteem and beliefs about exercise generally characterize psychological factors. In the biopsychosocial model of exercise addiction, social forces share a

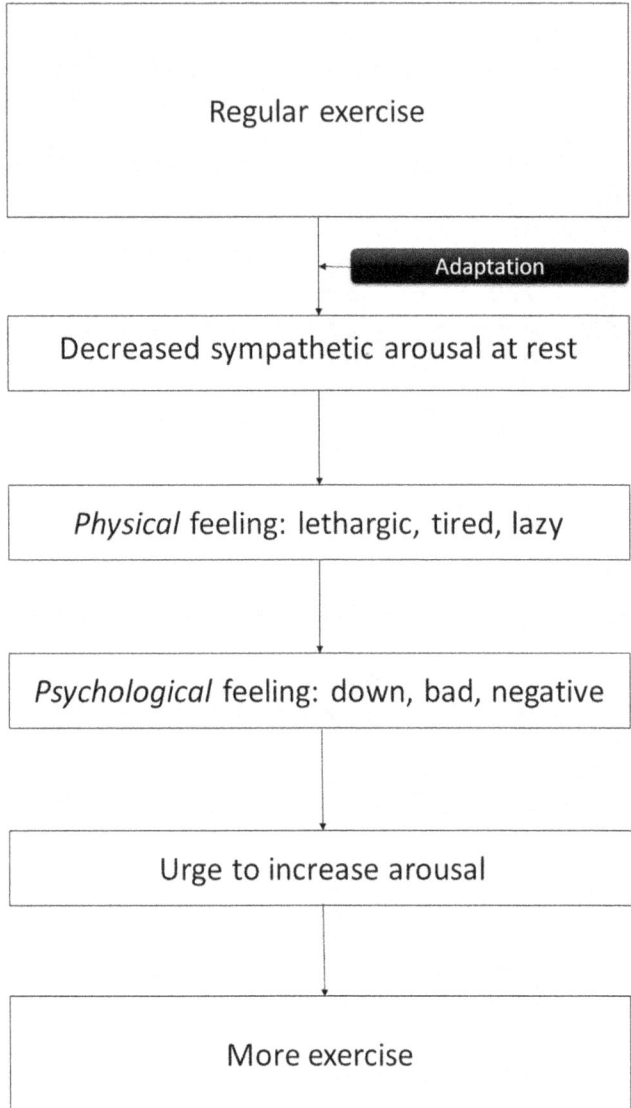

Figure 11.7 The sympathetic arousal hypothesis (Thompson & Blanton, 1987).

reciprocal relationship with psychological factors (Figure 11.8). It is conjectured that the social and psychological factors interact to mediate the onset and maintenance of exercise addiction. This model was forwarded to explain exercise addiction in elite athletes (McNamara & McCabe, 2012).

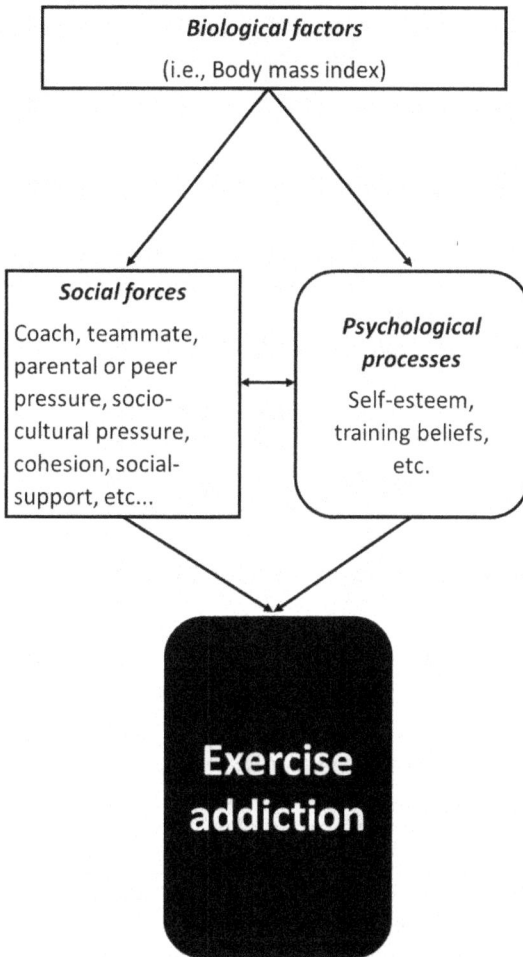

Figure 11.8 The biopsychosocial model (McNamara & McCabe, 2012).

At its core, BMI, as a biological factor, might be the route of the origin of exercise addiction in elite athletes. The interaction between social and psychological processes then determines whether exercise (sport) addiction occurs or not. This interaction is linked to socially and psychologically demanding athletic training at high levels of competition. However, Freimuth et al. (2011) clarified that hard training for long hours and ambitious strivings for a noble goal to become the best – which characterizes successful elite athletes – should not be confused with the symptoms of addiction. The model is illustrated in Figure 11.8.

11.2.3 The interleukin 6 model

Another physiological model has highlighted the possible role of interleukin 6 (IL-6) in exercise addiction (Hamer & Karageorghis, 2007). The IL-6 is a pro-inflammatory and anti-inflammatory cytokine secreted by T-cells and macrophages to increase the immune response to trauma, such as burning or other types of tissue damage leading to inflammation. The blood concentration level of IL-6 increases during exercise (Aguiló et al., 2014), and higher levels of IL-6 are often associated with increased cardiovascular mortality, depression, and negative affect (Puterman et al., 2013). Hamer and Karageorghis (2007) suggest that IL-6 links the periphery to the brain. This link may mediate the components of exercise addiction. For example, in people prone to dysfunctional exercise, a workout results in a momentary reduction in negative feeling states; However, at the same time, it raises the synthesis of IL-6 and activates the neuroendocrine pathways, which contribute to other negative feelings manifested through the experiencing of withdrawal symptoms. Therefore, exercise acts as a vicious circle by lowering and increasing negative affect. This model is based on a psycho-neuroimmunological relationship between the body and the brain that deserves further research attention. This model is presented in Figure 11.9.

11.2.4 The monoamine model

The monoamine model is based on the empirical observation that exercise triggers increased catecholamine levels in the peripheral circulation (Cousineau et al., 1977). For example, a 30-minute bout of medium- to high-intensity aerobic exercise was shown to increase the uric phenylacetic acid levels – reflecting the phenylethylamine concentration – in healthy males habituated to exercise (Szabo et al., 2001). While catecholamines, among other functions, are involved in the stress response, phenylethylamine is more closely linked to changes in mood. The monoamine hypothesis implies that in addition to an increase in monoamines in the peripheral circulation, the central aminergic activity may also rise in response to exercise. Since brain monoamines are involved in the regulation of mood and affect, their alteration by exercise seems to be an attractive explanation for the role of exercise in stress response. This monoamine model is a biological explanation for exercise addiction that is probably more closely linked to the positive mood-enhancing effects of exercise than exercise addiction *per se*. However, considering this model, exercise may act as a buffer of stress in the addiction process because the positive effects of exercise soak up the negative emotional experiences resulting from life stress.

11.2.5 The endorphin model

This endorphin model is perhaps the most popular in the literature. It posits that exercise leads to increased levels of β-endorphins in the brain,

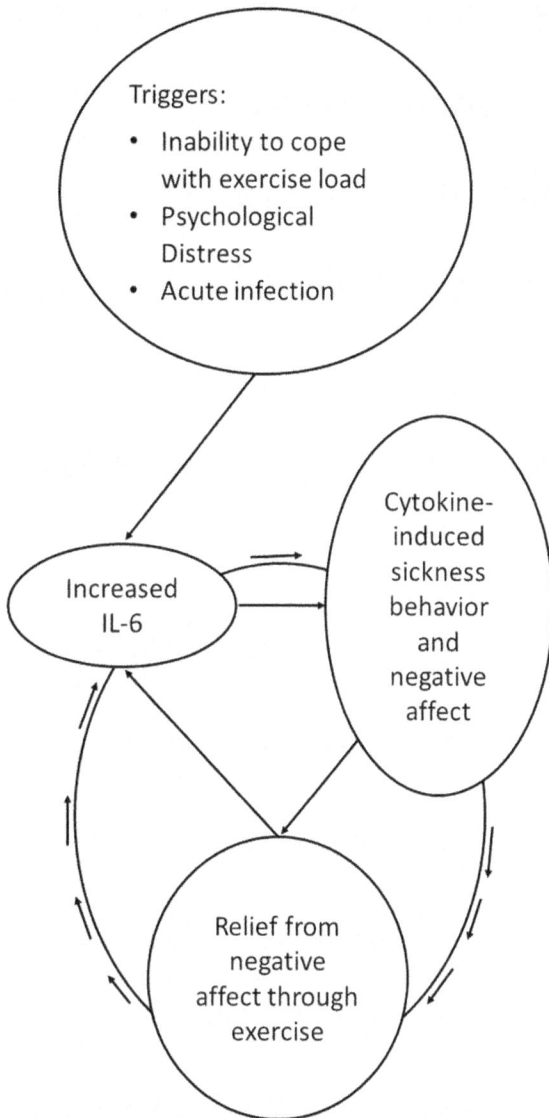

Figure 11.9 The interleukin 6 (IL-6) model (Hamer & Karageorghis, 2007).

which act as internal psychoactive agents by generating feelings of euphoria. This hypothesis may be analogous to the substance or recreational drug addiction (e.g., heroin and morphine) except that the psychoactive agent (β-endorphin) is generated *internally* during exercise instead of being administered externally. Endogenous opioids are involved in modulating several sensory, motivational, emotional, and mental functions (McNally & Akil, 2002). In support of the model, a study with positron emission tomography found that exercise performed between the aerobic and anaerobic threshold for 60 minutes increased the availability of μ-opioid receptors in the anterior cingulate cortex, prefrontal cortex, and temporal cortex of young, healthy recreational exercising men (Saanijoki et al., 2014). While further research in this area is needed, the opioid response to exercise is likely to be workload- or dose-dependent in addition to individual variability. It could be one of the several explanations for exercise addiction in relationship with stress management.

11.3 What do the models tell us about exercise addiction?

As noted at the beginning of this chapter, the presented models are not 'standalone' explanations for the etiology and persistence of exercise addiction. The cognitive arousal hypothesis explains the withdrawal symptoms-caused urges in the process of addiction. The sympathetic arousal hypothesis and the monoamine and endorphin models account for the feeling good effect of exercise that is universally reported. With adaptation to exercise, the various routines become easier, and the practitioner experiences feelings of mastery and success, which is complemented by changes in brain neurotransmitters exacerbating these good feelings. The bunch of positive feelings is paralleled by increased body temperature leading to physical (and consequently mental) relaxation, and based on a thermogenic hypothesis (Koltyn, 1997), this psychophysiological relief could mediate the stress-coping in exercise addiction. IL-6 is also produced to modulate mood and other feeling states. The stress-relieving effects of exercise emerge indirectly by making the exerciser feel good despite experiencing stress. The interactional model then predicts that personal factors will determine how these exercise benefits will be used in individual situations. For example, the addictive path to exercise would surface with significant stress and trauma and if personal factors facilitate that. Altogether, the complex changes in the psychophysiological system, experienced because of exercise, yield unique effects that interact with specific situational factors. This is the reason why the interactional model recommends an idiographic approach to the understanding of exercise addiction.

11.4 Key points

1. There are several psychological and physiological models for exercise addiction.
2. Models of exercise addiction complement each other but have a narrow focus.
3. None of the models can be generalized because exercise addiction is idiographic.

4. The interactional model accounts for the idiographic nature of exercise addiction.
5. The idiographic aspect of exercise addiction obscures its scientific investigation.

11.5 References

Aguiló, A., Monjo, MM., Moreno, C., Martinez, P., Martínez, S., & Tauler, P. (2014). Vitamin C supplementation does not influence plasma and blood mononuclear cell IL-6 and IL-10 levels after exercise'. *Journal of Sports Sciences, 32*(17), 1659–1669. Doi:10.1080/02640414.2014.912759.

Bircher, J., Kasos, K., Demetrovics, Z., Griffiths, M. D., & Szabo, A. (2017). Exercise addiction and personality: A two-decade systematic review of the empirical literature (1995–2016). *Baltic Journal of Sports and Health Sciences, 3*(106), 19–33.

Çakın, G., Juwono, I. D., Potenza, M. N., & Szabo, A. (2021). Exercise addiction and perfectionism: A systematic review of the literature. *Current Addiction Reports, 8*(1), 144–155. Doi:10.1007/s40429-021-00358-8

Coen, S. P., & Ogles, B. M. (1993). Psychological characteristics of the obligatory runner: A critical examination of the anorexia analogue hypothesis. *Journal of Sport and Exercise Psychology, 15*(3), 338–354. Doi:10.1123/jsep.15.3.338

Cook, B., Hausenblas, H., & Rossi, J. (2013). The moderating effect of gender on ideal-weight goals and exercise dependence symptoms. *Journal of Behavioral Addictions, 2*(1), 50–55. Doi:10.1556/jba.1.2012.010

Cook, C. A. (1996). *The psychological correlates of exercise dependence in aerobics instructors.* Unpublished master's thesis. University of Alberta, Alberta, Canada

Cook, R. H., Griffiths, M. D., & Pontes, H. M. (2020). Personality factors in exercise addiction: A pilot study exploring the role of narcissism, extraversion, and agreeableness. *International Journal of Mental Health and Addiction, 18*(1), 89–102. Doi:10.1007/s11469-018-9939-z

Cousineau, D., Ferguson, R. J., de Champlain, J., Gauthier, P., Cote, P., & Bourassa, M. (1977). Catecholamines in coronary sinus during exercise in man before and after training. *Journal of Applied Physiology, 43*(5), 801–806.

Csikszentmihalyi, M., & Csikzentmihaly, M. (1990). *Flow: The psychology of optimal experience.* New York, NY: Harper & Row.

Deci, E. L., & Ryan, R. M. (1980). Self-determination theory: When mind mediates behavior. *The Journal of Mind and Behavior,* 33–43.

De la Vega, R., Parastatidou, I. S., Ruíz-Barquín, R., & Szabo, A. (2016). Exercise addiction in athletes and leisure exercisers: The moderating role of passion. *Journal of Behavioral Addictions, 5*(2), 325–331. Doi:10.1556/2006.5.2016.043

Dinardi, J. S., Egorov, A. Y., & Szabo, A. (2021). The expanded interactional model of exercise addiction. *Journal of Behavioral Addictions, 10*(3), 626–631. Doi:10.1556/2006.2021.00061

Egorov, A. Y., & Szabo, A. (2013). The exercise paradox: An interactional model for a clearer conceptualization of exercise addiction. *Journal of Behavioral Addictions, 2*(4), 199–208. Doi:10.1556/jba.2.2013.4.2

Freimuth, M., Moniz, S., & Kim, S. R. (2011). Clarifying exercise addiction: Differential diagnosis, co-occurring disorders, and phases of addiction. *International Journal of Environmental Research and Public Health, 8*(10), 4069–4081. Doi:10.3390/ijerph8104069

Glasser, W. (1976). *Positive addiction*. New York, NY: Harper & Row.

Griffiths, M. D. (2005). A 'components' model of addiction within a biopsychosocial framework. *Journal of Substance Use, 10*(4), 191–197. Doi:10.1080/14659890 500114359

Hamer, M., & Karageorghis, C. I. (2007). Psychobiological mechanisms of exercise dependence. *Sports Medicine, 37*(6), 477–484. Doi:10.2165/00007256-2007370 60-00002

Hausenblas, H. A., & Giacobbi Jr, P. R. (2004). Relationship between exercise dependence symptoms and personality. *Personality and Individual Differences, 36*(6), 1265–1273. Doi:10.1016/S0191-8869(03)00214-9

Koltyn, K. F. (1997). The thermogenic hypothesis. In W. P. Morgan (Ed.), *Physical activity and mental health* (pp. 213–226). Washington, DC: Taylor and Francis.

Kovacsik, R., Griffiths, M. D., Pontes, H. M., Soós, I., de la Vega, R., Ruíz-Barquín, R., . . . Szabo, A. (2018a). The role of passion in exercise addiction, Exercise volume, and exercise intensity in long-term exercisers. *International Journal of Mental Health and Addiction, 17*(6), 1389–1400. Doi:10.1007/s11469-018-9880-1

Kovacsik, R., Soós, I., de la Vega, R., Ruíz-Barquín, R., & Szabo, A. (2018b). Passion and exercise addiction: Healthier profiles in team than in individual sports. *International Journal of Sport and Exercise Psychology, 18*(2), 176–186. Doi:10.1080/1612 197x.2018.1486873

Kovácsik, R., Tóth-Király, I., Egorov, A., & Szabo, A. (2020). A longitudinal study of exercise addiction and passion in new sport activities: The impact of motivational factors. *International Journal of Mental Health and Addiction.* Doi:10.1007/ s11469-020-00241-z

Leary, M. R., & Tangney, J. P. (Eds.). (2012). *Handbook of self and identity*. New York, NY: Guilford Press.

Lichtenstein, M. B., Hinze, C. J., Emborg, B., Thomsen, F., & Hemmingsen, S. D. (2017). Compulsive exercise: Links, risks and challenges faced. *Psychology Research and Behavior Management, 10*, 85–95. Doi:10.2147/PRBM.S113093

Lichtenstein, M. B., Jensen, E. S., Larsen, P. V., Omdahl, M. K., & Szabo, A. (2020b). Passion for exercise has three dimensions: Psychometric evaluation of The Passion Scale in a Danish fitness sample. *Translational Sports Medicine.* (Online first). Doi:10.1002/tsm2.173

Lichtenstein, M. B., Jensen, E. S., & Szabo, A. (2020a). Exercise addiction, obsessive passion, and the use of nutritional supplements in fitness center attendees. *Translational Sports Medicine, 3*(3), 188–195. Doi:10.1002/tsm2.131

McNally, G. P., & Akil, H. (2002). Role of corticotropin-releasing hormone in the amygdala and bed nucleus of the stria terminalis in the behavioral, pain modulatory, and endocrine consequences of opiate withdrawal. *Neuroscience, 112*(3), 605–617. Doi:10.1016/S0306-4522(02)00105-7

McNamara, J., & McCabe, M. P. (2012). Striving for success or addiction? Exercise dependence among elite Australian athletes. *Journal of Sports Sciences, 30*(8), 755–766. Doi:10.1080/02640414.2012.667879

Nogueira, A., Molinero, O., Salguero, A., & Márquez, S. (2018). Exercise addiction in practitioners of endurance sports: A literature review. *Frontiers in Psychology, 9*, 1484. doi:10.3389/fpsyg.2018.01484

Parastatidou, I. S., Doganis, G., Theodorakis, Y., & Vlachopoulos, S. P. (2014). The mediating role of passion in the relationship of exercise motivational regulations with exercise dependence symptoms. *International Journal of Mental Health and Addiction, 12*(4), 406–419. Doi:10.1007/s11469-013-9466-x

Puterman, E., Epel, E. S., O'Donovan, A., Prather, A. A., Aschbacher, K., & Dhabhar, F. S. (2013). Anger is associated with increased IL-6 stress reactivity in women, but only among those low in social support'. *International Journal of Behavioral Medicine, 21*(6), 936–945. Doi:10.1007/s12529-013-9368-0

Reifsteck, E. J., Gill, D. L., & Labban, J. D. (2016). "Athletes" and "exercisers": Understanding identity, motivation, and physical activity participation in former college athletes. *Sport, Exercise, and Performance Psychology, 5*(1), 25–38. doi:10.1037/spy0000046

Rejeski, W. J., Best, D. L., Griffith, P., & Kenney, E. (1987). Sex-role orientation and the responses of men to exercise stress. *Research Quarterly for Exercise and Sport, 58*(3), 260–264. Doi:10.1080/02701367.1987.10605459

Robbins, J. M., & Joseph, P. (1985). Experiencing exercise withdrawal: Possible consequences of therapeutic and mastery running. *Journal of Sport Psychology, 7*(1), 23–39. Doi:10.1123/jsp.7.1.23

Rodrigues, F., Teixeira, D. S., Neiva, H. P., Cid, L., & Monteiro, D. (2020). The bright and dark sides of motivation as predictors of enjoyment, intention, and exercise persistence. *Scandinavian Journal of Medicine & Science in Sports, 30*(4), 787–800. doi:10.1111/sms.13617

Saanijoki, T., Tuominen, L., Nummenmaa, L., Arponen, E., Kalliokoski, K., & Hirvonen, J. (2014). Physical exercise activates the μ-opioid system in human brain. *The Journal of Nuclear Medicine, 55*(1), 1909. Retrieved from: https://jnm.snm-journals.org/content/55/supplement_1/1909

Scanlan, T. K., Russell, D. G., Beals, K. P., & Scanlan, L. A. (2003). Project on elite athlete commitment (PEAK): II. A direct test and expansion of the sport commitment model with elite amateur sportsmen. *Journal of Sport and Exercise Psychology, 25*(3), 377–401. Doi:10.1123/jsep.25.3.377

Sicilia, Á., Alcaraz-Ibáñez, M., Lirola, M.-J., & Burgueño, R. (2017). Influence of goal contents on exercise addiction: Analysing the mediating effect of passion for exercise. *Journal of Human Kinetics, 59*(1), 143–153. Doi:10.1515/hukin-2017-0154

Simpson, D., Prewitt-White, T. R., Feito, Y., Giusti, J., & Shuda, R. (2017). Challenge, commitment, community, and empowerment: Factors that promote the adoption of CrossFit as a training program. *The Sport Journal, 1*, 1–14.

Spano, L. (2001). The relationship between exercise and anxiety, obsessive-compulsiveness, and narcissism. *Personality and Individual Differences, 30*(1), 87–93. Doi:10.1016/S0191-8869(00)00012-X

Sussman, S., Leventhal, A., Bluthenthal, R. N., Freimuth, M., Forster, M., & Ames, S. L. (2011). A framework for the specificity of addictions. *International Journal of Environmental Research and Public Health, 8*(8), 3399–3415. Doi:10.3390/ijerph8083399

Szabo, A. (1995). The impact of exercise deprivation on well-being of habitual exercisers. *The Australian Journal of Science and Medicine in Sport, 27*, 68–75.

Szabo, A. (2010). *Addiction to exercise: A symptom or a disorder?* New York, NY: Nova Science Publishers.

Szabo, A. (2018). Addiction, passion, or confusion? New theoretical insights on exercise addiction research from the case study of a female body builder. *Europe's Journal of Psychology, 14*(2), 296–316. Doi:10.5964/ejop.v14i2.1545

Szabo, A., Billett, E., & Turner, J. (2001). Phenylethylamine, a possible link to the antidepressant effects of exercise? *British Journal of Sports Medicine, 35*(5), 342–343. Doi:10.1136/bjsm.35.5.342

Szabo, A., Tóth, E., Kósa, L., Laki, Á., & Ihász, F. (2021). Increased exercise effort after artificially-induced stress: Laboratory-based evidence for the catharsis theory of stress. *Baltic Journal of Sport and Health Sciences, 4*(119), 24–30. Doi:10.33607/bjshs.v4i119.1016

Szabo, A., & Tsang, T. C. E. (2003). Motivation for increased self-selected exercise intensity following psychological distress: Laboratory based evidence for catharsis. *Journal of Psychosomatic Research, 55*(2), 133 (Abstract). Doi:10.1016/S0022-3999(03)00308-8

Thompson, J. K., & Blanton, P. (1987). Energy conservation and exercise dependence: A sympathetic arousal hypothesis. *Medicine and Science in Sports and Exercise, 19*, 91–97. Doi:10.1249/00005768-198704000-00005

Vallerand, R. J. (2000). Deci and Ryan's self-determination theory: A view from the hierarchical model of intrinsic and extrinsic motivation. *Psychological Inquiry, 11*(4), 312–318.

Woolf, J., & Lawrence, H. (2017). Social identity and athlete identity among Cross-Fit members: An exploratory study on the CrossFit Open. *Managing Sport and Leisure, 22*(3), 166–180. doi:10.1080/23750472.2017.1415770

12 Psychometric assessment of exercise addiction

Before developing reliable psychometrically validated tools for assessing exercise addiction, researchers used interviews to identify dysfunction (Sachs & Pargman, 1979). However, personal interviews are time-consuming and uneconomical. Therefore, other researchers adopted the Commitment to Running Scale (Carmack & Martens, 1979), later modified into the Commitment to Exercise Scale (Corbin et al., 1987) to fit a wide range of exercise forms in assessing exercise addiction. Although useful in nomothetic research, using a *commitment scale* for assessing *addiction* has been criticized (Szabo, 2010) because addiction and commitment to exercise are two very different constructs. While addiction is a dysfunction, commitment to exercise reflects the healthy involvement in the chosen form of training for mastery, enjoyment, and fun. Soon after a relatively slow but progressively growing interest in exercise addiction, researchers realized a need for more specific instruments in the investigation of the dysfunction. Consequently, several tools were developed over time, some being more popular than others and, therefore, more frequently used in research. We present these instruments in chronological order.

12.1 Negative Addiction Scale (Hailey & Bailey, 1982)

The Negative Addiction Scale (NAS) was developed with runners, but it was also used to measure exercise addiction in other exercisers (e.g., Furst & Germone, 1993; Modoio et al., 2011; Pierce et al., 1993). The scale has 14 equally weighted items that focus specifically on exercise addiction's psychological rather than physiological aspects. Its name is antithetical to *positive addiction* (Glasser, 1976) to specifically denote the assessment of morbid patterns of running or exercise. Its 14 items are rated with zero if a symptom is absent or one if it is present. Researchers use a cutoff score of five to classify the runners with negative addiction symptoms (Modoio et al., 2011). Its internal reliability (Cronbach's alpha) was .79 in Modoio et al.'s (2011) study. The scale is still in use in recent publications (e.g., de Brito Alexandria et al., 2021). In early research, this tool was relatively frequently

DOI: 10.4324/9781003173595-12

used, and some scholars use it in their studies even nowadays, but it is not a widely used instrument.

12.2 Obligatory Running Questionnaire (Blumenthal et al., 1984)

The Obligatory Running Questionnaire (ORQ) was developed to examine the analogy between running addiction and anorexia nervosa. It consists of 21 items, which are rated as either true or false. However, soon after its publications, researchers realized that some statements could not be accurately answered as simply true or false but rather in some gradients that better reflect the 'level' of presence or absence of a symptom. Also, its transformation into a more general exercise scale was warranted because the original scale could only be used with runners. This scale was extremely rarely adopted for research purposes in its original form, but it represents the infrastructure for later developed and more often adopted scales.

12.3 Obligatory Exercise Questionnaire (Pasman & Thompson, 1988)

Initially, the Obligatory Exercise Questionnaire (OEQ) was adopted from the ORQ (Blumenthal et al., 1984). Later the scale was further modified into a more general and shorter measure fitting a wide range of exercise activities (Thompson & Pasman, 1991). This scale consists of 20 exercise habits, rated on a four-point frequency scale: 1, never; 2, sometimes; 3, usually; and 4, always. Two of the items are rated inversely during the scoring. The psychometric properties of the scale have been supported (Coen & Ogles, 1993). The internal reliability of the OEQ was reported to be (Cronbach's alpha). 96 (Thompson & Pasman, 1991), but it was lower (.79) in a later study by Coen and Ogles (1993).

After performing a principal components analysis, Ackard et al. (2002) found that this tool has three subscales as reflected by 11 items loading on three factors. These subscales reflect three dimensions. The first is *exercise fixation*, which is mirrored by five items describing preoccupation with exercise, negative feelings when exercise is missed, and using exercise to compensate for overeating. The second is *exercise frequency*, which addresses the frequency and type of exercise. Finally, the third dimension is *exercise commitment*, which reflects an individual's sense that the routine exercise episodes cannot be missed. The internal reliabilities of the three subscales (Cronbach's alpha) were .78, .83, and .66. Consequently, Ackard et al. (2002) presented a valid, shorter, and more specific version of the OEQ.

Ten years later, the instrument was further validated by Duncan and her colleagues (2012). They presented a 10-item revised scale with good psychometric properties. The ten items, similarly to Ackard et al. (2002), comprised three factors. The first factor contains four items reflecting *a preoccupation with exercise.* The second factor has three items accounting for *typical exercise behavior.* Finally, the third factor also embeds three items mirroring *negative emotionality.* These factors are similar but not identical to the 11-item version (Ackard et al., 2002). All items are rated on a four-point frequency scale ranging from never to always, similarly to the original scale. The various versions of the OEQ are used relatively often in researching exercise addiction.

12.4 Running Addiction Scale (Chapman & De Castro, 1990)

Another running-specific tool, the Running Addiction Scale (RAS), is an 11-item instrument developed to assess the level of exercise addiction in runners. Its items are rated on a five-point agreement-disagreement Likert scale. Two sample items are: 'I would not reschedule activities with my friends in order to run' (reverse scored) and 'I feel that I need to run at least once every day.' Scoring ranges from 11 to 55. The psychometric properties of the RAS were reported to be adequate (Chapman & De Castro, 1990). The original scale has acceptable internal reliability (Cronbach's alpha = .82; Chapman & De Castro, 1990) similar to its later validated Spanish version (.79; Sancho & Ruiz-Juan, 2011). The 11 items of the original scale are openly available in the paper published by the developers (Chapman & De Castro, 1990). The scale is frequently adopted in research examining exercise addiction in runners.

12.5 Exercise Salience Scale (Kline et al. 1994)

Initially, the Exercise Salience Scale (ESS) was presented by Morrow and Harvey (1990) in a popular health magazine. These authors suggested six symptom-based criteria for identifying exercise addiction, including 1) the person engages in regular strenuous exercise; 2) the person experiences a dysphoric or anxious mood when exercise is not possible; 3) the person alters priorities, and exercise priorities are higher than those related to social and occupational activities; 4) the person holds irrational expectations regarding the amount of exercise needed to maintain the desired body shape or fitness level; 5) the individual persists in exercise behavior in the face of physical consequences, such as bad weather and physical injury; and 6) the person ruminates about the effects of any decrease in exercise level. Kline et al. (1994) attempted to validate the 40-item instrument in 74 university students. They showed that only two 10-item factors, one associated with anxiety of not exercising and the other with the determination to exercise in the face of adversity, could be identified. These two factors accounted for 38.4% of the variance. The remaining 20 items yielded four uninterpretable factors. The 40 items, which are rated on a one (1) to five (5) agreement-disagreement scale, are openly available in the validation paper published by Kline et al. (1994). The scale is very rarely used in exercise addiction research.

12.6 Exercise Dependence Questionnaire (Ogden et al., 1997)

The Exercise Dependence Questionnaire (EDQ) was developed with a sample of 449 participants who exercised for more than 4 hours a week. The scale consists of 29 items, and it has eight subscales: 1) interference with social/family/work life, 2) positive reward, 3) withdrawal symptoms, 4) exercise for weight control, 5) insight into the problem, 6) exercise for social reasons, 7) exercise for health reasons, and 8) stereotyped behavior. The EDQ is based on the criteria for exercise addiction of De Coverley Veale (1987) presented in Chapter 6. The instrument can be adopted in all forms of exercise and conceptualizes exercise addiction as a combination of traditional addiction models (i.e., withdrawal, tolerance, repetitive behavior, and excess) while also considering psychosocial perspectives (i.e., psychological consequences and effects on interpersonal relationships). While the internal reliability of the total items in the scale is good (Cronbach's alpha = .84), the eight subscales have lower reliabilities ranging from .52 to .81 (Allegre et al., 2006; Ogden et al., 1997). The complete scale is available in the original paper published by Ogden et al. (1997). The scale is relatively often used in research on exercise addiction.

12.7 Exercise Beliefs Questionnaire (Loumidis & Wells, 1998)

The Exercise Beliefs Questionnaire (EBQ) was developed to investigate problematic exercise from physical and psychological risk perspectives assuming that the emotional schema reflects beliefs and expectations associated with the behavior, which, in turn, have a major impact on the actual behavior. The tool assesses beliefs about exercise behavior considering four factors: 1) social desirability, 2) physical appearance, 3) mental and emotional functioning, and 4) vulnerability to disease and aging. The scale's internal reliability is relatively good, ranging between r = .67 and r = .89 and its test-retest reliability is acceptable ranging between r = .67 and r = .77 (Loumidis & Wells, 1998). The instrument aims to gauge the beliefs' strengths to differentiate those displaying and not displaying symptoms of exercise addiction despite performing high volumes of exercise, such as army personnel and athletes versus recreational exercisers. The tool has 21 items. Respondents' task is to rate each belief on a scale ranging from 0 to 100, where 0 means 'I do not believe this thought at all' and 100 means 'I am completely convinced this thought is true.' The 21 items of the original scale are openly available in the paper presenting the development of the instrument (Loumidis & Wells, 1998). Although the scale is frequently adopted in research on exercise behavior, its specific use for researching exercise addiction is more restricted.

12.8 Bodybuilding Dependency Scale (Smith et al., 1998)

The Bodybuilding Dependency Scale (BDS) was developed primarily to assess excessive workouts in bodybuilders. The scale contains three sub-scales: 1) social dependence (a person's need to be in a weightlifting environment), 2) training dependence (a person's compulsion to lift weights), and 3) mastery dependence (individuals' need to exert control over their training schedule). The instrument consists of nine items, which are rated on a seven-point agreement-disagreement type of Likert scale. The three subscales have acceptable or good internal reliabilities (Cronbach's alpha) .83, .70, and .89, respectively (Hale et al., 2013). The instrument is often used in the literature, especially in studying bodybuilders.

12.9 The Exercise Dependence Scale (Hausenblas & Downs, 2002)

The Exercise Dependence Scale (EDS) views dysfunctional (addictive) exercise as a craving for the adopted training that results in uncontrollable and excessive physical activity or sports performance and manifests in physiological symptoms, psychological symptoms, or both (Hausenblas & Downs, 2002). The tool's development relied on an earlier edition of the *Diagnostic and Statistical Manual of Mental Disorders* criteria for substance dependence (*DSM-4*; American Psychiatric Association, 1994). The EDS can differentiate between at-risk, nondependent-symptomatic, and nondependent-asymptomatic individuals. It can also specify whether people might have a physiological dependence (evidence of withdrawal) or no physiological dependence (no evidence of withdrawal). The original scale had 30 items, and then it was revised into a 28-item instrument. The items are rated on a six-point Likert frequency scale ranging from 1 (never) to 6 (always). Its evaluation is made on the basis of the *DSM-4* criteria, screening for the presence of three or more of the following symptoms: 1) tolerance, 2) withdrawal, 3) intention effects (exercise is often performed in larger volumes and longer duration than it was planned), 4) loss of control, 5) time (too much time is spent with activities conducive to the exercise performance), 6) conflict, and 7) continuance (exercise is maintained despite the knowledge of persistent or recurrent physical or psychological problems that are likely to have been caused or augmented by exercise).

The total score and subscale scores can be calculated for the EDS. Scoring is done with the aid of a scoring manual that comprises flowchart-format decision rules. The rules specify the items or combinations that help classify the individual as being at risk, nonaddicted symptomatic or nonaddicted asymptomatic on each criterion. Individuals who score in the addiction range, defined as 4–5 (out of 6) on the Likert scale on at least three of the seven criteria, are classified as being 'at risk' for exercise addiction. Those who fulfill at least three of the criteria in the nonaddicted symptomatic range by scoring around three on the Likert scale, or a combination of at least three criteria in the 'at risk' and nonaddicted symptomatic range, but do not meet the criteria for exercise addiction are classified as nonaddicted symptomatic. Finally, individuals who fit at least three of the criteria in the nonaddicted asymptomatic range (1–2 on the Likert scale) are classified as nonaddicted asymptomatic. The scale has good internal reliability (Cronbach's alpha, .78 to .92), and its test-retest reliability is .92. Not long after the release of the original scale, improvements in the scale were reported, in a revised 21-item version, by the developers (Downs et al., 2004). This scale is among the top two most widely used tools in studying exercise addiction, the other being the Exercise Addiction Inventory (EAI) (Terry et al., 2004), which is described later. The revised version has excellent psychometric properties, and it was validated in several languages. Despite its popularity, validity, and reliability, the scale is relatively challenging to score and interpret by non-clinicians or professionals lacking the expertise in psychological testing and evaluation.

12.10 Excessive Exercise Scale (McCabe & Vincent, 2002)

The Excessive Exercise Scale (EES) was adopted from a study combining three previous exercise habit scales (Long et al., 1993). The adopted version was aimed at assessing problematic exercise behavior related to the regulation of body shape and weight in adolescents. The scale is comprised of ten items. Answers to the first eight questions are rated on a five-point Likert-type scale ranging from 1 (never) to 5 (always). Sample items are: 'How often do you think about exercise?' and 'Do you feel angry or upset when you do not exercise?' Item nine requests that respondents indicate how often they exercise on each occasion, placed into one of five categories including 0, 15–30, 35–60, 65–90, and 95+ minutes. Finally, for item 10, participants are required to rank in order of preference their principal reasons for exercise from 1 (the strongest reason) to 7 (the least reason) for exercising. The possible alternative choices for the last question are: 1) to keep fit and healthy, 2) gain weight, 3) be attractive to the opposite sex, 4) have fun, 5) lose weight, 6) tone muscles, and 7) increase muscle size. The scale has two factors. One is exercise focus, and the other is the need to exercise. Considering the internal reliability of the EES, it was good for the whole sample (Cronbach's alpha = .86) and separately for girls (.86) and boys (.87). The items of the scale can be found in the published validation paper (McCabe & Vincent, 2002). This tool is very rarely used in exercise addiction research.

12.11 Exercise Addiction Inventory (Terry et al., 2004)

The EAI was developed for quick and easy use by both researchers and practitioners to screen the risk of exercise addiction. It is the shortest psychometrically validated instrument in this research area. It consists of only six statements that correspond to the six symptoms in the components model of addiction (Griffiths, 2005). Each statement is rated on a five-point agreement-disagreement Likert scale. The statements are 1) 'Exercise is the most important thing in my life' (salience), 2) 'Conflicts have arisen between me and my family and/or my partner about the amount of exercise I do' (conflict), 3) 'I use exercise as a way of changing my mood' (mood modification), 4) 'Over time I have increased the amount of exercise I do in a day' (tolerance), 5) 'If I have to miss an exercise session I feel moody and irritable' (withdrawal symptoms), and 6) 'If I cut down the amount of exercise I do, and then start again, I always end up exercising as often as I did before' (relapse).

The EAI's cutoff score for individuals considered at-risk of exercise addiction is 24. This cutoff value represents those individuals with scores in the top 20% of the total scale score. High scores reflect a high risk of addiction. A score of 13 to 23 is indicative of potential risk or symptomatic person, and a score of 0 to 12 mirrors an asymptomatic individual (Terry et al., 2004). The EAI was developed on the basis of a sample of 200 habitual exercisers. The internal reliability of the original scale was good (Cronbach's alpha = .84), and its concurrent validity was at least .80. A cross-cultural evaluation of the scale (Griffiths et al., 2015) supported the configural and metric but not the scalar invariance of the scale. Therefore, its factor scores from various nations are not comparable because of culture-related use or interpretation of the scale items. However, Griffiths et al. (2015) confirmed that the covariates of the risk of exercise addiction could be studied from a cross-cultural perspective because of the metric invariance of the scale. The internal reliability of the EAI varies from poor to good across various translations (Griffiths et al., 2015). A youth version of the EAI (EAI-Y) has also been validated (Lichtenstein et al., 2018). The internal reliability (Cronbach's α) of the EAI-Y was acceptable (.70). The developers found that the rate of the risk of exercise addiction was 4.0% in school athletes, 8.7% in fitness attendees, and 21% in youngsters affected by some eating disorders. However, it should be noted that we are not aware of any published case that has identified exercise addiction in a child or an adolescent. Still, the tool may help screen the potential current risk with extrapolation to the unfolding of the dysfunction in adulthood.

Recently, the EAI has been revised (Szabo et al., 2019). The six items did not change at all. Still, their rating range was expanded from a five-point to a six-point agreement-disagreement Likert scale to eliminate the neutral midpoint, which, according to the authors, has artificially increased the total score and consequently made the accuracy of the interpretation

questionable. The revised instrument was exposed to a principal component analysis, which confirmed that its six items represent a single component explaining 68.12% of the variance, which is larger than the value
reported for the original scale (55.9%). The internal consistency of the
revised scale is also higher (Cronbach's alpha = .90) than that reported in
the original scale development study (.84; Terry et al., 2004). The modified scale's concurrent validity with the revised EDS was also greater (.87)
than the original scale (.81). Finally, the new scale shares a larger variance
with the weekly exercise frequency (38%) than the original instrument
(29%). The revised EAI is presented in the paper by Szabo et al. (2019).
This instrument is frequently used in exercise addiction research, probably
because of its brevity, easy scoring, and theoretical underpinning. Indeed,
the EAI and the EDS are the two most often adopted tools in studying
exercise addiction.

12.12 Compulsive Exercise Test (Taranis et al., 2011)

The Compulsive Exercise Test (CET) was developed because the commonly
used exercise addiction measures could not isolate the specific aspects of
exercise connected with different facets of eating pathology (Taranis et al.,
2011). This test consists of 24 items assessing compulsive exercise's cognitive, behavioral, and emotional aspects. These items are rated on a six-point
Likert scale ranging from zero (0, never true) to five (5, always true). It has
five subscales: 1) avoidance and rule-driven behavior (e.g., *I feel extremely
guilty if I miss an exercise session*), 2) weight-control exercise (e.g., *I exercise to
burn calories and lose weight*), 3) mood improvement (e.g., *I feel less anxious
after I* exercise), 4) lack of exercise enjoyment (e.g., *I find exercise a chore*),
and 5) exercise rigidity (e.g., *I follow a set routine for my exercise*). Higher
scores are suggestive of a greater likelihood of dysfunctional exercise. The
CET has good psychometric properties. Its internal reliability was reported
to be (Cronbach's alpha) .72 in adolescents (Goodwin et al., 2011), .85 in
female university students (Taranis et al., 2011), and .93 in clinical patients
(all women) diagnosed with a form of eating disorder (Meyer et al., 2016).
The 24 items of the test are presented in a table in the original validation
paper (Taranis et al., 2011). The five-factor structure of the scale could not
be demonstrated in competitive athletes. Instead, a three-factor structure,
consisting of 1) weight control, 2) avoidance of negative affect, and 3)
mood improvement subscales, was proposed for this population (Plateau
et al., 2014). The internal reliabilities of these factors were (Cronbach's
alpha) .82, .87 and .71, respectively. A four-factor structure was also proposed for this scale in a study examining adolescents with eating disorders
(Swenne, 2016). This tool has been translated into several languages, and it
is relatively widely used in exercise addiction research, especially in eating
disorders.

12.13 Exercise Dependence and Elite Athletes Scale (McNamara & McCabe, 2013)

The Exercise Dependence and Elite Athletes Scale (EDEAS) was developed to measure exercise addiction symptoms in elite athletes. The scale has 24 items rated on a five-point frequency Likert scale ranging from 'never' to 'always.' Total scores range from 24 to 120. Preliminary analyses with a large sample of elite Australian athletes suggested that the scale has acceptable psychometric properties (McNamara & McCabe, 2013). It consists of six factors: 1) unhealthy eating behavior, 2) conflict and dissatisfaction, 3) more training, 4) withdrawal, 5) emotional difficulties, and 6) continuance behavior. The internal reliability of the scale is good (Cronbach's alpha = .82). A 26-item version of the scale is published in the appendix of the original validation paper. We are not convinced that all its items could be directly linked to exercise addiction, but we may be biased considering our skeptical view on exercise addiction in elite athletes (Juwono et al., 2021; Szabo et al., 2015; Szabo, 2018). The scale is relatively rarely used in exercise addiction research.

12.14 Strengths and limitations of using scales in exercise addiction research

Perhaps, we should start with a much-overlooked limitation that could be the reason for many inconsistent findings in the function of the sample studied and the pertinent exercise environment. It is important to keep in perspective that, without exception, all exercise addiction-assessing scales can only be used for surface screening or *risk assessment* but not for medical diagnosis. Therefore, the scale-based assessment estimates the likelihood of addiction in the respondent. Even individuals scoring above average or any cutoff value may not become addicted to exercise. Nevertheless, a score that is close to the maximum may suggest that there is a strong possibility of, or as many research papers call it, a high risk of addiction. For example, a score of 24 on the EAI, or 29 on the revised EAI (Appendix), should be considered a potential warning sign. However, scale-based research may never meet with the clinical practice, where the advanced morbid cases of exercise-related dysfunctions surface. Therefore, the proper and unambiguous assessment of exercise addiction could only be established after a deep interview with a qualified health professional cooperating with a research team.

12.15 Further research dilemmas

Serving well for screening purposes, exercise addiction scales direct the individual or those concerned in the right direction. In schools, sport, and leisure facilities, they are helpful for screening. However, many addicted exercisers perform their activity in an informal setting by simply going out for a run independently. Most exercise addicts are likely loners in some sense because no structured physical activity classes or exercising friends could keep up with the massive amount and busy schedule of exercise in which they engage daily. Assuming that only about 1% to 3% percent of the exercising population may be affected by exercise addiction (Szabo, 2010; Terry et al., 2004) and that most exercises addicts are 'lone wolfs,' the use of the scales may have further limited value in assessment.

By doing a database search, scholars can realize that there is a vast research diversity in studying exercise addiction. However, such an over-diversified, perhaps unfocused, effort may not be productive. Instead, the identification and then the closer examination of cases in which the morbidity can be established through a clear history of self-harm, arising as a consequence of the behavior, could be the way forward in this area of research. Twenty years ago, the first author of this book proposed a 'pyramid' approach to advance knowledge about exercise addiction (Szabo, 2001; Figure 12.1). This model is a bottom-to-top approach requiring orchestrated multidisciplinary collaboration at research and professional practice levels. It requires planning and organization to generate focused effort in work invested in better understanding, prevention, and treatment of exercise addiction.

According to the pyramid model, scholars with academic or research training can do the surface screening (see 'population' in Figure 12.1). Health professionals with clinical or medical training could then follow up the individuals 'at-risk' with in-depth clinical interviews. Subsequently, separate those who exercise in high volumes but maintain control over their exercise from those who have lost control over their exercise and exhibit maladaptive behavioral patterns (see 'group' in Figure 12.1). The primary incentive for exercise, with particular attention to 'wants to do it' and 'has to do it,' should be kept in perspective during these interviews. Once separation at the group level has taken place, professionals with clinical training should engage in treating the positively identified individuals. At the same time – with the patient's consent – maintain a confidential record about the causes and consequences of their addiction (see 'person' in Figure 12.1).

Data from case studies could then be compiled over time and analyzed inductively by using qualitative methods. This approach can reveal the commonalities between various cases and allow the testing of several models, including the interactional model (Egorov & Szabo, 2013), to understand the phenomenon of exercise addiction better. Indeed, perhaps the most significant shortcoming in the exercise addiction literature is a confounding interpretation of *nomothetic* research findings that do not emphasize that the findings only represent the likely or possible level of risk instead of a clinically established morbidity. The 'actual' dysfunction is unique to the person and, therefore, it is *idiographic* as suggested by the interactional model developed by Egorov and Szabo (2013), which presents a dilemma for its scientific investigation.

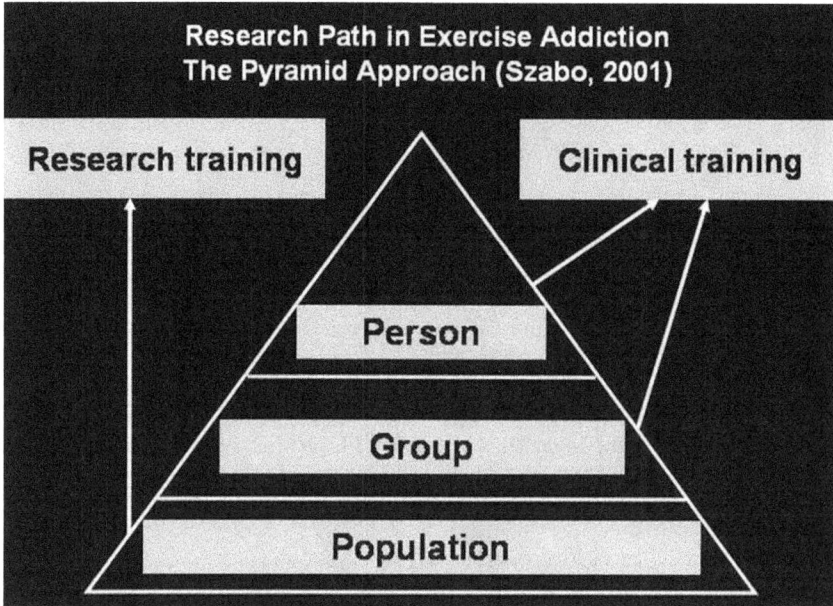

Figure 12.1 The interdisciplinary and collaboration-requiring 'pyramid' approach for the better understanding and treatment of exercise addiction (Szabo, 2001).

12.16 Key points

1. There are many scales developed for assessing the risk of exercise addiction.
2. The two most widely used, valid and reliable, instruments are the EDS and the EAI.
3. Scales are screening tools, merely assessing the risk of exercise addiction.
4. The 'risk scores,' even if high, may not reflect any psychological dysfunction.
5. Clinical diagnosis is only possible via in-depth clinical interviews by health professionals.

12.17 References

Ackard, D. M., Brehm, B. J., & Steffen, J. J. (2002). Exercise and eating disorders in college-aged women: Profiling excessive exercisers. *Eating Disorders: The Journal of Treatment & Prevention, 10*(1), 31–47. Doi:10.1080/106402602753573540

Allegre, B., Souville, M., Therme, P., & Griffiths, M. (2006). Definitions and measures of exercise dependence. *Addiction Research & Theory, 14*(6), 631–646. Doi:10.1080/16066350600903302

American Psychiatric Association. (1994). *Diagnostic and statistical manual of mental disorders* (4th ed.). Washington, DC: American Psychiatric Publishing, Inc.

Blumenthal, J. A., O'Toole, L. C., & Chang, J. L. (1984). Is running an analogue of anorexia nervosa? *Journal of the American Medical Association (JAMA), 252*(4), 520–523. Doi:10.1001/jama.1984.03350040050022

Carmack, M. A., & Martens, R. (1979). Measuring commitment to running: A survey of runners' attitudes and mental states. *Journal of Sport Psychology, 1*(1), 25–42. Doi:10.1123/jsp.1.1.25

Chapman, C. L., & De Castro, J. M. (1990). Running addiction: Measurement and associated psychological characteristics. *The Journal of Sports Medicine and Physical Fitness, 30*(3), 283–290.

Coen, S. P., & Ogles, B. M. (1993). Psychological characteristics of the obligatory runner: A critical examination of the anorexia analogue hypothesis. *Journal of Sport and Exercise Psychology, 15*(3), 338–354. Doi:10.1123/jsep.15.3.338

Corbin, C. B., Nielsen, A. B., Borsdorf, L. L., & Laurie, D. R. (1987). Commitment to physical activity. *International Journal of Sport Psychology, 18*(3), 215–222.

De Brito Alexandria, D., de de Macêdo Araújo, M. L., Malacarne, J. A. D., De Lima, J. D., & Palma, A. (2021). Prevalence of physical exercise addiction in people aged 50 or over living in Rio de Janeiro, Brazil. *Journal of Exercise Physiology Online, 24*(3), 110–118.

De Coverley Veale, D. M. W. (1987). Exercise dependence. *British Journal of Addiction, 82*(7), 735–740. doi:10.1111/j.1360-0443.1987.tb01539.x

Downs, D. S., Hausenblas, H. A., & Nigg, C. R. (2004). Factorial validity and psychometric examination of the Exercise Dependence Scale-Revised. *Measurement in Physical Education and Exercise Science, 8*(4), 183–201. Doi:10.1207/s15327841mpee0804_1

Duncan, L. R., Hall, C. R., Fraser, S. N., Rodgers, W. M., Wilson, P. M., & Loitz, C. C. (2012). Re-examining the dimensions of Obligatory Exercise. *Measurement in Physical Education and Exercise Science, 16*(1), 1–22. Doi:10.1080/1091367x.2012.641442

Egorov, A. Y., & Szabo, A. (2013). The exercise paradox: An interactional model for a clearer conceptualization of exercise addiction. *Journal of Behavioral Addictions, 2*(4), 199–208. Doi: 10.1556/JBA.2.2013.4.2

Furst, D. M., & Germone, K. (1993). Negative addiction in male and female runners and exercisers. *Perceptual and Motor Skills, 77*(1), 192–194. Doi:10.2466/pms.1993.77.1.192

Glasser, W. (1976). *Positive addiction.* New York, NY: Harper & Row.

Goodwin, H., Haycraft, E., Taranis, L., & Meyer, C. (2011). Psychometric evaluation of the compulsive exercise test (CET) in an adolescent population: Links with eating psychopathology. *European Eating Disorders Review, 19*(3), 269–279. Doi:10.1002/erv.1109

Griffiths, M. D. (2005). A 'components' model of addiction within a biopsychosocial framework. *Journal of Substance Use, 10*(4), 191–197. Doi:10.1080/14659890500114359

Griffiths, M. D., Urbán, R., Demetrovics, Z., Lichtenstein, M. B., de la Vega, R., Kun, B., . . . Szabo, A. (2015). A cross-cultural re-evaluation of the Exercise Addiction Inventory (EAI) in five countries. *Sports Medicine – Open, 1*(1). Doi:10.1186/s40798-014-0005-5

Hailey, B. J., & Bailey, L. A. (1982). Negative addiction in runners: A quantitative approach. *Journal of Sport Behavior, 5*(3), 150–153.

Hale, B. D., Diehl, D., Weaver, K., & Briggs, M. (2013). Exercise dependence and muscle dysmorphia in novice and experienced female bodybuilders. *Journal of Behavioral Addictions, 2*(4), 244–248. Doi:10.1556/jba.2.2013.4.8

Hausenblas, H. A., & Downs, D. S. (2002). How much is too much? The development and validation of the Exercise Dependence Scale. *Psychology and Health, 17*(4), 387–404. Doi:10.1080/0887044022000004894

Juwono, I. D., Tolnai, N., & Szabo, A. (2021). Exercise addiction in athletes: A systematic review of the literature. *International Journal of Mental Health and Addiction.* (Online first). Doi:10.1007/s11469-021-00568-1

Kline, T. J. B., Franken, R. E., & Rowland, G. L. (1994). A psychometric evaluation of the exercise salience scale. *Personality and Individual Differences, 16*(3), 509–511. Doi:10.1016/0191-8869(94)90078-7

Lichtenstein, M. B., Griffiths, M. D., Hemmingsen, S. D., & Støving, R. K. (2018). Exercise addiction in adolescents and emerging adults – Validation of a youth version of the Exercise Addiction Inventory. *Journal of Behavioral Addictions, 7*(1), 117–125. Doi:10.1556/2006.7.2018.01

Long, C. G., Smith, J., Midgley, M., & Cassidy, T. (1993). Over-exercising in anorexic and normal samples: Behaviour and attitudes. *Journal of Mental Health, 2*(4), 321–327. Doi:10.3109/09638239309016967

Loumidis, K. S., & Wells, A. (1998). Assessment of beliefs in exercise dependence: The development and preliminary validation of the Exercise Beliefs Questionnaire. *Personality and Individual Differences, 25*(3), 553–567. Doi:10.1016/S0191-8869(98)00103-2.

McCabe, M. P., & Vincent, M. A. (2002). Development of body modification and excessive exercise scales for adolescents. *Assessment, 9*(2), 131–141. Doi:10.1177/10791102009002003

McNamara, J., & McCabe, M. P. (2013). Development and validation of the Exercise Dependence and Elite Athletes Scale. *Performance Enhancement & Health, 2*(1), 30–36. Doi:10.1016/j.peh.2012.11.001

Meyer, C., Plateau, C. R., Taranis, L., Brewin, N., Wales, J., & Arcelus, J. (2016). The compulsive exercise test: Confirmatory factor analysis and links with eating psychopathology among women with clinical eating disorders. *Journal of Eating Disorders, 4*(1), 1–9. Oi: 10.1186/s40337-016-0113-3

Modoio, V. B., Antunes, H. K. M., Gimenez, P. R. B. De, Santiago, M. L. D. M., Tufik, S., & Mello, M. T. De. (2011). Negative addiction to exercise: Are there differences between genders? *Clinics, 66*(2), 255–260. Doi:10.1590/s1807-59322011000200013

Morrow, J., & Harvey, P. (1990, November). Exermania! *American Health*, 31–32.

Ogden, J., Veale, D., & Summers, Z. (1997). The development and validation of the Exercise Dependence Questionnaire. *Addiction Research, 5*(4), 343–355. Doi:10.3109/16066359709004348

Pasman, L., & Thompson, J. K. (1988). Body image and eating disturbance in obligatory runners, obligatory weightlifters, and sedentary individuals. *International Journal of Eating Disorders, 7*(6), 759–777. Doi:10.1002/1098-108X(198811)7:6<759::AID-EAT2260070605>3.0.CO;2-G

Pierce, E. F., Daleng, M. L., & McGowan, R. W. (1993). Scores on exercise dependence among dancers. *Perceptual and Motor Skills, 76*(2), 531–535. Doi:10.2466/pms.1993.76.2.531

Plateau, C. R., Shanmugam, V., Duckham, R. L., Goodwin, H., Jowett, S., Brooke-Wavell, K. S. F., . . . Meyer, C. (2014). Use of the Compulsive Exercise Test with athletes: Norms and links with eating psychopathology. *Journal of Applied Sport Psychology, 26*(3), 287–301. Doi:10.1080/10413200.2013.867911

Sachs, M. L., & Pargman, D. (1979). Running addiction: A depth interview examination. *Journal of Sport Behaviour, 2*(3), 143–155.

Sancho, A. Z., & Ruiz-Juan, F. (2011). Psychometric properties of the Spanish version of the Running Addiction Scale (RAS). *The Spanish Journal of Psychology, 14*(2), 967–976.

Smith, D. K., Hale, B. D., & Collins, D. (1998). Measurement of exercise dependence in bodybuilders. *The Journal of Sports Medicine and Physical Fitness, 38*(1), 66–74. PMID: 9638035

Swenne, I. (2016). Evaluation of the compulsive exercise test (CET) in adolescents with eating disorders: Factor structure and relation to eating disordered psychopathology. *European Eating Disorders Review, 24*(4), 334–340. Doi:10.1002/erv.2439

Szabo, A. (2001, May 30) *The dark side of sports and exercise: Research dilemmas.* Paper presented at the 10th World Congress of Sport Psychology, Skiathos, Greece.

Szabo, A. (2010). *Addiction to exercise: A symptom or a disorder?* New York, NY: Nova Science Publishers.

Szabo, A. (2018). Addiction, passion, or confusion? New theoretical insights on exercise addiction research from the case study of a female body builder. *Europe's Journal of Psychology, 14*(2), 296–316. Doi:10.5964/ejop.v14i2.1545

Szabo, A., Griffiths, M. D., Marcos, R. D. L. V., Mervó, B., & Demetrovics, Z. (2015). Methodological and conceptual limitations in exercise addiction research. *The Yale Journal of Biology and Medicine, 88*(3), 303–308.

Szabo, A., Pinto, A., Griffiths, M. D., Kovácsik, R., & Demetrovics, Z. (2019). The psychometric evaluation of the Revised Exercise Addiction Inventory: Improved psychometric properties by changing item response rating. *Journal of Behavioral Addictions, 8*(1), 157–161. Doi: 10.1556/2006.8.2019.06

Taranis, L., Touyz, S., & Meyer, C. (2011). Disordered eating and exercise: Development and preliminary validation of the Compulsive Exercise Test (CET). *European Eating Disorders Review, 19*(3), 256–268. Doi:10.1002/erv.1108

Terry, A., Szabo, A., & Griffiths, M. (2004). The exercise addiction inventory: A new brief screening tool. *Addiction Research & Theory, 12*(5), 489–499. Doi:10.1080/16066350310001637363

Thompson, J. K., & Pasman, L. (1991). The obligatory exercise questionnaire. *The Behavior Therapist, 14*, 137.

13 Undiagnosed but real cases of exercise addiction

In this chapter, we present cases of exercise addiction reflecting dysfunctional exercise behavior. However, it should be remembered that, as discussed in Chapter 9, exercise addiction *cannot be diagnosed* because, at this time, there are no clinical criteria for the diagnosis of this morbidity. Therefore, although the symptoms are of clinical significance and personally annoying, the presented cases were not *formally* diagnosed as exercise addiction.

While reading the cases in this chapter, readers should focus on the idiographic nature from which generalizations are difficult to make. This difficulty hinders gathering solid and consistent evidence for the clinical classification of exercise addiction. A further barrier to establishing a clinical category for exercise addiction is the very few cases exposed in medical writings despite the possible existence of many instances, as shown by Juwono and Szabo (2020). The first published case study in exercise addiction, Anna's case (Veale, 1995), was presented in Chapter 6. Other published cases are presented in this chapter in chronological order.

13.1 Joanna (typical symptoms of addiction)

In the second published case study on exercise addiction, Griffiths (1997) described the story of a 25-year-old woman exhibiting problematic exercise behavior. Joanna had a good education and reported a stable background. She paid attention to her eating habits, which were deemed adequate and healthy. Joanna saw herself as being in an excellent physical condition. She had practiced a martial art known as jiujitsu, which was her primary hobby. She started the sport in her late teenage years, and she thought about herself to be good in her sport. Joanna did not use anabolic steroids or other forms of performance-enhancement agents. However, jiujitsu was the most important activity in Joanna's life, reflecting the *salience* component of the addictive behaviors. While doing other things, Joanna was thinking about her next training session or competition several times a day. She claimed that she spent about six hours a day in training, which included other forms of exercises too, like weight training, jogging, or general exercise.

DOI: 10.4324/9781003173595-13

A year before the interview, she walked out of a final exam to catch a train and travel to a jiujitsu competition. She got behind with her studies due to her high exercise volume that left little time for education. Joanna enjoyed exercising both in the morning and in the evening. When she missed a morning session, she had a longer or an extra-long evening session to compensate for it. Moreover, she started to go swimming during her lunch break. The increasing amounts of exercise illustrate how Joanna's behavior was affected by *tolerance*, another common component of exercise addiction and other addictions. Indeed, she started jiujitsu at an evening class once a week in her teens and built up progressively over several years. At the time of the interview, she exercised every day. The duration of each exercise session was getting longer and longer. When she could not practice jiujitsu, she had to do other forms of exercises.

Joanna said that she became highly agitated and irritable when she was unable to exercise, pointing to the presence of *withdrawal symptoms*. For example, when her arm was bandaged because of an injury, she went for a three-hour jog instead. She also exhibited physical symptoms, like headaches and nausea, if she had to go for more than one day without exercise or if she had to miss a planned exercise session. These symptoms point to strong *feelings of deprivation* when exercise is prevented for any reason, mimicking or being identical to withdrawal symptoms in chemical addictions. Joanna also experienced positive mood changes and *euphoria* in several ways. She was in an excellent mood if she had a good jiujitsu session or a successful competition as well as when she won. She also felt satisfied and euphoric after a hard and long training session. Furthermore, Joanna was productive in other life areas, like academic work, only if she fulfilled her exercise needs. She claimed that she often trained until very late at night, and upon fulfilling her exercise, she was able to study throughout the rest of the night.

Joanna's relationship with a long-term partner has ended as a result of her excessive exercise behavior. She admitted that she never spent enough time with him, leading to *conflict*, but apparently, she was not sad because of the breakup. Joanna felt that she had become 'a bit of a loner' (p. 165), having fewer and fewer friends due to her excessive exercise. She also felt that her studies have suffered because of the time constraint and significant difficulty in concentration. Joanna also admitted that she was spending too much time with her exercise and knew that she had other essential life obligations that she had neglected. She affirmed that she could not resist the urge to exercise, and her exercise sessions must last a minimum of a few hours. She claimed that she could not concentrate during her lectures at the university or study at home unless she had satisfied her need to exercise, reflecting the loss of control over the behavior (i.e., exercise).

The *relapse* aspect of the addiction was also present in Joanna's case. She could do only a few days without exercise before her day became unbearable. If she missed a competition, that was just as bad. She tried to cut down on her exercise, but she was unsuccessful. Joanna became anxious if she could not exercise and got better only after the next exercise session. She was aware that exercise had taken a toll on her life but felt powerless to control it. Joanna experienced many negative consequences stemming from her maladaptive exercise. She spent lots of money, beyond her means, to keep up with her exercise. Joanna was in financial debt because of her low income as a student and the significant cost associated with her exercise and traveling to, or participating in, jiujitsu competitions. She said that she had to resort to some socially unacceptable means of getting money for herself (the act is not disclosed).

Joanna suffered a sport-related reinjury at the time of the interview. She was much worried about her arm that was not given enough time to heal properly because of the urge to train. Her doctor has advised her to give up the sport before suffering permanent damage to her arm. However, Joanna felt that giving up was not an option and that she would not do that despite the risk of an irreversible loss. Griffiths (1997) published the account of Joanna because he saw the components of exercise addiction in her case. All typical symptoms were present, but the route or the cause (origin) of addiction was not identified. Therefore, the triggering cause(s) of the maladaptive exercise behavior in the 'black box' of the interactional model (Egorov & Szabo, 2013) could not be determined in Joanna's case.

13.2 Mr. M.Y. (comorbidities, psychopathology, and other addictions)

The story of this lonely man was reported by Kotbagi et al. (2014). Mr. M.Y. was a 50-year-old cyclist. He showed up at the Center for Support and Prevention of Athletes at Saint Andrew Hospital in Bordeaux, France, to seek help for his maladaptive exercise habits. His reason for seeking treatment was a conflict in personal affective partnerships that resulted in the breakup of his relationships. The conflict was due to his unavailability to nurture a relationship.

He started cycling at the age of 15 and continued without interruption. When interviewed, he trained 10 hours a week and participated in one or two races each month. His family had no history of athletic training, but his father supported and encouraged him in his training and competition. Between 1980 and 1987, M.Y. participated successfully in nearly 100 races each year. He had a short experience with a performance enhancer in 1982 but gave up the habit upon advice from his cycling mates and coaches.

His personal life was also fulfilled in this period that M.Y. remembered nostalgically. Due to his only average physical condition, he could not become a first-class professional cyclist. However, he still competed at a regional level, where he got good results. He trained hard to become a national champion in his age category. In his personal life, M.Y. worked at night to get more time for training. He has lived alone since his divorce.

He met a woman on the Internet, but the relationship failed, and he had a depressive relapse.

His exercise behavior was very stereotypical. He followed the same training program he started when he was 15 years old. He cycled on the same path, the same number of hours, and the same distance. His training logbook dated back to 1979. He followed the same warm-up rituals in preparing for competitions. All his life seemed to revolve around cycling. He planned his holidays in accord with the cycling races. M.Y. matched his cycling outfit to the color of his bicycle on which he spent large amounts of money. He derived pleasure from visual self-observation. While cycling, he enjoyed passing by a reflective window or mirror and seeing his reflection in it. He expressed tolerance in his cycling pattern because he needed more and more training to feel good about himself over the years. When he was unable to train, he experienced tension and anxiety that affected his work and performance in subsequent races. At the time of the interview, he also reported fear of aging and sadness. Mr. M.Y. had a poor social life because his life priorities revolved around cycling.

Symptoms of other behavioral addictions were present between 1980 and 1986. Part of these symptoms was suggestive of compulsive shopping. However, Mr. M.Y., at this time, also manifested behavior that was pointing to sexual addiction. For example, he had several sexual acts with different partners each day, and he experienced severe urges to masturbate that were no longer present at the time of the interview. While eating disorders were not evident in Mr. M.Y.'s case, he showed past concern for his body, especially concerning his shape and muscularity and weighed only 65 kg while his height was 1.80 m. Mr. M.Y. also had a history of psychiatric disorders. Apart from experiencing generalized anxiety disorder and being treated for depression, he also attempted suicide when he was younger. In addition, his score on an exercise addiction questionnaire was high.

Kotbagi et al. (2014) have approached the problem correctly. They have established a case history that showed most exercise addiction symptoms in conjunction with comorbidities. The stereotypical behavior, the following of the same routine over 35 years, shows the inherent need for stability and control. Mr. M.Y. had, in general, poor social life and a series of unsuccessful romantic relationships following his divorce. The discomfort, lack of control, and hindrance of repressed needs in this context may have been self-vindicated, at least temporarily, by training. Clearly, many major adverse events, like not making the professional team, divorce, loss of control over sexuality, all may have driven Mr. M.Y.'s exercise addiction and be either triggering or fueling 'items' in his 'black box' (subjective anguish requiring coping) considering the interactional model proposed by Egorov and Szabo (2013). Perhaps, the only stability in his life, since the age of 15, was his cycling.

In the case of Mr. M.Y., exercise addiction was an escape from the unknown, uncertain, or unreachable into the predictable, stable, and accessible. However, even cycling had to be performed in a stereotypical way to yield anticipated safety, stability, and reassurance. Cycling was a *controllable* mate to Mr. M.Y. His psychological condition has improved after a four-phase cognitive-behavioral therapy at the Center for Support and Prevention of Athletes. Like Anna (Chapter 6) and Joanna, in M.Y.'s case, there was no evidence of eating pathology, supporting the existence of exercise addiction *independently of eating disorders* (Veale, 1995).

13.3 Ludmilla (when too much exercise appears to be the solution)

Ludmilla was consulted for an over-devotion to her exercise and physical activity, without any current manifestation of psychological dysfunction, as part of an earlier collaborative project with A. Y. Egorov (Egorov & Felsendorff, personal communication on 29.10.2014). We summarize and evaluate this case in this section because it has a unique and paradoxical link with exercise addiction. Ludmilla was often sick during her childhood. She started gymnastics in school but dropped out. She also engaged in athletics, volleyball, skating, and long-distance running. All her exercises were done at the amateur level, with little success. However, she remembered the picture that hung on the board of honor in her school entitled: 'the best athletes.' By the age of 15, she had severe sports injuries. She quit sports after enrolling in college, but sometimes she played basketball. She got injured again.

All her sporting injuries may be linked to psychological problems. At age 7, her father died in a car crash. Her mother concealed the news from her for 40 days, but she knew it already the next day, from the kids at school. This event caused her severe psychological trauma. She hated the world and felt ugly. At that time, she wanted to die. Luda (Ludmilla's nickname) hated her mother for not telling her the truth. Even later, she had a complicated relationship with her mother because of this. The anguish resulted in her having tachycardia. The tachycardia attacks became frequent, and she could not do physical education. She left school at 19 years and got married. Soon she started to have 'paranoia attacks.' She felt that everyone laughed at her, and being jealous of her husband, she was afraid that he would divorce her. She also had severe migraine attacks and menstrual pain lasting for several days. At the age of 25, she had another significant injury needing surgery, but she refused the operation. A few years later, at the age of 29, she had an intense fear of death because her father died at that age.

At this time, she radically changed her lifestyle. Luda went back to school, started seeing a psychologist, and paid attention to her well-being. Eventually, she graduated with honors. Soon after that, she went to a country club known as 'Good Life.' She stayed there for several weeks, practiced vegetarianism, abstained from alcohol, and had massages. In the club, she met a woman who advised her to start up fitness. She was skinny and had

insufficient muscle and fat that may have been why she did not get preg-
nant, which led to conflicts with her husband concerning their childless
partnership.

Her life changed on September 30, 2011, when she joined a fitness club.
Since then, Luda has started to run regularly and has never missed a fitness class. All her thoughts and talks were about fitness. She also walked
three times a week and attended yoga classes on the weekend. Exercise
changed her life. Her menstruation ceased to be painful, the migraine
attacks have passed, and the tachycardia dissipated slowly. She had experienced improved movement coordination and posture. Luda became physically more robust, appeared more muscular, and she was in a good mood. If
there were no opportunities to train at the club, she would perform physical exercises at home, or run, because it has become a lifestyle. When her
friends went to a birthday party, Luda went to exercise. Her new friends
were from leisure and fitness clubs. She even helped the fitness instructors
by solving personal issues, leading workshops, and planning and organizing exercise sessions (Egorov & Felsendorff, personal communication on
29.10.2014).

Despite her life revolving around exercise, she scored very low on an
exercise addiction questionnaire. Was then Ludmilla affected by exercise
addiction? It seems that she had more losses and traumas before than after
her exercise life. Ludmilla has solved most, if not all, of her problems with
exercise efficiently and healthily. Indeed, her exercise addiction score was
low. She followed a large volume and possibly exaggerated but healthy
exercise pattern in that she did not experience adverse effects in her life
because of her exercise. Whether this pattern has changed since then is
unknown.

We have presented her case since, ironically, salience, tolerance, mood
modification, deprivation feelings, and possibly conflict (with her husband
and old friends who were going drinking) were all present in Luda's case.
Still, she has not lost control over her exercise, which resulted in positive
gains for Ludmilla. Other people may try to run away from stress by escaping into exercise and experience the opposite effects. The fact that exercise
is the solution to a problem for one person while it causes anguish instead
of a solution for another illustrates the paradox of exercise behavior that
is little understood. The next case covered below presents a story in which
even a lifelong pattern of excessive exercise presented no problem at all;
instead, it was rewarding.

13.4 Péter (exaggerated amounts of exercise do not imply addiction)

A misconception in the exercise addiction literature is that a high exercise volume is associated with pathological exercise. Like the mere

occurrence of withdrawal symptoms, exercise volume has little to do with exercise addiction. To illustrate this point, we need to present Péter Kropkó's case even though Péter was not tested for exercise addiction. 'My family is the most important,' claims Péter Kropkó (Kropkó & Bene, 2006, p. 149), a happily married man, father of four children. Péter is a world-class triathlete who completed the Ironman Triathlon 51 times (3.8 km swimming, 42 km running, and 180 km cycling). Until 2006, Péter was 16 times the 'Triathlete of the Year' in Hungary, and he was undefeated for 15 years in the country. He swam 70,000 km, ran 140,000 km, and cycled 650,000 km throughout his 37-year sporting career (Kropkó & Bene, 2006).

Is he sane? Of course, he is! The first author is privileged to know Péter in person. All his friends and the Hungarian sporting community can confirm that he is a well-balanced person, a great father, and an exemplary husband. He puts his family first and above everything else. The last time the first author met Péter in a swimming pool, he was organizing a training camp for young triathletes in the company of his supportive wife and children. We do not wish to make this story long, but we need to make a point clear. This point is that an obsessively passionate involvement in sports and exercise can be accompanied by a high harmonious passion and a well-balanced training regimen. A person who spent almost all his life exercising and competing in the world's most challenging endurance races is still able to have a well-balanced and psychologically sound personal and social life, without signs of pathological exercise behavior, even though the volume of his exercise may seem to be 'pathological' to the average person. His Hungarian book describing his athletic life, entitled *I did it because I believed it*, is no evidence of any maladaptive exercise behavior but rather a well-controlled training regimen that could be an inspiration to all.

It is essential to realize that exercise is a behavior that has healthy and unhealthy aspects, which depend on the person's approach to it, skills, and control over the activity. It also depends on the social and physical environment. Péter received maximal social support from his family and friends and had the physical ability that matched the challenges he undertook. For Péter, the word 'moderation' is inadequate as he expects(ed) to conquer the world, requiring the maximum possible. However, the *maximum possible* is the necessarily *recognized* self-limit in one's physical and psychological abilities. Such recognition is essential since if the actual ability/skill is lower than the perceived ability/skill, the person could push her or himself to the point of injury, reoccurring injuries, and eventually to the sports career's termination. Therefore, an athlete must always be aware of the 'breaking point' and stop just below that which is the 'personal best' they can do at a given time. Under the breaking point, even vast amounts of training do not necessarily imply morbidity.

13.5 Evelyn (when self-perceived addiction means positive change)

Evelyn (a pseudonym) responded to a call by the first author of this book (Szabo, 2018) seeking people addicted to exercise to volunteer for an interview. She contacted the author claiming that she was surely addicted to her exercise. At that time, she was 24 years and a young university graduate who lived in Budapest, Hungary. She worked as a managerial assistant for a private company. This job was essential to her. During her university studies, she attended a gym sporadically but gradually got involved in bodybuilding. After experiencing subjective and objective results, less than a year before the interview, she has started to compete under the guidance of a coach and took part in two national and one major international competition.

At this point, a shift from exercise to a sport has occurred. Her early athletic results were excellent, considering her brief sporting history. She became a highly successful athlete who has achieved three remarkable competition results within six months. She trained at least five times a week, for at least 90 minutes each time. Occasionally, Evelyn felt like working out in addition to her scheduled training. Guilt for not training enough or missing a training session, or lack of personal satisfaction with the progress toward the self-set goals were the reasons for the extra workouts. She received support and criticism from her friends on social media concerning her sport and athletic physical appearance. This change in her appearance, however, was perceived positively by Evelyn. However, she had little time left for socializing due to work and training commitments, which bothered her at the time of the interview.

Evelyn completed several psychometric scales, followed by the interview with Szabo (2018). On these tests, she scored 20 out of 30 of the maximum score on the Exercise Addiction Inventory, which classifies her as 'symptomatic,' but not 'at risk' based on Terry et al.'s (2004) criteria. On a passion scale (Marsh et al., 2013), she scored 33 out of the maximum of 42 on the harmonious passion and 40 out of 42 on obsessive passion. Her criterion passion score, reflecting her commitment to her sport, was 33 out of 35. On an exercise deprivation scale (Robbins & Joseph, 1985), Evelyn scored 44 out of 63. Finally, she reported six out of nine symptoms on the Nonsubstance-Related Disorders category of the *Diagnostic and Statistical Manual of Mental Disorders* (*DSM-5*; American Psychiatric Association, 2013), which would classify her as exhibiting *disordered exercise behavior* (based on the analogous classification of gambling disorder in *DSM-5*). In terms of percentages of the maximum possible scores (to illustrate the relative position [i.e., low, medium, high] of her answers on the various measures used in exercise addiction research), her relative scores were high, as summarized in Figure 13.1.

Evelyn scored in the upper third on all questionnaires, probably rendering her suspect at risk of exercise addiction. However, her high score

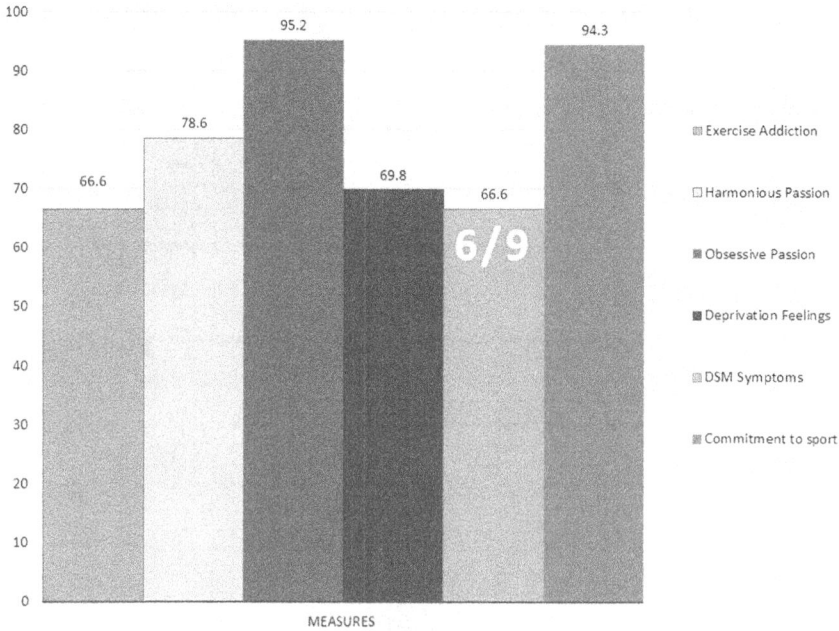

Figure 13.1 Evelyn's scores in percent (%) of the maximum possible (vertical axis range 0–100) on six measures of exercise behavior.

on both obsessive and harmonious passion was suggestive of a devotion and love for bodybuilding, to which Evelyn was highly committed (see her commitment/sport affinity scores). As discussed earlier in the context of Péter's story, athletes with ambitious goals could be expected to exhibit high obsessive passion along with high harmonious passion. Such an athletic profile, as based on Evelyn's scores on the passion scale, is illustrated in Figure 13.2.

The interview was centered around well-being in eight life domains: health (physical), environment, intellectual growth, occupation, health (emotional), social life, financial status, and spiritual life (Swarbrick, 2006). Initially, she had to consider the current aspect of well-being and then recall her well-being in these life domains before her involvement in bodybuilding. The outcome measure was the *perceived difference* between her past and present, recorded as a *positive change, no change,* or *negative change.* As illustrated in Table 13.1, Evelyn perceived her well-being better in six out of eight (75%) life domains at the time of the interview compared to the past when exercise was sporadic and for leisure only. The fact that work and exercise took a toll on her social life emerged as a negative change compared to the past, while no change has occurred in her

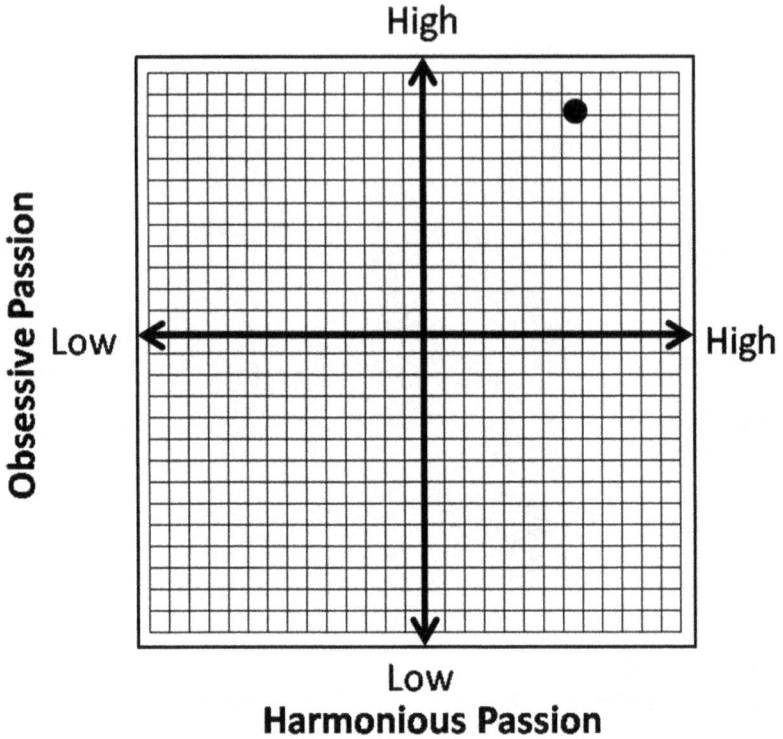

Figure 13.2 The conceptually expected association between obsessive and harmonious passion in athletes. The black dot reflects the intersecting position of Evelyn's scores.

spiritual life. This trend of improvement was also justified by her answer to a summary question asking her to *indicate on a ruler where her overall well-being is now and where was before her involvement in bodybuilding*; the current rating corresponded to a 7–8 on a 10-inch partition while the rating of her past well-being was only around 3–4. If we consider the middle point (5) as the separation between negative and positive appraisal, it might be assumed that the involvement in sport triggered *positive changes* in Evelyn's well-being.

Evelyn's case provides a real-life example of how self-perceived exercise addiction is only a reflection of both obsessive and harmonious passion along with the high commitment of an athlete. The parallel high scores of obsessive passion and commitment suggest that there is an internal pressure related to conformity with training. Research evidence reveals positive relationships between obsessive passion and commitment in work and sport (Forest et al., 2010; Kovácsik et al., 2021). Furthermore, high obsessive passion can be expected to co-occur with high harmonious passion in athletes, the latter reflecting the joy and satisfaction derived from the results of successful training and competition. The message from this case study is that questionnaire-based 'risk' scores may not reflect an actual risk for dysfunction, and therefore, their conceptual validity needs to be revisited.

It is possible that nomothetic (quantitative) research, assessing the risk for exercise addiction, embeds a confounding overlap between passion, commitment, and exercise addiction, yielding false estimates of the actual risk and prevalence of the dysfunction. Despite the self-perceived risk of exercise addiction that was also supported by questionnaire scores, no signs of dysfunction could be detected in the case of Evelyn. She perceived positive changes in the majority (75%) of life domains due to her involvement in sport. Considering this paradox between the negative perception of exercise addiction and positive perception of life changes due to exercise, the bulk of past research on exercise addiction might need to be reevaluated to understand this problematic behavior mirrored and overestimated by questionnaires.

13.6 More cases of exercise addiction

The cases presented in this chapter were selected to illustrate dysfunctional exercise and instances where exercise was a solution for the problem or helped the individual live a more satisfying life. We also presented a case where excessive exercise training was associated with a well-balanced personal life and the successful athletic career of a world-class athlete. Other cases of exercise addiction with dramatic outcomes are also reported. For example, Schreiber and Hausenblas (2015) published nine cases which they describe in detail in Chapter 7 of their book. The first case is one of the first authors who shares her dramatic experience with her readership in an authentic way with the uttermost credibility.

Similarly, Juwono and Szabo (2020) performed a search and content analysis on the Internet until they located 100 cases that fit the criteria of 'at risk' of exercise addiction based on the components model of addiction and at least one for physical, psychological, or social trauma suffered by the affected person. These cases project a heterogeneous spectrum of antecedents, exercise behavior, and consequences, further justifying the need for an idiographic approach in understanding exercise addiction better. The pyramid model, suggested in Chapter 12, could be a valuable path for expanding the current knowledge on this dysfunction. In addition, the interactional model (Dinardi et al., 2021; Egorov & Szabo, 2013) may account for the highly individual nature of the cases of exercise addiction.

Table 13.1 Evelyn's perceived well-being in eight life domains (Swarbrick, 2006) as compared to the recalled well-being before Evelyn's intense involvement in bodybuilding. The recall also reflects the current (at the time of the interview) appraisal of past events. Therefore, the critical outcome measure is the *current state of the mind* or thought. In boldface are the areas where changes have occurred in Evelyn's life domains.

Life domain	At the time of the interview	Before the heavy involvement in exercise training
Emotional	Appears balanced, self-confident, aware of the situation	**Experienced emotional distress due to family, financial, and relationship issues; had to seek professional help**
Physical	Perceives to be in good physical health	**Experienced stomach and cardiac problems**
Environmental	Lives independently, has control over her life	**Lived with a parent, was dependent on others**
Occupational	Works in a full-time job	**Studied, had no or part-time job only**
Intellectual	Faces work-related intellectual challenge at work	**Faced challenges related to student life and studies**
Financial	The financial situation is good or satisfactory, but it is not yet ideal	**It was very unsatisfactory, had a major financial hardship**
Social	**It is not satisfactory because work and training leave no time for socialization or developing a lasting relationship**	It was slightly better than now, but still not fully satisfactory
Spiritual	No change in this domain; she is a believer with some interest in astrology	It was not different before; she was a believer with some interest in astrology

13.7 Key points

1. Although exercise addiction cases are rarely identified, they exist.
2. Escape into exercise can be both dysfunction and a solution for some.
3. Exaggerated volumes of exercise do not necessarily imply exercise addiction.

4. Avid exercisers and athletes exhibit high harmonious and obsessive passion.
5. Athletes who would be classed as exercise addicts based on psychometric scales may project a healthy profile when interviewed.

13.8 References

American Psychiatric Association. (2013). *Diagnostic and statistical manual of mental disorders* (5th ed.). Arlington, VA: Author.

Dinardi, J., Egorov, A. & Szabo, A. (2021). The revised interactional model of exercise addiction. *Journal of Behavioral Addictions* (In Press).

Egorov, A. Y., & Felsendorff, O. (2014). *Personal communication.* E-mail. 29.10.2014.

Egorov, A. Y., & Szabo, A. (2013). The exercise paradox: An interactional model for a clearer conceptualization of exercise addiction. *Journal of Behavioral Addictions,* 2(4), 199–208. doi:10.1556/jba.2.2013.4.2

Forest, J., Mageau, G. A., Sarrazin, C., & Morin, E. M. (2010). "Work is my passion": The different affective, behavioural, and cognitive consequences of harmonious and obsessive passion toward work. *Canadian Journal of Administrative Sciences/ Revue Canadienne Des Sciences de l'Administration, 28*(1), 27–40. doi:10.1002/cjas.170

Griffiths, M. (1997). Exercise addiction: A case study. *Addiction Research, 5*(2), 161–168. doi:10.3109/16066359709005257

Juwono, I. D., & Szabo, A. (2020). 100 cases of exercise addiction: More evidence for a widely researched but rarely identified dysfunction. *International Journal of Mental Health and Addiction.* (Online first). doi:10.1007/s11469-020-00264-6

Kotbagi, G., Muller, I., Romo, L., & Kern, L. (2014). Pratique problématique d'exercice physique: un cas clinique. *Annales Médico-Psychologiques, Revue Psychiatrique, 172*(10), 883–887. doi:10.1016/j.amp.2014.10.011.

Kovácsik, R., Tóth-Király, I., Egorov, A., & Szabo, A. (2021). A longitudinal study of exercise addiction and passion in new sport activities: The impact of motivational factors. *International Journal of Mental Health and Addiction.* (Online first). doi:10.1007/s11469-020-00241-z

Kropkó, P., & Bene, J. (2006). Megtettem mert elhittem [*I did it because I believed it*]. Siófok, HU: Balatonpress Kft. ISBN 963-0606-275 (in Hungarian)

Marsh, H. W., Vallerand, R. J., Lafrenière, M.-A. K., Parker, P., Morin, A. J. S., Carbonneau, N., & Paquet, Y. (2013). Passion: Does one scale fit all? Construct validity of two-factor Passion Scale and psychometric invariance over different activities and languages. *Psychological Assessment, 25*(3), 796–809. doi:10.1037/a0032573

Robbins, J. M., & Joseph, P. (1985). Experiencing exercise withdrawal: Possible consequences of therapeutic and mastery running. *Journal of Sport Psychology, 7*(1), 23–39. doi:10.1123/jsp.7.1.23

Schreiber, K., & Hausenblas, H. A. (2015). What it feels like – Exercise addicts' true stories. In *The truth about exercise addiction: Understanding the dark side of thinspiration* (Chapter 7, pp. 77–116). London, UK: Rowman & Littlefield.

Swarbrick, M. (2006). A wellness approach. *Psychiatric Rehabilitation Journal, 29*(4), 311–314. doi:10.2975/29.2006.311.314

Szabo, A. (2018). Addiction, passion, or confusion? New theoretical insights on exercise addiction research from the case study of a female body builder. *Europe's Journal of Psychology, 14*(2), 296–316. doi:10.5964/ejop.v14i2.1545

Terry, A., Szabo, A., & Griffiths, M. (2004). The Exercise Addiction Inventory: A new brief screening tool. *Addiction Research & Theory, 12*(5), 489–499. doi:10.1080/1 6066350310001637363

Veale, D. (1995). Does primary exercise dependence really exist? In J. Annett, B. Cripps, & H. Steinberg (Eds.), *Exercise addiction: Motivation for participation in sport and exercise: Proceedings of British Psychology, Sport and Exercise Psychology Section* (pp. 71–75). Leicester, UK: British Psychological Society.

14 Is exercise addiction a symptom or a disorder?

14.1 Classification of exercise addiction

Currently, exercise addiction cannot be classified as a psychiatric *disorder*. The 5th edition of the *Diagnostic and Statistical Manual of Mental Disorders* (American Psychiatric Association, 2013) states that 'at this time there is insufficient peer-reviewed evidence to establish the diagnostic criteria and course descriptions needed to identify these behaviors as mental health disorders' (p. 481). Furthermore, the World Health Organization's *International Classification of Diseases* (ICD-11) uses a category of *impulse control disorders* for some behavioral addictions, which does not include exercise addiction specifically. These behaviors

> are characterised by the repeated failure to resist an impulse, drive, or urge to perform an act that is rewarding to the person, at least in the short-term, despite consequences such as longer-term harm either to the individual or to others, marked distress about the behaviour pattern, or significant impairment in personal, family, social, educational, occupational, or other important areas of functioning. Impulse Control Disorders involve a range of specific behaviours, including fire-setting, stealing, sexual behaviour, and explosive outbursts
>
> (World Health Organization, 2019).

Based on these characteristics, it may be tempting to describe exercise addiction as an impulse control disorder.

14.2 Impulse control disorder or obsessive-compulsive disorder?

Impulsivity refers to fast, abrupt, unplanned reactions to stimuli like an internal urge that arises from an outside trigger. For example, stress resulting from an argument can trigger the urge to exercise. Impulsive actions lack the consideration of their consequences. Instead, they narrowly focus on the reward, which fuels them (Grant & Potenza, 2006). Exercise for

DOI: 10.4324/9781003173595-14

most is an enjoyable activity. In its addictive form, it is carried out despite the possible negative consequences (Szabo, 2010). Indeed, an addicted runner with an injury might still run despite knowing that it could aggravate the injury. However, unlike in most impulse control disorders, the runner thinks about the possible consequences but decides to ignore them (Cook et al., 2011). Another reason why considering exercise addiction an impulse control disorder might be inadequate is that with time, tolerance and withdrawal effects occur, which are characteristic symptoms in most addictions (Griffiths, 2005) but are less characteristic of impulse control disorders.

Therefore, scholars believe that exercise addiction can be described as an obsessive-compulsive disorder, such as anxiety-associated disorders fueled by negative reinforcement through anxiolytic effects (Freimuth et al., 2011). Indeed, research shows that exercise addiction, like compulsive disorders, is maintained by its mood-mediating effects (Cox & Orford, 2004; Demetrovics & Kurimay, 2008; Iannos & Tiggemann, 1997; Weinstein & Weinstein, 2014). Furthermore, considering the interactional model (Dinardi et al., 2021; Egorov & Szabo, 2013), it can be argued that exercise addiction is a compulsive disorder because it functions to reduce stress. However, critics argue that compulsive behaviors do not yield pleasure, while exercise, in addition to decreasing anxiety, has a mood-improving effect (Szabo, 2003). Indeed, Goodman (2001) differentiates addictions from impulsive and compulsive behaviors by their dual capacity to alleviate anxiety and negative affective states while also triggering positive changes in feeling states.

Consequently, exercise performed for stress management, based on the interactional model (Dinardi et al. 2021; Egorov & Szabo, 2013), can be compulsive. Accordingly, the interactional model accounts for compulsive exercise more than for addiction because it considers the etiology of addiction as a result of stress. However, the interactional model does not exclude the positive effects of exercise because mastery exercisers in the model can get addicted by wishing to achieve increasingly better performance results (associated with positive feelings of accomplishment) that might exceed their physical ability (Egorov & Szabo, 2013). Still, the model imparts that exercise addiction is compulsive when it is therapeutically oriented because it acts as a coping strategy with stress. This conjecture agrees with the classification of exercise addiction (Demetrovics & Kurimay, 2008) on the obsessive-compulsive disorder spectrum (Hollander & Wong, 1995), where it assumes a 'risk avoiding' position toward the compulsive end of the spectrum (Figure 14.1).

14.3 Risk avoidance and brain activity in compulsive disorders and exercise addiction

It is important to note that exercise addiction involves physical effort and time investment (delayed gratification) compared to drugs or alcohol,

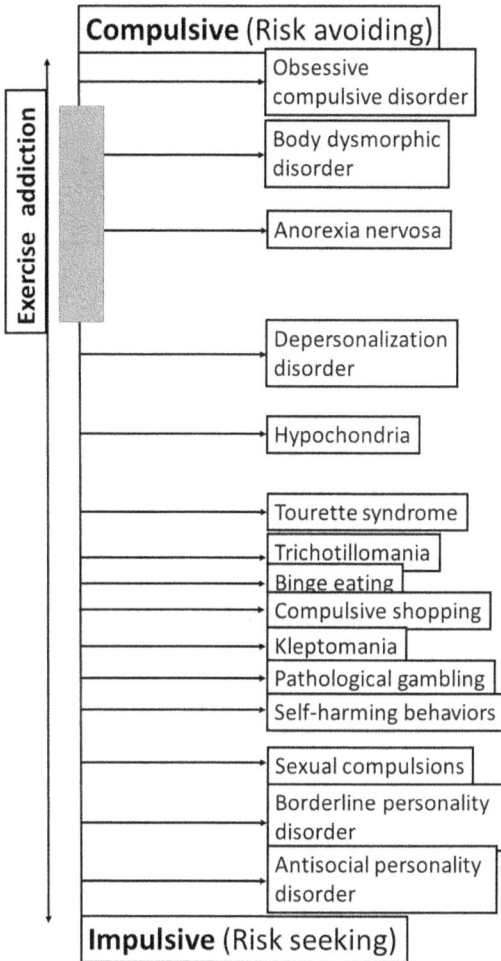

Figure 14.1 The hypothetical position (grey square) of exercise addiction on Hollander and Wong's (1995) obsessive-compulsive disorders spectrum. The figure was drafted on the basis of Demetrovics and Kurimay (2008) and Hollander and Wong (1995).

which provide relatively effortless and instant rewards. However, the latter have strong social stigmas, while exercise is a *socially perceived positive activity*. It is an activity behind which it is easy to hide if one becomes addicted. This choice of investing effort and waiting for delayed reward suggests a tendency of *risk avoidance* characteristic of compulsive behaviors on the spectrum proposed by Hollander and Wong (1995). These authors have also associated compulsive disorders with increased frontal lobe activity and increased serotonin in the brain. This relationship is supported by empirical data suggesting that serotonin levels increase in the brain because of exercise (Melancon et al., 2014; Young, 2007). There is also evidence for increased frontal lobe activity resulting from exercise (Shin, 2009; Yuki et al., 2012). These empirical results, along with the risk avoidance presumption in exercise addiction, support the placement of exercise addiction toward the compulsive end of the obsessive-compulsive disorders' spectrum (Demetrovics & Kurimay, 2008). However, addictions based on Goodman (1990) comprise both compulsion and dependence. Because the exercise addict also *depends* on exercise to cope with stress, for example, and trains to lower stress or anxiety (compulsive aspect), it fulfills the criteria of addiction. Consequently, exercise addiction is the best term for the dysfunction, which also accounts for tolerance and withdrawal effects in this morbidity.

14.4 Further possible reason for risk avoidance in exercise addiction

There are certain personality traits associated with exercise addiction. Among such traits, perfectionism has been the most closely associated with exercise addiction (Bircher et al., 2017; Çakın et al., 2021). Given that obsessions and compulsions are linked to perfectionism (Myers et al., 2008), classifying exercise addiction within the obsessive-compulsive disorders' spectrum (Demetrovics & Kurimay, 2008) appears to be further justified.

Perfectionism involves tendencies to set extremely high personal standards, strive for often unrealistic excellence, set overambitious goals, and be overly critical of oneself (Bieling et al., 2004). Perfectionism has been described as maladaptive psychopathology. However, it was also associated with positive tendencies to improve performance, experience satisfaction, and achieve goals (cf. Çakın et al., 2021). Hewitt et al. (1991) have described three dimensions of perfectionism: 1) self-oriented perfectionism or setting high and unrealistic standards for the self, 2) other-oriented perfectionism or setting unrealistic expectations of others, and 3) socially prescribed perfectionism, or believing that others expect perfect performance from them.

Exercise addiction appears to be related to self-oriented perfectionism and socially prescribed perfectionism (Çakın et al., 2021). This finding suggests that exercise addicts may have high expectancy from themselves, not only in the context of their exercise behavior but also to conform to others' expectancies. Such tendencies can be associated with risk and harm avoidance behavior (Grandi et al., 2011) and conformity, lending further support for placing exercise addiction toward the compulsive end of the obsessive-compulsive disorders' spectrum (Demetrovics & Kurimay, 2008). However, the empirical examination of the mediating role of risk-taking and risk avoidance between perfectionism and exercise addiction, and their direct relationship to exercise addiction, is still needed.

14.5 Personality characteristics and exercise addiction

14.5.1 Perfectionism

Most scholars examining the link between the risk of exercise addiction and perfectionism report a positive relationship (Coen & Ogles, 1993; Cook, 1997; Hagan & Hausenblas, 2003; Hall et al., 2007, 2009; Hausenblas & Downs, 2002; Miller & Mesagno, 2014). In our recent literature review (Çakın et al., 2021), we found that out of the 22 studies examined, only one did not yield a positive association between perfectionism or one of its domains and the risk of exercise addiction. Another recent systematic literature review (González-Hernández et al., 2021) also reported a positive link between exercise addiction and perfectionism. This personality trait was then identified as a risk factor in the etiology of exercise addiction.

14.5.2 Narcissism

Vanity, self-love, and self-admiration are characteristics of narcissism in the psychoanalytic view (Freud, 1957). Lasch (1979) described narcissism as an endemic to modern society, mirrored in the media-promoting preoccupation with bodily appearance that is manageable through diet, exercise, or cosmetic surgery. Consequently, exercise can act as a means of control for body shape. Lowen (1983) highlighted that while exercise for many is a health-promoting or mastery activity, for some people it is a means of conforming to the media's fashion ideal of 'a lean, tight, hard body, like that of a young Adonis or Venus' (p. 34), and uses bodybuilders as an example. Therefore, like in eating disorders, excessive exercise in narcissistic people can be *instrumental* in achieving an objective related to a body concern.

Research confirms the relationship between narcissism and exercise addiction. For example, Spano (2001) reported a correlation between the frequency of physical activity and narcissism. More recent research supported the relationship between narcissism and exercise addiction (Bruno et al., 2014; Miller & Mesagno, 2014). Our literature review (Bircher et al., 2017) has shown that narcissism may be a fundamental personality feature in exercise addiction. Indeed, several studies confirm the relationship between exercise addiction and narcissism (Bruno et al., 2014; Cook et al., 2018; Miller & Mesagno, 2014; Zeigler-Hill et al., 2021). The relationship appears to be stronger in men than in women (Brown, 2000; Carroll, 1989; Cook et al., 2018; Nogueira et al., 2019).

Collectively, the studies examining the link between the risk of exercise addiction and narcissism suggest an association between these factors. However, its strength may vary according to exercise volume and form of training, which requires more experimental scrutiny. The positive correlation between the risk of exercise addiction and narcissism does not reveal causality. Therefore, it is unclear whether narcissism is a symptom of excessive exercise behavior or vice versa. Exercise can be *instrumental* in narcissism, but future studies should examine the extent to which excessive exercise is prevalent among individuals diagnosed with narcissism.

14.5.3 Self-esteem

People at risk of exercise addiction appear to demonstrate lower levels of self-esteem than asymptomatic individuals (Ackard et al., 2002; Chittester & Hausenblas, 2009; Cook, 1997; Grandi et al., 2011; Hall et al., 2009). However, labile self-esteem (unstable self-esteem) appears to be the key mediator in this relationship (Bruno et al., 2014; Hall et al., 2009). For example, labile self-esteem mediated the relationship between unconditional self-acceptance and the risk for exercise addiction (Hall et al., 2009). A positive correlation between the latter and labile self-esteem indicated that the two shared 15.2% of the variance. These findings were supported by Bruno et al. (2014), who found that both labile self-esteem and narcissism predicted the risk of exercise addiction. On the contrary, another study showed that self-esteem is a positive predictor of exercise addiction when controlling for body shame (Ertl et al., 2017). Therefore, the link between self-esteem and exercise addiction is not straightforward, and the mediating factors should be further explored in future research.

Given that exercise is a socially accepted and appreciated behavior, its adoption for coping with adversities may be perceived to *preserve one's self-esteem* in contrast to destructive forms of coping like drug or alcohol abuse. The individual using exercise for coping with stress or anxiety may be convinced that exercise is the right and healthy path in dealing with such personal hardship. This form of coping behavior is unlikely to damage the potentially already fragile self-esteem of the individual.

14.5.4 Neuroticism and extroversion

Neuroticism is defined as a predisposition to experience negative affect mirroring labiality in mood states (McCrae, 1990). Extroversion can be defined as a broad personality dimension composed of positive orientation, sensation or attention-seeking, activity, reduced or absent social inhibition, and sociability (Dumitrache et al., 2017). Research shows that neuroticism is positively related to the risk of exercise addiction (Adams & Kirkby, 1997; Andreassen et al., 2013; Bamber et al., 2000; Costa & Oliva, 2012; Hausenblas & Giacobbi, 2004; Jibaja-Rusth, 1989; Kern, 2010; Yates et al., 1992). This association, in accord with the interactional model, may be linked to using or relying on exercise as a means of coping with labile affective or mood state characteristics of neuroticism.

In the context of extroversion, the research findings are less consistent. Mathers and Walker (1999) found that exercisers were more extroverted than non-exercisers, but extroversion was unrelated to the risk of exercise addiction. Similar negative findings were disclosed earlier by Davis (1990) in a study of 96 exercising women. Kern (2010) also could not disclose a relationship between extroversion and exercise addiction. However, a few years later, Danish researchers (Lichtenstein et al., 2014) failed to reveal a difference in neuroticism between those at risk for exercise addiction and a control group but found that the two differed statistically significantly in their extroversion scores. Still, the effect size was only small to moderate.

Similarly, a later study of 531 college students showed a significant but very weak correlation between compulsive exercise and extroversion (Martin & Racine, 2017). In contrast, in a more recent inquiry, Cook et al. (2018) found that, after exercise frequency, extroversion was the strongest predictor of the risk of exercise addiction. Finally, a recent study has also disclosed a positive association between extroversion and the risk of exercise addiction, but only in men (Strahler et al., 2021).

It appears that findings concerning the link between the risk for exercise addiction and extroversion are inconsistent. The reason for the controversial results could be blamed on the different participants studied in various studies and their forms of exercise. For example, a recent literature review (Allen et al., 2020) showed that 1) athletes are more extroverted than non-athletes, 2) team-sport athletes are more extroverted than individual-sport athletes, and 3) female athletes exhibit greater extroversion than their male counterparts. Another recent study divulged that player position is linked to extroversion in that offensive players are more extroverted than defensive players (Terwiel & Kritzler, 2021). Furthermore, team sports players appear to exhibit greater extroversion than physical education students (Rogowska, 2020). University students pursuing different interests also score differently on extroversion measures, with sports-oriented students scoring higher than the others (Sethi & Mehta, 2020).

Consequently, studying psychology students (i.e., Martin & Racine, 2017) is very likely to yield different results from studying physically active or athlete students. Overall, research participants' heterogeneity may be the main reason for inconsistent findings concerning the relationship between the risk of exercise addiction and extroversion. A stronger link between these two can be assumed for neuroticism because a higher score on this negative personality trait is more consistently associated with the risk of exercise addiction.

14.6 Exercise addiction as a clinical symptom

In Chapter 10, we elaborated on the concept of secondary exercise addiction in which high volumes of training are instrumental in achieving a weight management-related goal. In this case, excessive exercise is recognized as a *diagnostic symptom* for restricting subtypes of anorexia nervosa and bulimia nervosa in the *Diagnostic and Statistical Manual of Mental Disorders* (American Psychiatric Association, 2013). Therefore, as noted earlier, excessive exercise is an established *symptom* of eating disorders from a clinical perspective.

14.7 Is exercise addiction a symptom or a disorder?

Therefore, from a clinical perspective, excessive exercise, which is not necessarily identical to exercise addiction, is a *symptom* of certain eating disorders. Szabo (2010) also thought that exercise addiction is likely a symptom of another psychological hardship. The interactional model (Dinardi et al., 2021; Egorov & Szabo, 2013) also suggests that exercise addiction is a result (again a symptom) of intolerable stress or trauma when it surfaces as a result of therapeutic exercise, or alternately could be the result of the Dunning–Kruger symptom (overestimation of one's ability) when it surfaces as a result of mastery exercise. Since the antecedent of mental health history is not always evident in the few case studies published in the literature, developing exercise addiction often remains unclear. In Chapter 13, Mr. M.Y. had several other psychological problems, which permits the assumption that his addiction to cycling was a symptom of, or a co-dysfunction with, the other psychological dysfunctions he experienced in the past. Therefore, most of the evidence points toward exercise addiction being a *symptom* of another disorder, which might be the reason why insufficient evidence could be obtained for its inclusion in the latest edition (5th) of the *Diagnostic and Statistical Manual of Mental Disorders* (American Psychiatric Association, 2013) as a distinct category of mental disorder.

   The link between the risk of exercise addiction and personality traits like narcissism, perfectionism, and neuroticism is not directional, and, therefore, it is unclear whether narcissistic individuals suffer more of exercise addiction than their healthy counterparts. Nevertheless, prevalence studies could reveal whether exercise addiction is a symptom of narcissistic behavior or vice versa. The close relationship is established to maladaptive personality traits only because exercise addiction's link to extroversion, and other positive personality traits, have not been empirically established.

   Therefore, in accord with the current clinical standpoints, it is difficult to argue that exercise addiction is a distinct category of mental disorder. The pyramid approach proposed in Chapter 12 could be the way for generating evidence for its distinctiveness. This method requires the use of deep interviews, too, not merely *risk assessment* as done in nomothetic questionnaire-based research representing the bulk of work in the field. A starting point could be the 100 cases identified by Juwono and Szabo (2020). However, these cases reveal only part of the story approved or disclosed by the affected individual. Further questions concerning the antecedent of the dysfunctional exercise behavior need to be answered to distinguish between the symptom of excessive exercising and its distinctiveness as a mental or psychological disorder.

14.8 Key points

1. Exercise addiction is compulsive but not impulsive behavior.
2. Exercise addiction is positively associated with perfectionism.
3. Exercise addiction is positively associated with narcissism.
4. Exercise addiction is positively related to neuroticism and low self-esteem.
5. Exercise addiction appears to be a symptom of another mental dysfunction.

14.9 References

Ackard, D. M., Brehm, B. J., & Steffen, J. J. (2002). Exercise and eating disorders in college-aged women: Profiling excessive exercisers. *Eating Disorders: The Journal of Treatment & Prevention, 10*(1), 31–47. doi:10.1080/106402602753573540

Adams, J., & Kirkby, R. J. (1997). Exercise dependence: A problem for sports physiotherapists. *Australian Journal of Physiotherapy, 43*(1), 53–58. doi:10.1016/S0004-9514(14)60402-5

Allen, M. S., Mison, E. A., Robson, D. A., & Laborde, S. (2020). Extraversion in sport: A scoping review. *International Review of Sport and Exercise Psychology*, 1–31. (Online first). doi:10.1080/1750984x.2020.1790024

American Psychiatric Association (2013). *Diagnostic and statistical manual of mental disorders* (5th ed.). doi:10.1176/appi.books.9780890425596

Andreassen, C. S., Griffiths, M. D., Gjertsen, S. R., Krossbakken, E., Kvam, S., & Pallesen, S. (2013). The relationships between behavioral addictions and the five-factor model of personality. *Journal of Behavioral Addictions, 2*(2), 90–99. doi:10.1556/JBA.2.2013.003

Bamber, D. J., Cockerill, I. M., & Carroll, D. (2000). The pathological status of exercise dependence. *British Journal of Sports Medicine, 34*(2), 125–132. doi:10.1136/bjsm.34.2.125

Bieling, P. J., Israeli, A. L., & Antony, M. M. (2004). Is perfectionism good, bad, or both? Examining models of the perfectionism construct. *Personality and Individual Differences, 36*(6), 1373–1385. doi:10.1016/s0191-8869(03)00235-6

Bircher, J., Griffiths, M. D., Kasos, K., Demetrovics, Z., & Szabo, A. (2017). Exercise addiction and personality: A two-decade systematic review of the empirical literature (1995–2015). *Baltic Journal of Sports and Health Sciences, 3*(106), 19–33. doi:10.33607/bjshs.v3i106.30

Brown, L. B. (2000). Powerful physiques, vulnerable psyches: Narcissism, body image and masculinity in male bodybuilders. *Dissertation Abstracts International: Section B: The Sciences and Engineering, 61*(7 – B), 3833.

Bruno, A., Quattrone, D., Scimeca, G., Cicciarelli, C., Romeo, V. M., Pandolfo, G., . . . Muscatello, M. R. A. (2014). Unraveling exercise addiction: The role of narcissism and self-esteem. *Journal of Addiction, 987841*, 1–6. doi:10.1155/2014/987841

Çakın, G., Juwono, I. D., Potenza, M. N., & Szabo, A. (2021). Exercise addiction and perfectionism: A systematic review of the literature. *Current Addiction Reports*, *8*(1), 144–155. doi:10.1007/s40429-021-00358-8

Carroll, L. (1989). A comparative study of narcissism, gender, and sex-role orientation among bodybuilders, athletes, and psychology students. *Psychological Reports*, *64*(3), 999–1006. doi:10.2466/pr0.1989.64.3.999

Chittester, N. I., & Hausenblas, H. A. (2009). Correlates of drive for muscularity: The role of anthropometric measures and psychological factors. *Journal of Health Psychology*, *14*(7), 872–877. doi:10.1177/1359105309340986

Coen, S. P., & Ogles, B. M. (1993). Psychological characteristics of the obligatory runner: A critical examination of the anorexia analogue hypothesis. *Journal of Sport and Exercise Psychology*, *15*(3), 338–354. doi:10.1123/jsep.15.3.338

Cook, B., Hausenblas, H., Tuccitto, D., & Giacobbi, P. R. (2011). Eating disorders and exercise: A structural equation modelling analysis of a conceptual model. *European Eating Disorders Review*, *19*(3), 216–225. doi:10.1002/erv.1111

Cook, C. A. (1997). *The psychological correlates of exercise dependence in aerobics instructors.* Unpublished master's thesis. University of Alberta, Alberta, Canada. Retrieved from: https://bac-lac.on.worldcat.org/v2/oclc/46533891

Cook, R. H., Griffiths, M. D., & Pontes, H. M. (2018). Personality factors in exercise addiction: A pilot study exploring the role of narcissism, extraversion, and agreeableness. *International Journal of Mental Health and Addiction*, *18*(1), 89–102. doi:10.1007/s11469-018-9939-z

Costa, S., & Oliva, P. (2012). Examining relationship between personality characteristics and exercise dependence. *Review of Psychology*, *19*(1), 5–11. Retrieved from: https://hrcak.srce.hr/91383

Cox, R., & Orford, J. (2004). A qualitative study of the meaning of exercise for people who could be labelled as "addicted" to exercise – can "addiction" be applied to high frequency exercising? *Addiction Research & Theory*, *12*(2), 167–188. doi:10.1080/1606635310001634537

Davis, C. (1990). Body image and weight preoccupation: A comparison between exercising and non-exercising women. *Appetite*, *15*(1), 13–21.

Demetrovics, Z., & Kurimay, T. (2008). Exercise addiction: A literature review. *Psychiatria Hungarica*, *23*(2), 129–141. PMID: 18956613

Dinardi, J. S., Egorov, A. Y., & Szabo, A. (2021). The expanded interactional model of exercise addiction. *Journal of Behavioral Addictions*, *10*(3), 626–631. doi:10.1556/2006.2021.00061

Dumitrache, C. G., Rubio, L., & Rubio-Herrera, R. (2017). Extroversion, social support and life satisfaction in old age: A mediation model. *Aging & Mental Health*, *22*(8), 1069–1077. doi:10.1080/13607863.2017.1330869

Egorov, A. Y., & Szabo, A. (2013). The exercise paradox: An interactional model for a clearer conceptualization of exercise addiction. *Journal of Behavioral Addictions*, *2*(4), 199–208. doi:10.1556/jba.2.2013.4.2

Ertl, M. M., Longo, L. M., Groth, G. H., Berghuis, K. J., Prout, J., Hetz, M. C., & Martin, J. L. (2017). Running on empty: High self-esteem as a risk factor for exercise addiction. *Addiction Research & Theory*, *26*(3), 205–211. doi:10.1080/16066359.2017.1347257

Freimuth, M., Moniz, S., & Kim, S. R. (2011). Clarifying exercise addiction: Differential diagnosis, co-occurring disorders, and phases of addiction. *International*

Journal of Environmental Research and Public Health, 8(10), 4069–4081. doi:10.3390/ijerph8104069

Freud, S. (1957). On narcissism: An introduction (1914). In J. Strache (Ed., Transl.), *The standard edition of the complete psychological works of Sigmund Freud* (Vol. 6, 14). London: Hogarth.

Goodman, A. (1990). Addiction: Definition and implications. *British Journal of Addiction, 85*(11), 1403–1408. doi:10.1111/j.1360-0443.1990.tb01620.x

Goodman, A. (2001). What's in a name? Terminology for designating a syndrome of driven sexual behavior. *Sexual Addiction & Compulsivity: The Journal of Treatment and Prevention, 8*(3–4), 191–213. doi:10.1080/107201601753459919

González-Hernández, J., Nogueira, A., Zangeneh, M., & López-Mora, C. (2021). Exercise addiction and perfectionism, joint in the same path? A systematic review. *International Journal of Mental Health and Addiction.* (Online first). doi:10.1007/s11469-020-00476-w

Grandi, S., Clementi, C., Guidi, J., Benassi, M., & Tossani, E. (2011). Personality characteristics and psychological distress associated with primary exercise dependence: An exploratory study. *Psychiatry Research, 189*(2), 270–275. doi:10.1016/j.psychres.2011.02.025

Grant, J. E., & Potenza, M. N. (2006). Compulsive aspects of impulse-control disorders. *Psychiatric Clinics of North America, 29*(2), 539–551. doi:10.1016/j.psc.2006.02.002

Griffiths, M. D. (2005). A 'components' model of addiction within a biopsychosocial framework. *Journal of Substance Use, 10*(4), 191–197. doi:10.1080/14659890500114359

Hagan, A., & Hausenblas, H. A. (2003). The relationship between exercise dependence symptoms and perfectionism. *American Journal of Health Studies, 18*(2/3), 133–137.

Hall, H. K., Hill, A. P., Appleton, P. R., & Kozub, S. A. (2009). The mediating influence of unconditional self-acceptance and labile self-esteem on the relationship between multidimensional perfectionism and exercise dependence. *Psychology of Sport and Exercise, 10*(1), 35–44. doi:10.1016/j.psychsport.2008.05.003

Hall, H. K., Kerr, A. W., Kozub, S. A., & Finnie, S. B. (2007). Motivational antecedents of obligatory exercise: The influence of achievement goals and multidimensional perfectionism. *Psychology of Sport and Exercise, 8*(3), 297–316. doi:10.1016/j.psychsport.2006.04.007

Hausenblas, H. A., & Downs, S. D. (2002). How much is too much? The development and validation of the exercise dependence scale. *Psychology and Health, 17*(4), 387–404. doi:10.1080/0887044022000004894

Hausenblas, H. A., & Giacobbi Jr, P. R. (2004). Relationship between exercise dependence symptoms and personality. *Personality and Individual Differences, 36*(6), 1265–1273. doi:10.1016/S0191-8869(03)00214-9

Hewitt, P. L., Flett, G. L., Turnbull-Donovan, W., & Mikail, S. F. (1991). The Multidimensional Perfectionism Scale: Reliability, validity, and psychometric properties in psychiatric samples. *Psychological Assessment, 3*(3), 464–468. doi:10.1037/1040-3590.3.3.464

Hollander, E., & Wong, C. M. (1995). Obsessive-compulsive spectrum disorders. *The Journal of Clinical Psychiatry, 56*(suppl. 4), 3–6. PMID: 7713863

Iannos, M., & Tiggemann, M. (1997). Personality of the excessive exerciser. *Personality and Individual Differences, 22*(5), 775–778. doi:10.1016/s0191-8869(96)00254-1

Jibaja-Rusth, M. L. (1989). *The development of a psycho-social risk profile for becoming an obligatory runner.* Doctoral dissertation. University of Houston, Houston, TX.

Juwono, I. D., & Szabo, A. (2020). 100 cases of exercise addiction: More evidence for a widely researched but rarely identified dysfunction. *International Journal of Mental Health and Addiction.* (Online first). doi:10.1007/s11469-020-00264-6

Kern, L. (2010). [Relationship between exercise dependence and big five personality]. *L'Encephale, 36*(3), 212–218. doi:10.1016/j.encep.2009.06.007 (in French)

Lasch, C. (1979). *The culture of narcissism.* New York, NY: Norton.

Lichtenstein, M. B., Christiansen, E., Elklit, A., Bilenberg, N., & Støving, R. K. (2014). Exercise addiction: A study of eating disorder symptoms, quality of life, personality traits and attachment styles. *Psychiatry Research, 215*(2), 410–416. doi:10.1016/j.psychres.2013.11.010

Lowen, A. (1983). *Narcissism: Denial of the true self.* New York, NY: Macmillan.

Martin, S. J., & Racine, S. E. (2017). Personality traits and appearance-ideal internalization: Differential associations with body dissatisfaction and compulsive exercise. *Eating Behaviors, 27*, 39–44. doi:10.1016/j.eatbeh.2017.11.001

Mathers, S., & Walker, M. B. (1999). Extraversion and exercise addiction. *The Journal of Psychology, 133*(1), 125–128. doi:10.1080/00223989909599727

McCrae, R. R. (1990). Controlling neuroticism in the measurement of stress. *Stress Medicine, 6*(3), 237–241. doi:10.1002/smi.2460060309

Melancon, M. O., Lorrain, D., & Dionne, I. J. (2014). Changes in markers of brain serotonin activity in response to chronic exercise in senior men. *Applied Physiology, Nutrition, and Metabolism, 39*(11), 1250–1256. doi:10.1139/apnm-2014-0092

Miller, K. J., & Mesagno, C. (2014). Personality traits and exercise dependence: Exploring the role of narcissism and perfectionism. *International Journal of Sport and Exercise Psychology, 12*(4), 368–381. doi:10.1080/1612197x.2014.932821

Myers, S. G., Fisher, P. L., & Wells, A. (2008). Belief domains of the Obsessive Beliefs Questionnaire-44 (OBQ-44) and their specific relationship with obsessive – compulsive symptoms. *Journal of Anxiety Disorders, 22*(3), 475–484. doi:10.1016/j.janxdis.2007.03.012

Nogueira, A., Tovar-Gálvez, M., & González-Hernández, J. (2019). Do it, don't feel it, and be invincible: A prolog of exercise addiction in endurance sports. *Frontiers in Psychology, 10.* doi:10.3389/fpsyg.2019.02692. Retrieved from: www.frontiersin.org/articles/10.3389/fpsyg.2019.02692/full

Rogowska, A. M. (2020). Personality differences between academic team sport players and physical education undergraduate students. *Physical Education of Students, 24*(1), 55–62. doi:10.15561/20755279.2020.0107

Sethi, P. K., & Mehta, V. (2020). Topography of personality traits among university students pursuing different interest. *Journal of Sports Science and Nutrition, 1*(2), 29–31.

Shin, M. K. (2009). Effects of an exercise program on frontal lobe cognitive function in elders. *Journal of Korean Academy of Nursing, 39*(1), 107. doi:10.4040/jkan.2008.39.1.107

Spano, L. (2001). The relationship between exercise and anxiety, obsessive-compulsiveness, and narcissism. *Personality and Individual Differences, 30*(1), 87–93. doi:10.1016/S0191-8869(00)00012-X

Strahler, J., Wachten, H., Stark, R., & Walter, B. (2021). Alike and different: Associations between orthorexic eating behaviors and exercise addiction. *International Journal of Eating Disorders, 54*(8), 1415–1425. doi:10.1002/eat.23525

Szabo, A. (2003). The acute effects of humor and exercise on mood and anxiety. *Journal of Leisure Research, 35*(2), 152–162. doi:10.1080/00222216.2003.11949988

Szabo, A. (2010). *Addiction to exercise: A symptom or a disorder?* New York, NY: Nova Science Publishers.

Terwiel, S., & Kritzler, S. (2021). Introverted goalie versus extraverted center? Comprehensive investigation of Big Five personality traits within and between team sports. *PsyArXix Preprints.* doi:10.31234/osf.io/h28ct Retrieved from: https://psyarxiv.com/h28ct/

Weinstein, A., & Weinstein, Y. (2014). Exercise addiction- diagnosis, bio-psychological mechanisms and treatment issues. *Current Pharmaceutical Design, 20*(25), 4062–4069. doi:10.2174/13816128113199990614

World Health Organization (2019). *International statistical classification of diseases and related health problems* (11th ed.). Retrieved from: https://icd.who.int/

Yates, A., Shisslak, C. M., Allender, J., Crago, M., & Leehey, K. (1992). Comparing obligatory to nonobligatory runners. *Psychosomatics, 33*(2), 180–189. doi:10.1016/s0033-3182(92)71994-x

Young, S. N. (2007). How to increase serotonin in the human brain without drugs. *Journal of Psychiatry & Neuroscience, 32*(6), 394–399. PMID: 18043762

Yuki, A., Lee, S., Kim, H., Kozakai, R., Ando, F., & Shimokata, H. (2012). Relationship between physical activity and brain atrophy progression. *Medicine & Science in Sports & Exercise, 44*(12), 2362–2368. doi:10.1249/mss.0b013e3182667d1d

Zeigler-Hill, V., Besser, A., Gabay, M., & Young, G. (2021). Narcissism and exercise addiction: The mediating roles of exercise-related motives. *International Journal of Environmental Research and Public Health, 18*(8), Article 4243. (Online first). doi:10.3390/ijerph18084243

15 Treatment of exercise addiction

Specific treatment for exercise addiction does not exist because there are no diagnostic criteria for the dysfunction. The various symptoms of exercise addiction are treated together with the comorbidities or related dysfunctions using *multiple* psychological interventions. At moderate levels of exercise addiction, a potential treatment method is the patient's guidance and education (Berczik et al., 2012). The teaching of self-control is the primary focus of such treatment. While parents or teachers can help in the patient's education, a psychologist or a qualified mental health professional should set up a systematic learning strategy.

15.1 Cognitive-behavioral therapy

This treatment focuses on incorrect information processing as a source of dysfunction (Beck & Weishaar, 2000). Therefore, it aims to change the person's *schema* associated with the erroneously processed information. According to the schema theory (Axelrod, 1973), stored information forms schemas or blueprints in the memory to be retrieved later. This cognitive model expands the Pavlovian conditioning by highlighting that weak associations form labile schemas while strong mental associations form robust and instantly retrievable schemas. Furthermore, mental access to schemas is sequential so that easily accessible robust schemas are processed first, whereas less accessible (weak or labile) schemas are processed last.

In exercise addiction, the mental schema connected to exercise behavior is strongly conditioned. Such a robust schema is challenging to alter. However, the therapeutic aim is to change the information processing strategy or modify how people think about exercise. Therefore, the newly acquired schemas, generated through progressive education of the person (Berczik et al., 2012), are usually weak in the early stages. Cognitive-behavioral therapy aims to strengthen the schema associated with a new adaptive or healthy information through progressive practice and reinforcement. A new schema's solidification occurs through repeated practice (frequency) or impactful events (intensity). For example, an exercise addict may attend a year-long therapy before the new healthy schema overtakes the old maladaptive

DOI: 10.4324/9781003173595-15

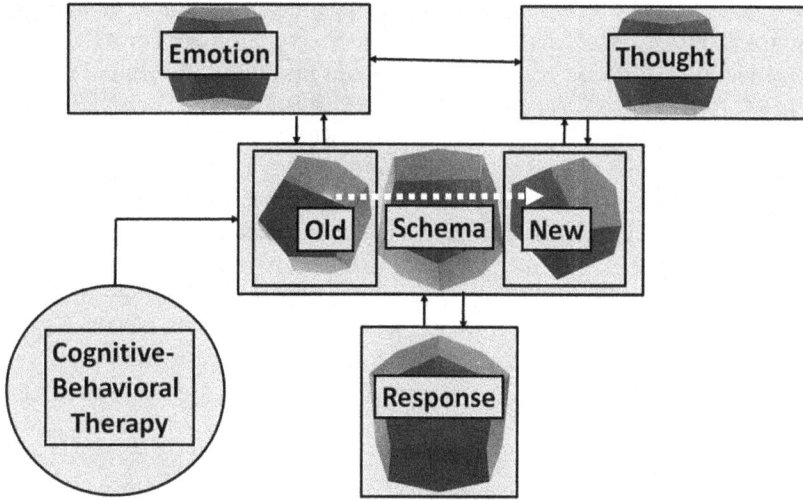

Figure 15.1 A cognitive-behavioral therapy model. It aims to change how information is processed (shaping the mental schema) to elicit an adaptive response.

schema. Alternately, a very emotional or intense experience (high impact), such as the threat of life, can induce an almost instantaneous schema modification. The cognitive-behavioral therapy is illustrated in Figure 15.1.

Consequently, the objective of this treatment method is to replace the old maladaptive or unhealthy schema with a new adaptive schema. Schema is the trigger for action. The correct schema will trigger the right action. Avid exercisers are usually convinced that their schema of exercise behavior is adequate, and they might not think about changing it. Still, when they experience some damage, the faulty trigger is forcefully recognized. Various related schemas are retrieved to justify the correctness of the schema connected to the exercise behavior. At this stage, a set of competing schemas influence the thoughts and emotions of the involved person. Their complex central interactions determine whether the person will seek help or not. Unfortunately, it appears that there is relatively little empirical or clinical evidence for the effectiveness of cognitive-behavioral therapy for treating exercise addiction (Weinstein & Weinstein, 2014). Adherence to the long-lasting treatment might be the main reason for the low success rate of this method (Maher et al., 2012).

15.2 Cue exposure therapy

Cue exposure therapy, which encompasses a reaction stop or response prevention strategy, has been used to treat patients wishing to control their alcoholism and those who want to abstain from drinking. As Rosenberg (2002) described, there is a general assumption on which the cue exposure therapy is based. Accordingly, over time, diverse cues are connected with the craving for the object of addiction. Consequently, cues that are paired with exercise deprivation or reward of exercising form mental schemas that trigger a conditioned urge or craving when the addicted person perceives one or more of these cues. These cues vary from person to person. They may include scenarios like seeing a jogger or a cyclist on the street, or passing before the window of a sports equipment shop, or seeing a gym in the area, or feeling an emotional state like anger (if anger management is paired with exercise), or being in the company of other athletes or exercisers and attending sports contests.

Cue exposure therapy assumes that the repeated exposure to these cues (retrieval of schemas) without engaging in the conditioned exercise behavior can break the connection to the exercise. The process involves a mental dissociation. According to Axelrod (1973), the mental schema could be altered by sufficiently important and impactful information. Such an altered mental schema, as illustrated in Figure 15.1, is also the objective of the cue exposure therapy. For individuals who wish to exert greater control over their excessive exercise, cue exposure therapy helps to resist the urges triggered by various exercise cues. Even if the resistance is not always successful, more and more control might be exerted concerning the timing, volume, and intensity of exercise.

Cue exposure therapy aimed at moderate or early exercise addiction consists of repeated sessions during and after exercise. In these sessions, the person is exposed to those cues that trigger the urge to exercise more often or in greater volumes. Therefore, they take place after exercise sessions to try to prolong the interval between two exercise sessions. The cues are also delivered during exercise (i.e., recorded audio or chat contact with the therapist) to help attain and maintain control over the exercise volume. Each therapy session typically involves several cue exposure episodes and assessment of craving, resistance, expected withdrawal symptoms, self-efficacy, and should be combined with the learning and practice of coping skills to deal with the craving for the exercise. The therapy continues until the client reports that exposure to cues no longer provokes painful cravings. In the treatment, exercise addicts are encouraged to face and work through their cravings, instead of fearing, avoiding, or giving in to them. Cue *replacement*, or cue reconfiguration (Cubillas et al., 2017) during the therapy, is an expanded method in which the cues triggering the urge for exercise are paired with another behavior, such as relaxation, social interaction, or family interactions. The aim is that the new pairing is mentally strengthened until it outcompetes the wrong (exercise triggering) cue. Although, in essence, this approach is a sort of cognitive-behavioral therapy, in substance addictions, especially alcoholism, it is less effective (Mellentin et al., 2017).

15.3 Systematic desensitization

Systematic desensitization therapy accompanied by reinforcement of the newly emerging behavior are two other possible interventions for exercise addiction. It is similar to cue exposure therapy, and when it comprises substitution therapy too, it is a form of cue-replacement therapy. Systematic desensitization (McGlynn, 2010) is based on the mental vision and acceptance of progressively lower exercise volumes while teaching how to take and maintain control over the exercise behavior. Successful reductions are subsequently placed in practice and are rewarded. There is ongoing consultation with the individual to make a fair and reasonable plan for reducing and controlling the exercise volume. Goal-setting is a regular part of the treatment with an emphasis on short-term goals. Personal tangible and intangible rewards are encouraged at all stages of the short-term goal achievements. It is expected that over time, the affected person gradually takes control and decreases the exercise volume, with the result being the cessation of exercise dependence. In none of the therapies should complete exercise cessation be the aim. Instead, moderate and controlled pleasurable exercise should be the set goal.

15.4 Substitution therapy

Another alternative, substitution therapy, aims to help the exercise-addicted individual to see, appreciate, and enjoy other activities that could become habitual, such as another form of exercise, cultural programs like concerts, theater or movies, social interaction with others, board games, voluntary work, helping the needy, or discovering new places. Basically, the therapy's objective is to help addicts improve their social skills and encourage them to get involved more and more in group and other personally rewarding activities so that their social and spiritual life is improved, and their exercise dependence is reduced (Eisenberg et al., 1998). The factors determining the clinical framework of substitution therapy are known as *treatment thresholds*. The treatment threshold reflects the objective difficulties and barriers patients face before and during their treatment. These barriers affect treatment efficacy and the overall success rate (Stöver, 2011). Consequently, despite its efficacy proven in substance abuse disorders, substitution therapy may not work in all cases of exercise addiction. Cognitive-behavioral therapy combined with systematic desensitization followed by substitution therapy may be a more efficient treatment in severe cases.

15.5 Acceptance and commitment therapy

Hayes et al. (2006) define acceptance commitment therapy as 'a psychological intervention based on modern behavioral psychology, including relational frame theory, that applies mindfulness and acceptance processes, and commitment and behavior change processes, to the creation of psychological flexibility' (p. 10). In their paper, the authors describe in detail this therapy, which is beyond the scope of the current discussion. Instead, we delineate how it may be applied to treating exercise addiction. Acceptance and commitment therapy teaches the affected person to face and more importantly to accept the urge and craving that triggers impulsive need to exercise. The treatment is aimed at changing the way in which the individual interacts with, or relates to, thoughts (schemas) by creating new contexts (new schema associations) in which their dysfunctional behavior diminishes or ceases altogether (Hayes et al., 2006). This treatment method has been used effectively in the treatment of other behavioral addictions, such as Internet pornography (Twohig et al., 2010), and a relatively recent literature review concluded that the method is also effective in managing substance use disorders (Osaji et al., 2020).

One of the six components of acceptance commitment therapy is the mental or cognitive *diffusion* denoting *the actual meaning* of the *correct* mental schemas representing thoughts and emotions instead of the harmful schemas focusing on the threat of what might happen if one misses an exercise session. Therefore, the exercise-addicted person must reconsider and relearn the feelings associated with the fear of missing a workout. Again, like in cognitive-behavioral therapy, cue exposure therapy, and other interventions, this method's mechanism functions by inducing a change in the maladaptive mental schema. In general, psychological help, regardless of the treatment approach, comes from the *change* in the person's relationship to their exercise behavior, which implies a change in the mental schema connecting the two (Axelrod, 1973). The phase of addiction is an essential determinant of the progress, duration, and efficacy (outcome) of the treatment because the weaker schemas (involving uncertainty and doubt) are easier altered than older, more strongly conditioned, schemas (Axelrod, 1973; Szabo, 2020).

15.6 Meditation

Perhaps alone or in combination with a form of cognitive-behavioral therapy (depending on the stage of addiction), meditation, and similar self-awareness-enhancing interventions could be effective in the prevention or treatment of exercise addiction. Meditation was used in the treatment of various addictions. A relatively recent review of the literature concluded that spiritual meditation is a promising treatment for drug addiction (Kadri et al., 2020). Its efficacy in treating behavioral addictions was also shown. For example, Yoo et al. (2019) demonstrated that mind subtraction meditation (a form of spiritual meditation) effectively manages smartphone addiction in elementary school children. These results were corroborated in a later study with adolescents (Choi et al., 2020). Subsequently, a recent literature review (Lakshmi, 2021), based on 32 studies, concluded that meditation could be an effective therapy for reversing smartphone addiction.

Although exercise addiction is a behavioral addiction like smartphone addiction, the two differ in many respects. No focused studies were conducted on the effects of meditation techniques on exercise addiction. However, several investigations have demonstrated that meditation is an effective method for stress management (Heckenberg et al., 2018; Huberty et al., 2019). Among them, mindfulness meditation was shown to generate physiological benefits in addition to its positive mental health effects (Heckenberg et al., 2018; Ponte Márquez et al., 2018). Based on the interactional model (Dinardi et al., 2021), exercise addiction surfaces as a coping response to the accumulating stress or sudden trauma on the therapeutic path. If meditation yields stress relief, it is conceivable that the exercise-addicted person might perceive it as an additional method of coping and manage to balance the two, consequently reducing the excessive and harmful exercise behavior.

Nevertheless, meditation must be first accepted before practicing by the person addicted to exercise, which depends on the phase of addiction. Meditation can be employed in substitution therapy, too, in which the excessive part of the dysfunctional behavior is substituted with meditation. Consequently, creating a novel mental schema (through acceptance, trust, and experience) associated with meditation and complementing (even competing with) the schema connected to the exercise behavior might be effective in treating exercise addiction. Since hatha yoga (comprised of body postures, breathing exercises, and meditation; Riley, 2004) involves power and flexibility exercises and benefits fitness, endurance, and strength (Boraczyński et al., 2020), it can be an alternative form of exercise to the habitual (addicted form) exercise by the affected person. In this sense, hatha yoga is an excellent candidate for substitution therapy in treating exercise addiction, and its meditation component (Riley, 2004) could exacerbate its therapeutic effect.

15.7 Mindfulness

Given that compulsive behaviors are characterized by execution of the behaviors in response to 'instinctual' or automatic cravings and urges, mindfulness interventions, which could help individuals to relate more consciously with their exercise environment, might help develop a more adaptive relationship with exercise behavior. Mindfulness can be described as 'paying attention in a particular way: on purpose, in the present moment, and non-judgmentally' (Kabat-Zinn, 1994, p. 4). Therapies using mindfulness appear to be effective in treating a variety of mental health problems, including anxiety, depression, and several behavioral addictions (Quinones & Griffiths, 2019). Mindfulness-based interventions rely on meditation awareness training, so they may be considered as a specific form of meditation (Van Gordon et al., 2017). During regular meditation sessions, patients engage in guided sitting meditation, walking meditation, and work (exercise) meditation (i.e., achieving meditative awareness while exercising). The various meditative techniques used aim to foster 1) citizenship, 2) perceptive clarity, 3) ethical and compassionate awareness, 4) meditative insight, 5) patience, 6) generosity, and 7) life perspective (Van Gordon et al., 2017). Mindfulness has already been used successfully in treating symptoms of exercise addiction along with other treatment methods (Anandkumar et al., 2018) and is worth further investigating in this clinical domain.

15.8 Pharmacological intervention

The pharmacological treatment of exercise addiction is uncommon because the dysfunction is not classified as a clinical disorder, and, consequently, prescription medication is not available for it. Nevertheless, a study provided promising evidence for employing a pharmaceutical agent to manage the dysfunction (Di Nicola et al., 2010). This work used Quetiapine to treat bipolar type I disorder (which is characterized by full-blown and long-lasting manic episodes often requiring hospitalization). In addition, exercise addiction and compulsive shopping were identified comorbidities. After four weeks on the medication, the 47-year-old male patient exhibited a slight improvement in his compulsive shopping behavior and a more significant improvement in his addiction to exercise. After 12 weeks of treatment, his behavioral symptoms have improved markedly. Finally, after 24 weeks, the symptoms vanished utterly. His exercise addiction scores on the Exercise Addiction Inventory (Terry et al., 2004) dropped by 50% from 24 to 12, representing a shift from the 'at-risk category' into the 'asymptomatic category.' This case is incidental because the drug treatment was offered for the comorbidity, not for exercise addiction *per se*. Still, the possibility for the pharmaceutical therapy of the dysfunction was unveiled. Yet, until exercise addiction cannot be classified as a distinct category of mental dysfunction, its pharmacological treatment remains unlikely.

15.9 What to treat and how to treat?

Since exercise addiction currently is not a clinical dysfunction, only its symptoms could be treated. Treatment options involve some cognitive intervention based on learning and practice. At their core is the *change* in the mental schema or the rewiring of the maladaptive relationship between thoughts and emotions and exercise behavior. Therefore, all therapies should focus on the change in this mental association using a sequential intervention: 1) have the person *recognize and admit* that the symptoms cause problems; 2) identify the *stage* and *severity* of the problem(s); 3) *teach* the individual about the *value* of exercise along with the *threats* of its morbid practice; 4) let the person find *attractive alternatives* that should not replace but complement the habitual exercise behavior; 5) *reinforce* and teach the person to appreciate the pleasure of the alternative action (sport, culture, social, etc.); 6) adopt a *balance sheet* of gains and losses as a consequence of the additional or alternative action; 7) focus on the *gains* and use *goal-setting* to amplify and expand the gains; 8) *evaluate* goals, changes in feeling states, and intention effects; 9) if necessary, *adjust* the therapy by stepping back one stage; and 10) *generate social support* for the new (changed) adaptive behavior.

15.10 Key points

1. There is no proven specific treatment for exercise addiction.
2. Cognitive-behavioral therapy can be used to treat symptoms of exercise addiction.
3. A combination of several therapies may be the most efficient for morbid exercise.
4. Meditation and yoga could be attractive alternative therapies for exercise addiction.
5. Pharmacological interventions may prove efficient in treating exercises addiction through its comorbidities.

15.11 References

Anandkumar, S., Manivasagam, M., Kee, V. T. S., & Meyding-Lamade, U. (2018). Effect of physical therapy management of nonspecific low back pain with exercise addiction behaviors: A case series. *Physiotherapy Theory and Practice, 34*(4), 316–328. doi:10.1080/09593985.2017.1394410

Axelrod, R. (1973). Schema theory: An information processing model of perception and cognition. *The American Political Science Review, 67*(4), 1248–1266. doi:10.2307/1956546

Beck, A. T., & Weishaar, M. E. (2000). Cognitive therapy. In R. J. Corsini & D. Wedding (Eds.), *Current psychotherapies* (6th ed., pp. 241–272). Itasca, IL: F. E. Peacock.

Berczik, K., Szabó, A., Griffiths, M. D., Kurimay, T., Kun, B., Urbán, R., & Demetrovics, Z. (2012). Exercise addiction: Symptoms, diagnosis, epidemiology, and etiology. *Substance Use & Misuse, 47*(4), 403–417. doi:10.3109/10826084.2011.639120

Boraczyński, M. T., Boraczyński, T. W., Wójcik, Z., Gajewski, J., & Laskin, J. J. (2020). The effects of a 6-month moderate-intensity Hatha yoga-based training program on health-related fitness in middle-aged sedentary women: A randomized controlled study. *The Journal of Sports Medicine and Physical Fitness, 60*(8). doi:10.23736/s0022-4707.20.10549-8

Choi, E.-H., Chun, M. Y., Lee, I., Yoo, Y.-G., & Kim, M.-J. (2020). The effect of mind subtraction meditation intervention on smartphone addiction and the psychological wellbeing among adolescents. *International Journal of Environmental Research and Public Health, 17*(9), 3263. doi:10.3390/ijerph17093263

Cubillas, C. P., Vadillo, M. A., & Matute, H. (2017). Changes in cue configuration reduce the impact of interfering information in a predictive learning task. *Frontiers in Psychology, 7*. doi:10.3389/fpsyg.2016.02050

Dinardi, J. S., Egorov, A. Y., & Szabo, A. (2021). The expanded interactional model of exercise addiction. *Journal of Behavioral Addictions.* (Online first). doi:10.1556/2006.2021.00061

Di Nicola, M., Martinotti, G., Mazza, M., Tedeschi, D., Pozzi, G., & Janiri, L. (2010). Quetiapine as add-on treatment for bipolar I disorder with comorbid compulsive buying and physical exercise addiction. *Progress in Neuro-Psychopharmacology and Biological Psychiatry, 34*(4), 713–714. doi:10.1016/j.pnpbp.2010.03.013

Eisenberg, D. M., Davis, R. B., Ettner, S. L., Appel, S., Wilkey, S., Van Rompay, M., & Kessler, R. C. (1998). Trends in alternative medicine use in the United States, 1990–1997: Results of a follow-up national survey. *JAMA, 280*(18), 1569–1575.

Hayes, S. C., Luoma, J. B., Bond, F. W., Masuda, A., & Lillis, J. (2006). Acceptance and commitment therapy: Model, processes and outcomes. *Behaviour Research and Therapy, 44*(1), 1–25. doi:10.1016/j.brat.2005.06.006

Heckenberg, R. A., Eddy, P., Kent, S., & Wright, B. J. (2018). Do workplace-based mindfulness meditation programs improve physiological indices of stress? A systematic review and meta-analysis. *Journal of Psychosomatic Research, 114*, 62–71. doi:10.1016/j.jpsychores.2018.09.010

Huberty, J., Green, J., Glissmann, C., Larkey, L., Puzia, M., & Lee, C. (2019). Efficacy of the mindfulness meditation mobile app "Calm" to reduce stress among college students: Randomized controlled trial. *JMIR mHealth and uHealth, 7*(6), e14273. doi:10.2196/14273. Retrieved from: https://mhealth.jmir.org/2019/6/e14273

Kabat-Zinn, J. (1994). *Wherever you go, there you are: Mindfulness meditation in everyday life.* New York, NY: Hyperion.

Kadri, R., Husain, R., & Omar, S. H. S. (2020). Impact of spiritual meditation on drug addiction recovery and wellbeing: A systematic review. *International Journal of Human and Health Sciences, 4*(4), 237. doi:10.31344/ijhhs.v4i4.208

Lakshmi, R. (2021). Meditation and smartphone addiction – A short review. *Journal of Research in Traditional Medicine.* (Online first). doi:10.5455/jrtm.2021/77885

Maher, M. J., Wang, Y., Zuckoff, A., Wall, M. M., Franklin, M., Foa, E. B., & Simpson, H. B. (2012). Predictors of patient adherence to cognitive-behavioral therapy for obsessive-compulsive disorder. *Psychotherapy and Psychosomatics, 81*(2), 124–126. doi:10.1159/000330214

McGlynn, F. D. (2010). Systematic desensitization. In I. B. Weiner & W. E. Craighead (Eds.), *Corsini encyclopedia of psychology.* New York, NY: John Wiley & Sons.

Mellentin, A. I., Skøt, L., Nielsen, B., Schippers, G. M., Nielsen, A. S., Stenager, E., & Juhl, C. (2017). Cue exposure therapy for the treatment of alcohol use disorders: A meta-analytic review. *Clinical Psychology Review, 57*, 195–207. doi:10.1016/j.cpr.2017.07.006

Osaji, J., Ojimba, C., & Ahmed, S. (2020). The use of acceptance and commitment therapy in substance use disorders: A review of literature. *Journal of Clinical Medicine Research, 12*(10), 629–633. doi:10.14740/jocmr4311

Ponte Márquez, P. H., Feliu-Soler, A., Solé-Villa, M. J., Matas-Pericas, L., Filella-Agullo, D., Ruiz-Herrerias, M., ... Arroyo-Díaz, J. A. (2018). Benefits of mindfulness meditation in reducing blood pressure and stress in patients with arterial hypertension. *Journal of Human Hypertension, 33*(3), 237–247. doi:10.1038/s41371-018-0130-6

Quinones, C., & Griffiths, M. D. (2019). Reducing compulsive Internet use and anxiety symptoms via two brief interventions: A comparison between mindfulness and gradual muscle relaxation. *Journal of Behavioral Addictions, 8*(3), 530–536. doi:10.1556/2006.8.2019.45

Riley, D. (2004). Hatha yoga and the treatment of illness. *Alternative Therapies in Health and Medicine, 10*(2), 20–21.

Rosenberg, H. (2002). Controlled drinking. In *Encyclopaedia of psychotherapy* (pp. 533–544). New York, NY: Elsevier Science. doi:10.1016/b0-12-343010-0/00061-1

Stöver, H. (2011). Barriers to opioid substitution treatment access, entry and retention: A survey of opioid users, patients in treatment, and treating and non-treating physicians. *European Addiction Research, 17*(1), 44–54. doi:10.1159/000320576

Szabo, A. (2020). Immediate and persisting effects of controversial media information on young people's judgement of health issues. *Europe's Journal of Psychology, 16*(2), 249–261. doi:10.5964/ejop.v16i2.1929

Terry, A., Szabo, A., & Griffiths, M. (2004). The exercise addiction inventory: A new brief screening tool. *Addiction Research & Theory, 12*(5), 489–499. doi:10.1080/16066350310001637363

Twohig, M. P., & Crosby, J. M. (2010). Acceptance and commitment therapy as a treatment for problematic internet pornography viewing. *Behavior Therapy, 41*(3), 285–295. doi:10.1016/j.beth.2009.06.002

Van Gordon, W., Shonin, E., Dunn, T. J., Garcia-Campayo, J., Demarzo, M. M., & Griffiths, M. D. (2017). Meditation awareness training for the treatment of workaholism: A controlled trial. *Journal of Behavioral Addictions, 6*(2), 212–220. doi:10.1556/2006.6.2017.021

Weinstein, A., & Weinstein, Y. (2014). Exercise addiction- diagnosis, bio-psychological mechanisms and treatment issues. *Current Pharmaceutical Design, 20*(25), 4062–4069. doi:10.2174/13816128113199990614

Yoo, Y. G., Lee, M. J., Yu, B., & Yun, M. R. (2019). The effect of mind subtraction meditation on smartphone addiction in school children. *Global Journal of Health Science, 11*(10), 16. doi:10.5539/gjhs.v11n10p16

16 Untangling passion from exercise addiction

Shaping the knowledge

16.1 Passion, a brief refresher

Passion was discussed in Chapter 2. Its gist is refreshed in this brief section to facilitate the understanding of its relationship with exercise addiction. Accordingly, passion toward an activity reflects the avid engagement in a beloved activity that one finds attractive, important, and shows commitment by investing attention, time, and energy. Vallerand et al. (2003) presented a dual model of passion consisting of two forms: harmonious and obsessive passion. According to Vallerand (2008), passion develops when one likes the activity, freely selects to engage in it, and identifies herself with it. Harmonious passion surfaces when the adopted activity is internalized into the self automatically when one engages in the activity with flexibility, which is positively related to positive affect but has an inverse relationship with negative affect (Stenseng et al., 2011; Vallerand et al., 2003; 2006; Vallerand & Miquelon, 2007). In contrast, obsessive passion arises when one internalizes the activity in controlled ways, which is positively linked to negative affect (Stenseng et al., 2011; Vallerand et al., 2003; Vallerand et al., 2007; Vallerand & Miquelon, 2007). Furthermore, an obsessively passionate person attaches importance to activity contingencies, such as self-esteem and escape from problems, which makes it difficult for one to stop the passionate activity (Vallerand, 2010).

16.2 The association between exercise addiction and passion

There are an increasing number of scholastic publications on the relationship between exercise addiction and passion. In general, these reports suggest that obsessive passion is positively related to exercise addiction in endurance sports and leisure physical activities (Schipfer & Stoll, 2015; Stenseng et al., 2011). For example, Paradis et al. (2013) showed that obsessive passion is associated with all the dimensions of exercise addiction (i.e., time, reduction in other activities, tolerance, withdrawal, continuance, intention effects, and lack of control). However, no relationship has

DOI: 10.4324/9781003173595-16

emerged for harmonious passion, which was only related to time and tolerance. Furthermore, harmoniously passionate athletes and exercisers could augment the time spent on exercise without decreasing the time spent on other essential life activities. In contrast, obsessively passionate exercisers devote excessive time to exercise while reducing the time spent with other life activities (Paradis et al., 2013). The general finding that obsessive passion has a stronger relationship to the risk of exercise addiction than harmonious passion was also shown by Parastatidou et al. (2014) and other later studies.

16.3 Passion and exercise addiction in athletes

Empirical studies on the link between athletic involvement and passion are still limited. Early work has shown that highly competitive athletes scoring high on obsessive passion reported higher levels of well-being than athletes scoring high on harmonious passion (Amiot et al., 2006). In contrast, low-competitive athletes scoring high on obsessive passion reported lower levels of well-being than those scoring high on harmonious passion. Later, an inquiry examining 100 professional dancers (Akehurst & Oliver, 2013) reported that exercise addiction had a stronger relationship with obsession passion than with harmonious passion. The shared variance with the former was 52% while only 18% with the latter.

Another work by de la Vega et al. (2016) investigated regional- and national-level competitive athletes in contrast to noncompetitive leisure exercisers using a cross-sectional design. The authors found that, in general, obsessive passion and commitment to sports emerged as strong predictors of exercise addiction. Competitive athletes scored higher than leisure exercisers on all measures. Athletes competing at regional and national levels only differed in their commitment to their sport, with the latter group scoring higher than the former. Team sports athletes reported greater harmonious and obsessive passion and commitment to their sports, but not different levels of exercise addiction, than athletes involved in individual sports. At the same time, a study with 669 marathon runners (Lucidi et al., 2016) did not investigate exercise addiction but reported a weak positive correlation between training frequency and both obsessive and harmonious passion.

Finally, a study of 190 athletes involved in six different sports (Kovacsik, Soós et al., 2018) showed that both obsessive and harmonious passion were strong predictors of the risk of exercise addiction, and together, they accounted for 39% of the variance in it. Separate analyses for athletes involved in team and individual sports showed that passion accounted for 25% of the variance in the risk of exercise addiction in the former group, but for twice as much in those who practiced an individual sport (50%). However, harmonious passion had a weak contribution in both cases (3%–4%). Athletes in team sports scored higher on harmonious passion than those in individual sports. Overall, the few studies examining the relationship between the risk of exercise addiction and passion in athletes yield relatively consistent results, showing that obsessive passion is strong, whereas harmonious passion is a weak predictor of the risk of exercise addiction.

16.3 Passion and exercise addiction in leisure exercisers

A study by Back (2015) testing 106 leisure exercisers found a positive correlation between the risk of exercise addiction and obsessive passion, which explained 22.1% of the variance in the former. A later survey of 360 leisure exercisers (Kovacsik, Griffiths, et al., 2018) showed that obsessive passion was a strong predictor of the risk of exercise addiction by accounting for 32% of the variance, while harmonious passion only accounted for 1.8% of the variance. Comparatively, an extensive study of 1,255 fitness attendees (Lichtenstein et al., 2020b) reported that obsessive passion predicted an even more significant proportion of variance (48%) in the risk of exercise addiction. Furthermore, a study of 485 university students showed a stronger correlation between the risk of exercise addiction and obsessive passion than harmonious passion on two measures of the risk of exercise addiction (Sicilia et al., 2018). In this work, both forms of passion and, primarily, obsessive passion mediated the relationship between motivational regulations and the risk of exercise addiction. In an earlier study performed by the same research team (Sicilia et al., 2017), a statistically significant correlation emerged between the risk of exercise addiction and obsessive passion, accounting for 27% of common variance, while harmonious passion was unrelated to the risk of exercise addiction. However, both forms of passion mediated the relationship between goal contents and the risk of exercise addiction.

16.4 A longitudinal study

A recent longitudinal study of 149 young people who just started practicing a new sport (Kovacsik et al., 2020) has also reported statistically significant positive correlations between obsessive passion and the risk of exercise addiction. The two variables shared 27% of the variance at baseline (coinciding with the beginning of the first training session in the new sport), 30% after four weeks of practice, and 36% after 12 weeks of training. In this beginner (of a new passionate activity) sample, harmonious passion also shared relatively large proportions of the variances with the risk of exercise addiction at three sampling times: 30% at the beginning of the study (no experience with the activity at all), 38.4% after four weeks of practice, and 31% after 12 weeks of training, after the study. Despite these relatively strong relationships between passion and the risk of exercise addiction, motivational factors predicted passion. In contrast, exercise addiction was predicted by gender, team-sport involvement, exercise volume, and identified motivation. The findings of this study suggest that the development of passion and risk of exercise addiction, both being associated with sport motivations, appear to manifest independent patterns. Therefore, despite the repeatedly reported relationship between passion and the risk of exercise addiction, they may represent independent constructs. However, this independence may still involve a *symbiotic relationship* because when there is experimental control for passion, the results associated with the risk of exercise addiction vanish, as discussed below.

16.5 Controlling for passion in exercise addiction

Szabo and Kovacsik (2019) further tested the relationship between passion and exercise addiction by combining data from two previous studies and reanalyzing them. They showed that high- and low-exercise volume groups differed in the risk of exercise addiction even after controlling for age and gender. As expected, the former group scored higher than the latter. However, when they added obsessive and harmonious passion as continuous predictor variables (covariates), the statistical significance between high and low volume exercise groups has vanished. At the same time, the two forms of passion, as predictors, emerged to be statistically significant. Moreover, when controlling for the effect of passion, examining the correlation between exercise addiction and the weekly exercise volume turned out to be negative. This finding was unexpected because exercise addiction is associated with too much or exaggerated volumes of exercise in the literature. But the results of this study indicate that perhaps passion is more closely related to excessive exercise. It is logical to expect that a passionate activity is undertaken for an extended period, as the definition of passion (see Section 16.1) implies. But there are two forms of passion that could influence differently one's involvement level in exercise.

A cross-sectional study examining a large sample (n = 1,002) of Spanish and Hungarian volunteer research participants (Szabo et al., 2018) found cultural and gender differences in passion. For the sake of the current discussion, we looked again at these data from a different perspective and categorized exercise behavior as high and low volume using the cutoff value of ten hours per week. Subsequently, we subjected the data to a multivariate analysis of variance. The results showed that both harmonious passion and obsessive passion were statistically significantly higher in those who exercised more than 10 hours per week, on average, compared to those who exercised up to ten hours per week. As illustrated in Figure 16.1, these results were demonstrated in both Spanish and Hungarian samples.

Therefore, although there is a consensus in the literature that obsessive passion is a stronger predictor of exercise addiction than harmonious passion, both forms of passion differentiate the individuals who exercise in low volumes from those who exercise in higher volumes. However, the relationship between exercise volume, in terms of weekly hours of exercise, with

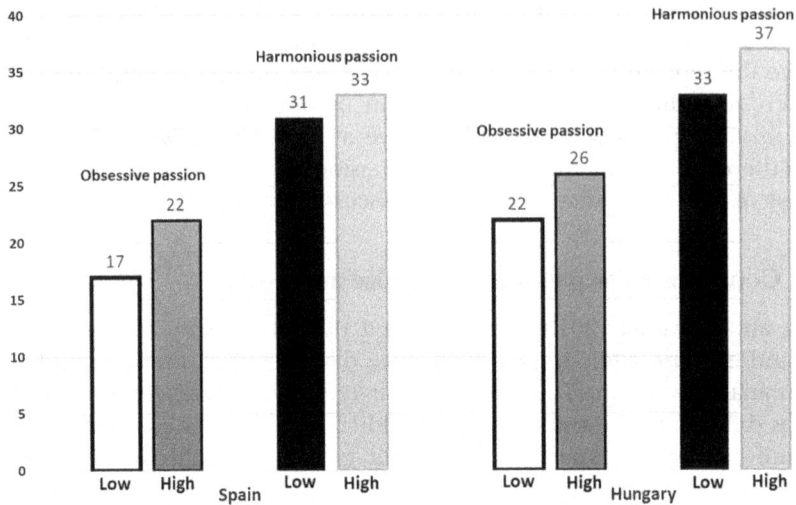

Figure 16.1 Differences in obsessive and harmonious passion between those who exercise up to 10 hours per week (low) and those who exercise more than 10 hours per week (high), the Spanish sample (left) and the Hungarian sample (right). The figure presents unpublished results from Szabo et al.'s (2018) data.

harmonious and obsessive passion is weak as based on correlation results, which reveal that the shared variances are less than 10% (8.41% and 5.76%, respectively). Yet exercise intensity is more closely associated with both forms of passion (shared variance 12.25% and 15.21%, respectively). Perhaps exercise volume is better defined as frequency, duration, and intensity in this context, yielding more accurate results concerning the passion exercise volume relationship.

Another large study (n > 1,000) conducted in eight Spanish-speaking nations (de la Vega et al., 2020) showed that the risk of exercise addiction was inversely related to changes in exercise volume during COVID-19 isolation. Still, after controlling for passion and perfectionism, this relationship has vanished. For the sake of the current discussion, we have repeated the grouping into low and high exercise volume categories based on up to 10 hours (low) and 10 hours or more (high) reported weekly exercise. Again, like in the aforementioned analyses of the data obtained by Szabo et al. (2018), we found that the high-volume exercise group reported greater obsessive and harmonious passion than the low volume exercise group (Figure 16.2). The findings were similar in all eight nations and were not connected to the gender of the participants.

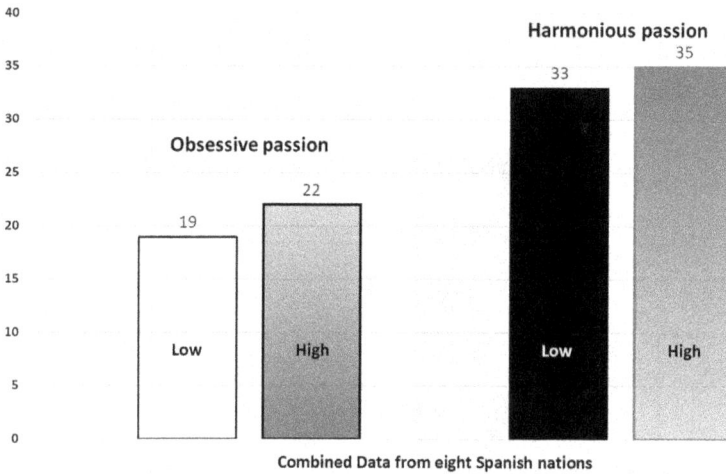

Figure 16.2 Illustration of the statistically significant differences (p < .001) in obsessive and harmonious passion between those who exercise up to 10 hours per week (low) and those who exercise more than 10 hours per week (high). The sample size (n) was 1,079. The figure presents unpublished results from de la Vega et al.'s (2020) data.

We then further examined the data from the study of de la Vega et al. (2020) by looking to passion (both forms) in three groups classified as being at no risk, low risk, or high risk as based on the classification recommended by Terry et al. (2004). Subsequently, we compared obsessive and harmonious passion in the three groups by using a multivariate analysis of variance. This test yielded statistically significant results, and the three groups differed from each other on both measures (p < .001, in all instances), with the group classified as being at risk for exercise addiction scoring the highest on both measures of passion (Figure 16.3).

Like in the data gathered by Szabo et al. (2018), the correlation between exercise volume and obsessive and harmonious passion was statistically significant but weak (.20 in both cases), suggesting that only a small proportion of the variance was shared by exercise volume and passion. When partial correlation was used to control for the effects of passion, the relationship between the risk of exercise addiction and weekly exercise volume was no longer significant, confirming the findings of Szabo and Kovacsik (2019). In contrast, the correlations with the risk of exercise addiction were higher, revealing common variances of 32.5% with obsessive passion and 17.65% with harmonious passion. When controlling for exercise volume by calculating the partial correlations, the association between the risk of exercise addiction and both forms

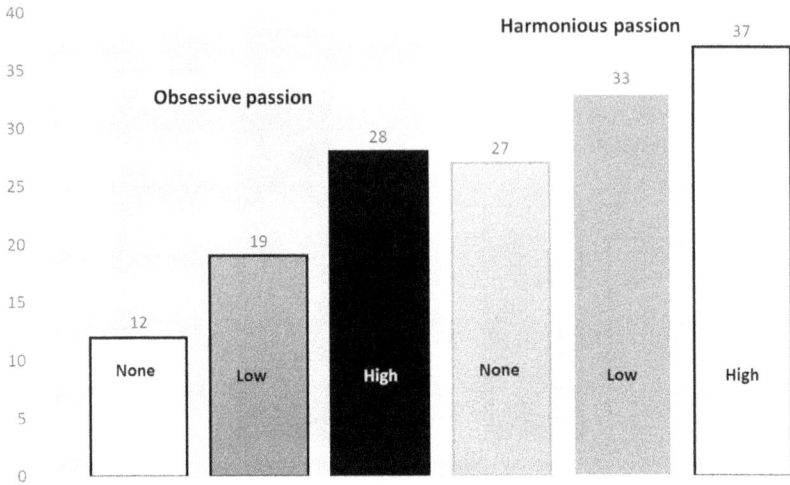

Figure 16.3 Illustration of the statistically significant differences (p < .001) in obsessive and harmonious passion between individuals showing no risk, low
risk, and high risk of exercise addiction. The figure presents unpublished results from de la Vega colleagues' (2020) data.

of passion remained virtually unchanged, as shown by a slight decrease (.02
and .03) in the two correlation coefficients. Therefore, exercise volume, heav-
ily implicated in exercise addiction in the literature, is unlikely to mediate the
relationship between the risk of exercise addiction and passion. This finding
is in accord with Szabo and Kovacsik (2019), who disclosed a small negative
association between the risk of exercise addiction and exercise volume.

16.6 Can exercise addiction be separated from passion?

The scope of this chapter is to critically evaluate and, based on empirical evidence, discuss the close relationship between addiction (to exercise)
and passion. Therefore, it is essential to answer the question posed in this
section. To accomplish this task, we first turn to Krüger (2016). At first,
one can observe addiction and passion in those who fail, which in exercise
addiction manifests as self-harm and those who excel, for example, the passionate athletes. Second, failing or excelling might often embed another
person within the person, one conforming to the social role and the other
driven by controlling urges. Such doubling of the person involves both
actual (new) and played (old) roles. This doubling, however, may not be
predominant when the preexisting and the new roles match each other,
such as a harmonious passion for work, exercise, or relationship. In addictions, life becomes eccentric because the affected person identifies more

with the new (controlling) than old roles and rules. Third, changes in the bio-psychological structure of the person may also occur. In exercise addiction, the changes surface as symptoms such as urges, cravings, or even withdrawal symptoms, but not in the harmoniously passionate exercise. Fourth, the person compelled to play roles dissociates several feelings from the manifested behavior. Fifth, there may be a conflict between fundamental roles and played roles. This conflict is like a double-edged sword: one compelling the person to give in to urges of addiction or obsessive passion and the other compelling them to fit into the social norms.

Theoretically, it would be easier to distinguish between passion as a positive driving force and addiction as a negative one. Perhaps this contrasting was Glassers's (1976) general idea when initiating the concept of 'positive addiction.' Indeed, if the term addiction is taken away from this two-word expression, the remaining term would suggest a desirable, pleasurable outcome or relationship to an activity. But, by definition, addiction is a harm-inducing behavior. Therefore, passion and addiction are not opposites. Instead, passion can change its emotional components. According to Lichtenstein et al. (2020a), after adopting, liking, and loving an activity (exercise) that can fit well into the person's life, with time and experience, the activity's new potentials, interacting with the person's needs, skills, and abilities, are discovered. The harmonious passion turns into discovery passion characterized by the person trying out and taking advantage of the new potentials. This phase can become harmonious again with the person's life or turn into obsessive passion. The direction of the change depends on the discovered aspect and rewards of the activity. For example, more excellent skills yield greater rewards, making the activity more attractive for the person who maintains control over it, and the activity is positively reinforced. Alternately, the stress-mediating effect of exercise can control the person and 'force' to exercise to avoid or manage stress, in which case the behavior becomes negatively reinforced.

Chapter 11 presents the model of Lichtenstein et al. (2020b) but in its original unidirectional way, indicating that discovery passion leads to obsessive passion. In contrast, as discussed earlier, discovery passion may switch back to harmonious passion. For example, after I discover that I am good at golf, I may not change my golf-related habits but enjoy more the activity than before. In contrast, if golf gives me time out from the stress of work or family life (or both), I may engage more and more frequently and become obsessed with the activity assuming progressively greater priority in my life. Still, obsessive passion is not the same as addiction because, despite the obsession with the action, there is still some control over it, and no harm or severe withdrawal symptoms should be present. When the control is lost, psychobiological symptoms appear, and the person experiences harm due to the activity; there is a transition from obsessive passion into addiction (discussed in the next chapter).

Szabo (2010) argues that not the presence of withdrawal symptoms but their severity or intensity is crucial in exercise addiction. Indeed, the harmoniously passionate person can have feelings of deprivation when the beloved activity is not accessible for some reason. For example, early research showed that even bowlers attending one bowling session per week reported experiencing deprivation sensation when they could not participate in bowling. Still, the severity of their symptoms was lower than that of aerobic dancers, weight trainers, cross-trainers, and fencers (Szabo et al., 1996). Therefore, the seriousness of feelings varying from deprivation to withdrawal may parallel the spectrum of harmonious passion and addiction.

Consequently, passion and addiction are not separable, as also suggested by research data. Higher passion seems to be associated with a greater risk of exercise addiction. Furthermore, obsessive passion can account for up to 47% of the variance in the risk of exercise addiction, while harmonious passion may only account for a mere 3% (Kovacsik, Soós et al., 2018), supporting the three-dimensional model for passion (Lichtenstein et al., 2020b). de la Vega et al. (2020) and Szabo and Kovacsik (2019) suggested that the risk of exercise addiction should be studied along with passion. To shape knowledge in this area, the testing of the model proposed by Lichtenstein et al. (2020b) deserves experimental scrutiny.

16.7 Key points

1. Obsessive passion is a stronger predictor of exercise addiction than harmonious passion.
2. Athletes in team sports score higher on harmonious passion than athletes in individual sports.
3. When controlling for passion, group differences in exercise addiction often vanish.
4. Greater exercise frequency is associated with greater passion, both obsessive and harmonious.
5. Exercise addiction and passion have a symbiotic relationship with each other.

16.8 References

Akehurst, S., & Oliver, E. J. (2013). Obsessive passion: A dependency associated with injury-related risky behaviour in dancers. *Journal of Sports Sciences, 32*(3), 259–267. doi:10.1080/02640414.2013.823223

Amiot, C., Vallerand, R. J., & Blanchard, C. M. (2006). Passion and psychological adjustment: A test of the person-environment fit hypothesis. *Personality and Social Psychology Bulletin, 32*(2), 220–229. doi:10.1177/0146167205280250

Back, J. (2015). *Profiles of exercise dependence – A person centred approach to study potential mechanisms.* Master's thesis. School of Health and Welfare: Halmstad

University, Halmstad, Sweden. Retrieved from: www.diva-portal.org/smash/get/diva2:940447/FULLTEXT02

de la Vega, R., Almendros, L. J., Barquín, R. R., Boros, S., Demetrovics, Z., & Szabo, A. (2020). Exercise addiction during the COVID-19 pandemic: An international study confirming the need for considering passion and perfectionism. *International Journal of Mental Health and Addiction.* doi:10.1007/s11469-020-00433-7

de la Vega, R., Parastatidou, I. S., Ruíz-Barquín, R., & Szabo, A. (2016). Exercise addiction in athletes and leisure exercisers: The moderating role of passion. *Journal of Behavioral Addictions, 5*(2), 325–331. doi:10.1556/2006.5.2016.043

Glasser, W. (1976). *Positive addiction.* New York, NY: Harper and Row.

Kovacsik, R., Griffiths, M. D., Pontes, H. M., Soós, I., de la Vega, R., Ruíz-Barquín, R., . . . Szabo, A. (2018). The role of passion in exercise addiction, exercise volume, and exercise intensity in long-term exercisers. *International Journal of Mental Health and Addiction, 17*(6), 1389–1400. doi:10.1007/s11469-018-9880-1

Kovacsik, R., Soós, I., de la Vega, R., Ruíz-Barquín, R., & Szabo, A. (2018). Passion and exercise addiction: Healthier profiles in team than in individual sports. *International Journal of Sport and Exercise Psychology, 18*(2), 176–186. doi:10.1080/1612197x.2018.1486873

Kovacsik, R., Tóth-Király, I., Egorov, A., & Szabo, A. (2020). A longitudinal study of exercise addiction and passion in new sport activities: The impact of motivational factors. *International Journal of Mental Health and Addiction.* (Online first). doi:10.1007/s11469-020-00241-z

Krüger, H. P. (2016). Passion and addiction. The approach by Helmuth Plessner's philosophical anthropology. *Studi di Estetica, 5,* 167–190.

Lichtenstein, M. B., Jensen, E. S., Larsen, P. V., Omdahl, M. K., & Szabo, A. (2020a). Passion for exercise has three dimensions: Psychometric evaluation of The Passion Scale in a Danish fitness sample. *Translational Sports Medicine, 3*(6), 638–648. doi:10.1002/tsm2.173

Lichtenstein, M. B., Jensen, E. S., & Szabo, A. (2020b). Exercise addiction, obsessive passion, and the use of nutritional supplements in fitness center attendees. *Translational Sports Medicine, 3*(3), 188–195. doi:10.1002/tsm2.131

Lucidi, F., Pica, G., Mallia, L., Castrucci, E., Manganelli, S., Bélanger, J. J., & Pierro, A. (2016). Running away from stress: How regulatory modes prospectively affect athletes' stress through passion. *Scandinavian Journal of Medicine & Science in Sports, 26*(6), 703–711. doi:10.1111/sms.12496

Paradis, K. F., Cooke, L. M., Martin, L. J., & Hall, C. R. (2013). Too much of a good thing? Examining the relationship between passion for exercise and exercise dependence. *Psychology of Sport and Exercise, 14*(4), 493–500. doi:10.1016/j.psychsport.2013.02.003

Parastatidou, I., Doganis, G., Theodorakis, Y., & Vlachopoulos, S. (2014). The mediating role of passion in the relationship of exercise motivational regulations with exercise dependence symptoms. *International Journal of Mental Health and Addiction, 12*(4), 406–419. doi:10.1007/s11469-013-9466-x

Schipfer, M., & Stoll, O. (2015, July). *Exercise-addiction/exercise commitment- model (EACOM).* Paper presented at the 14th European Congress of Sport Psychology, Bern, Switzerland.

Sicilia, Á., Alcaraz-Ibáñez, M., Lirola, M.-J., & Burgueño, R. (2017). Influence of goal contents on exercise addiction: Analysing the mediating effect of passion for exercise. *Journal of Human Kinetics, 59*(1), 143–153. doi:10.1515/hukin-2017-0154

Sicilia, Á., Alcaraz-Ibáñez, M., Lirola, M.-J., Burgueño, R., & Maher, A. (2018). Exercise motivational regulations and exercise addiction: The mediating role of passion. *Journal of Behavioral Addictions, 7*(2), 482–492. doi:10.1556/2006.7.2018.36

Stenseng, F., Rise, J., & Kraft, P. (2011). The dark side of leisure: Obsessive passion and its covariates and outcomes. *Leisure Studies, 30*(1), 49–62. doi:10.1080/02614361003716982

Szabo, A. (2010). *Addiction to exercise: A symptom or a disorder?* New York, NY: Nova Science Publishers.

Szabo, A., Frenkl, R., & Caputo, A. (1996). Deprivation feelings, anxiety, and commitment to various forms of physical activity: A cross-sectional study on the Internet. *Psychologia: An International Journal of Psychology in the Orient, 39*(4), 223–230.

Szabo, A., Griffiths, M. D., Demetrovics, Z., de la Vega, R., Ruíz-Barquín, R., Soós, I., & Kovacsik, R. (2018). Obsessive and harmonious passion in physically active Spanish and Hungarian men and women: A brief report on cultural and gender differences. *International Journal of Psychology, 54*(5), 598–603. doi:10.1002/ijop.12517

Szabo, A., & Kovacsik, R. (2019). When passion appears, exercise addiction disappears. *Swiss Journal of Psychology, 78*(3–4), 137–142. doi:10.1024/1421-0185/a000228

Terry, A., Szabo, A., & Griffiths, M. (2004). The exercise addiction inventory: A new brief screening tool. *Addiction Research & Theory, 12*(5), 489–499. doi:10.1080/16066350310001637363

Vallerand, R. J. (2008). On the psychology of passion: In search of what makes people's lives most worth living. *Canadian Psychology, 49*(1), 1–13. doi:10.1037/0708-5591.49.1.1

Vallerand, R. J. (2010). On passion for life activities: The dualistic model of passion. In M. P. Zanna & J. M. Olson (Eds.), *Advances in experimental social psychology* (pp. 97–133). San Diego, CA: Academic Press.

Vallerand, R. J., Blanchard, C., Mageau, G. A., Koestner, R., Ratelle, C., Leonard, M., Gagne, M., & Marsolais, J. (2003). Les passions de l'ame: On obsessive and harmonious passion. *Journal of Personality and Social Psychology, 85*(4), 756–767. doi:10.1037/0022-3514.85.4.756

Vallerand, R. J., & Miquelon, P. (2007). Passion for sport in athletes. In D. Lavallee & S. Jowett (Eds.), *Social psychology in sport* (pp. 249–262). Champaign, IL: Human Kinetics.

Vallerand, R. J., Rousseau, F. L., Grouzet, F. M. E., Dumais, A., Grenier, S., & Blanchard, C. M. (2006). Passion in sport: A look at determinants and affective experiences. *Journal of Sport and Exercise Psychology, 28*(4), 454–478.

Vallerand, R. J., Salvy, S. J., Mageau, G. A., Elliot, A. J., Denis, P., Grouzet, F. M. E., & Blanchard, C. (2007). On the role of passion in performance. *Journal of Personality, 75*(3), 505–534. doi:10.1111/j.1467-6494.2007.00447.x

17 Novel conceptualization of passion and addiction is sport and exercise

To date, research on passion in sports and exercise has primarily been conceptualized on the basis of the dual model of passion (Vallerand et al., 2003; Chapter 2). Recently, it was found that passion has three dimensions (Lichtenstein et al., 2020). This third dimension, *discovery passion*, rests somewhere between harmonious passion and obsessive passion and fits into the dualistic model. Discovery passion can be connected to human nature (Brand, 2009) and the self-determination theory (Deci & Ryan, 2000). Discovery is the answer (and the reward) to innate curiosity, characteristic of human and animal nature. Three of the essential functions that are assigned to curiosity – 1) incentive for reducing negative states including uncertainty; 2) inner motivation to explore and learn for one's own sake; and 3) unique motivational goals or orientations that differentiate people's knowledge, experiences, objectives, ideals, and achievements – are elaborated by Silvia (2012). All three aspects fit into sport and exercise activities and are directly related to discovery passion.

17.1 Discovery as a mediator of stress and anxiety

Discovery is the reward of learning and curiosity. There is the transition between the often subconscious curiosity (Aarts & Custers, 2012) and conscious curiosity characterized by the need to know or learn something. For example, beginners' low abilities and not well-learned skills harm sports performance. They act as barriers to performance, causing inner stress and anxiety; improving the skills through practice, and discovering new techniques, alleviates the stress and anxiety associated with inadequate and often self-intimidating performance. Alternatively, in social relationships, learning about teammates and coaches' habits and personality characteristics could lessen the stress in personal relationships, especially in the early phases of integration into a new sporting or exercise environment (Côté et al., 2010).

Learning and discovering adequate methods that facilitate physical effort and performance also reduces competitive anxiety. Researchers have reported that the players' willingness to learn before engaging in a

DOI: 10.4324/9781003173595-17

competitive situation could increase interest to engage in play and reduce competitive anxiety (Hong et al., 2013). Furthermore, athletes who turn to sports psychologists wish to learn (discover) new mental frames for handling difficulties. In all these and similar situations self- and aided learning is expected to lead to a *discovery* that reduces a negative state while providing an incentive for further discovery. This incentive fits into the concept of discovery passion, reflecting the inner drive to become better.

17.2 Discovery as a mediator of positive experience

While in the previous section, the drive to reduce a negative state(s) reflects a form of inner motivation, another form is the desire to succeed or excel in sports and exercise. On the basis of competence motivation theory (Harter, 1978, 1981), individuals tend to engage in skilled performances if they believe they can execute the task successfully. The theory posits that feelings of competence yield intrinsic pleasure as a form of inner reward. The personal sense of competence stems from good performance on successive mastery attempts. Successful mastery attempts are associated with social approval reinforcing perceptions of competence and control, generating positive affect and inner motivation to continue and demonstrate even higher competence.

The core of the competence motivation theory is the perceived competence, which is the person's self-assessment of their ability to learn (discover) new skills and accomplish the tasks involved in performance demands. In addition to relatedness and autonomy, the inner need for competence is also part of the self-determination theory (Deci & Ryan, 1991). Furthermore, in the achievement goal theory (Kaplan & Maehr, 2007), the activity is undertaken for learning new skills and discovering techniques through which one can manifest competence and avoid showing incompetence in an achievement situation. But competence is the result of *discovering* new performance-related facilitators, including skills, techniques, mental training and performance, imagery, relaxation, and many others all interacting with each other. Therefore, discovery passion can be present throughout the sporting career of an athlete. It is not necessarily linear or continuous, as it may be at the beginning of the commitment stage, but rather stepwise, with a pause between the various stages of growth and development. At the early stage of an athletic career, discovery passion, characterized by continuous learning, could merge and coexist with harmonious passion in a symbiotic context. Still, when it becomes an independent motivational fuel for acquiring new aspects of performance enhancement, it becomes a unique form of passion, like obsessive passion.

17.3 Discovery as a mediator of unique personal objectives and experiences

Accepting the proposition that discovery is the answer, as well as the reward, for exploration and learning (also to chance learning), it becomes evident that learning and experience also shape the direction of interest in new discoveries. Given that the directions of interests are different among people, the focused curiosity and discovery are also vastly different. This difference can be illustrated by comparing two youngsters starting to play soccer at a club level at the same time. One will demonstrate excellent competence in running and passing the ball while the other may be more competent in defense and fast positioning on the field. Based on the competence theories, the feelings associated with their competence will gravitate the two players in different directions. Still, both youngsters will try to minimize stress and anxiety related to performing and increase the skills and techniques that aid in their performance. To achieve these objectives, they need to explore, experience, practice, and learn, all leading to *discoveries* which, at the initial stages of the sporting career, mold into the pleasure of the sport because they occur several times during training. As the discoveries cease to become part of everyday training, they start to become rarer and rarer but could have a progressively greater impact (they follow the typical learning curve). Although athletes differ in what and how they learn and discover, every discovery can be a great reward via improved performance and fuel the passion for further discovery. On the contrary, discovery passion can turn into obsessive passion, as discussed below.

17.4 Discovery passion as the switch between harmonious and obsessive passion

When starting a new sport, the feelings of competence will substantially impact the intensity and direction of the individual's motivation. Successive successful mastery attempts (Harter, 1978, 1981) can lead to setting unrealistic goals in terms of personal abilities or skills or the selected interval for achieving the goals. In such goal pursuits, apart from the extraordinary commitment, the individual may become obsessed with the activity. The unrealistically set plan starts to control the individual progressively to a greater extent when the individual feels compelled to do the exercise (train harder and harder) or else the goal cannot be reached. At this point, the athletic behavior becomes negatively reinforced, reflecting the beginning of the transition from harmonious passion to obsessive passion. Then the obsessive passion, along with the failure to recognize personal limits, may lead to a total loss of control and, consequently, addiction via a self-coerced mastery path, based on the interactional model of exercise addiction (Dinardi et al., 2021).

Recreational exercisers could also discover many beneficial rewards associated with their exercise. Initially, as part of harmonious passion, the discovery is ongoing due to practice, experience, and learning. However, the rewards interacting with the personality, situation, and personal needs generate special attention (unique, high-value discovery) to the most needed reward. For example, discovering the social recognition associated with bodybuilding (Hutchinson et al., 2015) has different reinforcing values for those with high and low self-confidence (Macho et al., 2021). People with low self-confidence will experience the desired reward, which then acts as a strong incentive that could turn into controlling power, switching from discovery passion to obsessive passion and finally to addiction that is also characterized by the use of performance-enhancing drugs (Hutchinson et al., 2015; Macho et al., 2021). Alternately, runners may *discover* the stress-relieving properties of running (Major, 2001), which they will use in difficult times. If the stress becomes traumatic, running becomes obligatory, and the runner will be obsessed with running as a solution for their problem. However, the obsession can turn into addiction at a certain point when the perceived life events are not manageable without running.

In the aforementioned situations, there may be a shift from positive reinforcement of the sport or exercise behavior in which the person *gains* a reward to negative reinforcement in which the reward is the *avoidance* of something noxious (Szabo, 2010). This shift is through the *discovery* of a much-needed aspect of sport or exercise on which the person relies more and more. The shift, then, mirrors the transition from harmonious passion into an obsessive passion. Yet transition does not occur all the time. For example, the two forms of passion, with discovery passion between them, can coexist in competitive athletes (Szabo, 2018) who always gain and discover something in every training session and *avoid* failure or drawbacks in their sport by training correctly and in sufficient volume. In leisure athletes, the coexistence of the three forms of passion may be present without necessarily involving addiction. One is serving the enjoyment (*gain*) of the activity, the other the reward of learning new things through the exercise (*discovery*), and the third by assuring discipline (*avoid* lax attitude and the impact of mood fluctuation) over the training to achieve specific goals.

Then what is the difference between obsessive passion and addiction? First, it must be admitted that there is a very narrow boundary between the two, considering that they share a large proportion of the variance (Kovacsik et al., 2018). Second, the obsessively passionate activity is controlling, but the affected person may not have lost *total control* over the action (Szabo, 2018), which is the case in an addiction. According to this proposition, the obsessively passionate individual may recognize the dangers of their action and adjust the activity level. In contrast, the addicted person will go to the extent of self-injury. Therefore, obsessive passion may fit the sport and exercise behavior of the person without pathology and harm to the self. In contrast, by definition, addiction is a dysfunction involving physical, psychological, or social injury (Juwono & Szabo, 2020).

17.5 A novel conceptualization of passion and addiction is sport and exercise

Based on the aforementioned discussion, which implies the acceptance of the research-based premise that passion has three dimensions (Lichtenstein et al., 2020), a conceptual model illustrating interrelationship of passion and exercise addiction is presented in Figure 17.1. First, after the commitment phase, exercise is adapted. In its early stages, the activity embeds all components of passion, with discovery passion being primarily part of harmonious passion. The discipline of regular training and commitment or other controlling external influences manifested through obsessive passion is also present but does not dominate the exercise behavior. With increasingly more experience, the self-enhancing (the mastery path) or self-helping (the therapeutic path) aspects of exercise reward may receive special attention.

For example, skill improvement, muscle increase, or anxiety/stress relief could receive *special attention and priority* (based on personal needs) and act as special and additional incentives to the already experienced joy and enjoyment of the activity, which characterizes harmonious passion. After discovering these especially self-rewarding effects of exercise, repeated experience and a possible shift in the primary motivation (from enjoyment to stress relief) segregate discovery passion from harmonious passion. However, the two coexist and influence exercise behavior. With time, the initially secondary now primary reward may become obligatory because the person *must experience* it to feel good. This transition leads to a dominating controlling, obsessive passion, while harmonious and

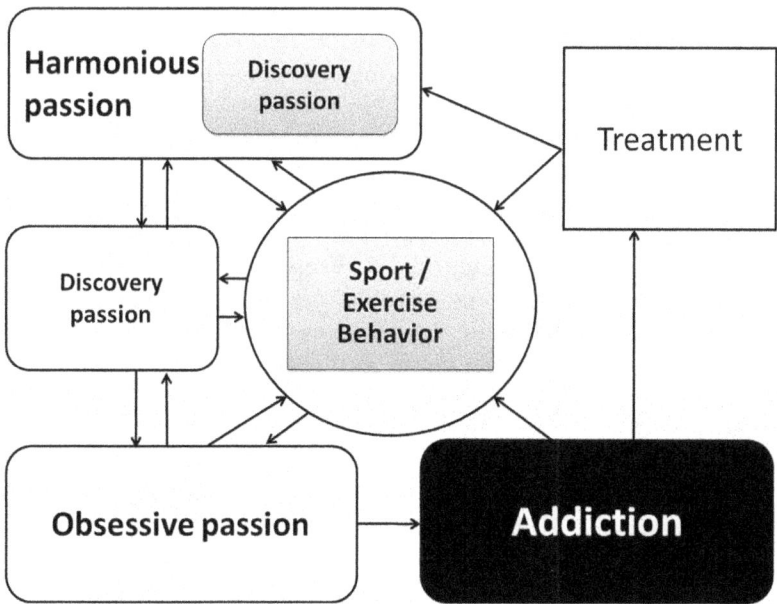

Figure 17.1 The passion–addiction model of exercise behavior (modified from Lichtenstein et al., 2020).

discovery passion are still part of one's exercise but have a lesser impact than obsessive passion.

The relationship between the three forms of passion is unlikely to be sequential, as Lichtenstein et al. (2020) suggested but reciprocal. Indeed, discovery passion can enhance harmonious passion, and the latter could lead to discovery passion. For example, discovering a new and more efficient technique to pass the ball or run more economically can enhance the enjoyment of the activity and increase harmonious passion while both influence the exercise behavior. The *discovery* of weight loss, for example, after regular exercise, can make the reward act as a primary motive replacing the initial reason(s) for training. If exercise is adopted for weight management, then it becomes obligatory, externally controlled, and the surfacing of obsessive passion may occur. Obsessively passionate exercise, leading to loss of time with friends and missing obligations, can also influence discovery passion positively by teaching the person to adjust and moderate the exercise behavior. If the lesson is not learned or the craving for the reward is too intense so that the person cannot resist, loss of control over exercise behavior may occur, which eventually leads to some sort of harm or unfavorable consequence (Szabo, 2010; Szabo et al., 2018). At this stage, treatment is necessary, which, if successful, positively affects exercise behavior. Therefore, while the risk of exercise addiction is not part of exercise behavior, the three forms of passion are constantly present in various proportions that shape exercise behavior.

The transition from obsessive passion into exercise addiction, in some cases, is still unidirectional, as implied by Lichtenstein et al. (2020) and Figure 11.6, because when control over the behavior is lost and the behavior controls the individual, professional help is needed to reestablish a healthy pattern of exercise behavior. Still, the three forms of passion cannot be separated from each other as they all have a distinct role in exercise behavior and the psychological effects of exercise. Future studies should develop psychometrically valid instruments for assessing the three forms of passion and use them to determine how they relate to exercise behavior and their mediators. Based on actual knowledge, while obsessive passion shares a large proportion of variance with the risk of exercise addiction, harmonious passion has a negligible predictive power on the risk of addiction. Still, the two forms of passion strongly correlate with each other and exercise addiction. The symbiotic relationship between the three forms, and two dimensions of passion (Szabo, 2018), and addiction needs idiographic scrutiny by relying on the pyramid approach (Figure 12.1) to identify the triggering cause of the shift from passion to addiction, or from healthy to unhealthy exercise.

17.6 Key points

1. Passion might have three dimensions in sports and exercise.
2. The dimensions of passion are dynamic.

3. Discovery passion is essential in learning and motivation.
4. Passion and addiction are inseparable.
5. Obsessive passion can turn into addiction.

17.7 References

Aarts, H., & Custers, R. (2012). Unconscious goal pursuit: Nonconscious goal regulation and motivation. In R. M. Ryan (Ed.), *The Oxford handbook of human motivation* (pp. 231–247). New York, NY: Oxford University Press. doi:10.1093/oxfordhb/9780195399820.013.0014

Brand, W. (2009). Hume's account of curiosity and motivation. *The Journal of Value Inquiry, 43*(1), 83–96. doi:10.1007/s10790-008-9142-8

Côté, J., Bruner, M., Erickson, K., Strachan, L., & Fraser-Thomas, J. (2010). Athlete development and coaching. In J. Lyle & C. Cushion (Eds.), *Sport coaching: Professionalism and practice* (pp. 63–83). Oxford, UK: Elsevier.

Deci, E. L., & Ryan, R. M. (1991). A motivational approach to self: Integration in personality. In R. Deinstbier (Ed.), *Nebraska symposium on motivation* (Vol. 38, pp. 237–288). Lincoln: University of Nebraska Press.

Deci, E. L., & Ryan, R. M. (2000). The "what" and "why" of goal pursuits: Human needs and the self-determination of behavior. *Psychological Inquiry, 11*, 227–268. doi:10.1207/s15327965pli1104_01

Dinardi, J. S., Egorov, A. Y., & Szabo, A. (2021). The expanded interactional model of exercise addiction. *Journal of Behavioral Addictions.* (Online first). doi:10.1556/2006.2021.00061

Harter, S. (1978). Effectance motivation reconsidered: Toward a developmental model. *Human Development, 21*(1), 34–64. doi:10.1159/000271574

Harter, S. (1981). A model of mastery motivation in children: Individual differences and developmental change. In W. A. Collins (Ed.), *Aspects of the development of competence.* Hillsdale, NJ: Erlbaum.

Hong, J.-C., Hwang, M.-Y., Liu, Y.-T., Lin, P.-H., & Chen, Y.-L. (2013). The role of pre-game learning attitude in the prediction to competitive anxiety, perceived utility of pre-game learning of game, and gameplay interest. *Interactive Learning Environments, 24*(1), 239–251. doi:10.1080/10494820.2013.841263

Hutchinson, B., Moston, S., & Engelberg, T. (2015). Social validation: A motivational theory of doping in an online bodybuilding community. *Sport in Society, 21*(2), 260–282. doi:10.1080/17430437.2015.1096245

Juwono, I. D., & Szabo, A. (2020). 100 cases of exercise addiction: More evidence for a widely researched but rarely identified dysfunction. *International Journal of Mental Health and Addiction.* (Online first). doi:10.1007/s11469-020-00264-6

Kaplan, A., & Maehr, M. L. (2007). The contributions and prospects of goal orientation theory. *Educational Psychology Review, 19*(2), 141–184. Doi: 10.1007/s10648-006-9012-5

Kovacsik, R., Soós, I., de la Vega, R., Ruíz-Barquín, R., & Szabo, A. (2018). Passion and exercise addiction: Healthier profiles in team than in individual sports. *International Journal of Sport and Exercise Psychology, 18*(2), 176–186. doi:10.1080/1612197x.2018.1486873

Lichtenstein, M. B., Jensen, E. S., Larsen, P. V., Omdahl, M. K., & Szabo, A. (2020). Passion for exercise has three dimensions: Psychometric evaluation of the Passion

Scale in a Danish fitness sample. *Translational Sports Medicine, 3*(6), 638–648. doi:10.1002/tsm2.173

Macho, J., Mudrak, J., & Slepicka, P. (2021). Enhancing the self: Amateur bodybuilders making sense of experiences with appearance and performance-enhancing drugs. *Frontiers in Psychology, 12.* doi:10.3389/fpsyg.2021.648467

Major, W. F. (2001). The benefits and costs of serious running. *World Leisure Journal, 43*(2), 12–25. doi:10.1080/04419057.2001.9674226

Silvia, P. J. (2012). Curiosity and motivation. In R. M. Ryan (Ed.), *The Oxford handbook of human motivation* (pp. 155–166), New York, NY: Oxford University Press. doi:10.1093/oxfordhb/9780190666453.013.9

Szabo, A. (2010). *Addiction to exercise: A symptom or a disorder?* New York, NY: Nova Science Publishers.

Szabo, A. (2018). Addiction, passion, or confusion? New theoretical insights on exercise addiction research from the case study of a female body builder. *Europe's Journal of Psychology, 14*(2), 296–316. doi:10.5964/ejop.v14i2.1545

Szabo, A., Demetrovics, Z., & Griffiths, M. D. (2018.). Morbid exercise behavior: Addiction or psychological escape? In H. Budde & M. Wegner (Eds.), *The exercise effect on mental health: Neurobiological mechanisms* (pp. 277–311). New York, NY: Routledge. doi:10.4324/9781315113906-11

Vallerand, R. J., Blanchard, C., Mageau, G. A., Koestner, R., Ratelle, C., Léonard, M., . . . Marsolais, J. (2003). Les passions de l'ame: On obsessive and harmonious passion. *Journal of Personality and Social Psychology, 85*(4), 756–767. doi:10.1037/0022-3514.85.4.756

Index

Note: Page numbers in *italics* indicate a figure and page numbers in **bold** indicate a table on the corresponding page.

For Product Safety Concerns and Information please contact our EU
representative GPSR@taylorandfrancis.com
Taylor & Francis Verlag GmbH, Kaufingerstraße 24, 80331 München, Germany

9 7 8 1 0 3 2 0 0 3 0 1 6